Diagnostic Histopathology of the Breast

TO WILLIAM M. SHELLEY

Director of Surgical Pathology at the Johns Hopkins
Hospital, 1960–1970; Director of Laboratories at
Charlotte Memorial Hospital, 1971–1974

He lived and taught the clinical role of the surgical
pathologist, and continues to inspire those fortunate
enough to have learned with him.

Diagnostic Histopathology of the Breast

David L. Page
MD
Professor of Pathology and Director of Anatomic Pathology,
Vanderbilt University Medical Center, Nashville, Tennessee, USA

Thomas J. Anderson
MB ChB FRCPath PhD
Senior Lecturer, Department of Pathology,
University of Edinburgh; Consultant, Royal Infirmary of
Edinburgh, Edinburgh, UK

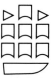

CHURCHILL LIVINGSTONE
EDINBURGH LONDON MELBOURNE AND NEW YORK 1987

CHURCHILL LIVINGSTONE
Medical Division of Longman Group UK Limited

Distributed in the United States of America by
Churchill Livingstone Inc., 1560 Broadway, New
York, N.Y. 10036, and by associated companies, branches
and representatives throughout the world.

First published 1987
  Reprinted 1988
  Reprinted 1989

ISBN   0-443-02240-2

British Library Cataloguing in Publication Data
Page, David L.
  Diagnostic histopathology of the breast.
  1. Breasts — Diseases — Diagnosis
  2. Histology, Pathological
  I. Title   II. Anderson, Thomas J.
  618.1'907583   RG493.5.H5

Library of Congress Cataloging in Publication Data
Diagnostic histopathology of the breast.
  Includes index.
  1. Breast — Diseases — Diagnosis.   2. Breast — Cancer —
Diagnosis.   3. Diagnosis, Cytologic.   4. Histology,
Pathological.   I. Page, David L.   II. Anderson,
Thomas J.   [DNLM: 1. Breast — pathology.   2. Breast
Neoplasms — pathology.   WP 870 D5365]
RG493.5.C97D53   1987   616.99'449075   87-6612

Printed and bound in Great Britain by
William Clowes Limited, Beccles and London

Preface

This book is written in order to promote the use of histopathology in the study and clinical management of breast disease. This may be most efficiently done by fostering consistency in diagnosis. Those who manage breast disease clinically have only recently departed from an era in which all that was asked of the histopathologist was a decision between benign and malignant. We are now in an era of change with new diagnostic and therapeutic approaches and an active debate between the 'lumpers' and 'splitters'. We have attempted to accept newly proposed diagnostic categories ('splitter') only when clinical importance may be demonstrated. This book attempts to make concepts in terminology consistent, recognizing the many contributions of students in the field. Specifically recognizable patterns and their currently appreciated clinical significance are presented throughout the book.

We are grateful to our Chairmen, Sir Alastair Currie and William H. Hartmann as well as to Sir Tom Symington, for their support and who made possible the sabbatical leave which initiated the cooperative effort of the two authors. We are also grateful to the many colleagues, clinicians and pathologists, who as teachers and students have taught and questioned us, helping to forge our understanding. Drs Richard Buchanan, Richard Oldham and Louis Graham aided us by providing access to their case material. Michael Dixon provided special stimulus and helped us with access to the material from the Royal Infirmary of Edinburgh. Many histotechnologists and secretaries have been of inestimable help in this effort and without them the book would not have been possible. We particularly wish to mention Carolyn Brown, Annelle Johnson, Robena Ross, Julia Smith, Caroline Nolen and LaDonna Creech. The photographs are the combined effort of the care and skill of Jim Paul of Edinburgh University and Mayhew Koellein, Geoffrey Hartmann and Michael Souviron of Vanderbilt University; the artwork is by Ian Lennox of Edinburgh University. The staff of Churchill Livingstone, our publishers, provided critical aid and support during the development and final production of this work.

We are grateful to the many surgeons, mammographers, medical oncologists, statisticians, surgical pathologists (histopathologists) and epidemiologists who have helped us in our understanding of breast disease. To the teachers who guided us and medical students and residents who have questioned and challenged us, we are particularly grateful. We record our gratitude to our wives, Lauren and Margaret, for their understanding and support.

We acknowledge the support of the National Cancer Institute, American Cancer Society, Burroughs-Wellcome, the Medical Research Council and the Scottish Home and Health Department.

D.L.P.
T.J.A.

Nashville and Edinburgh
1987

Contributors

James L. Connolly MD Associate Pathologist, Beth Israel Hospital; Assistant Professor of Pathology, Harvard Medical School; Consultant in Pathology, Dana-Farber Cancer Institute, Boston, Massachusetts, USA

Christopher W. Elston MD, FRCPath Department of Pathology, City Hospital, Nottingham; Clinical teacher, University of Nottingham Medical School, Nottingham, UK

Robert E. Fechner MD Royster Professor of Pathology, Director, Division of Surgical Pathology, University of Virginia Medical Center, Charlottesville, Virginia, USA

Richard L. Johnson MD Associate Pathologist, Laboratory of Surgical Pathology, Huntington Memorial Hospital, Pasadena, California; Formerly Assistant Professor of Pathology, Vanderbilt University, Nashville, Tennessee, USA

Lowell W. Rogers MD Pathologist, Carraway Methodist Medical Center, Birmingham, Alabama; Clinical Assistant Professor of Pathology, University of Alabama, Birmingham and Vanderbilt University; Formerly Director of Surgical Pathology, Vanderbilt University Medical Center, Nashville, Tennessee, USA

Goi Sakamoto MD Chief Pathologist, Cancer Institute (Japanese Foundation for Cancer Research), Tokyo, Japan

Stuart J. Schnitt MD Associate in Pathology, Beth Israel Hospital; Instructor in Pathology, Harvard Medical School; Consultant in Pathology Dana-Farber Cancer Institute, Boston, Massachusetts, USA

Dennis M. Smith Jr MD Director of Laboratories, Memorial Medical Center, Jacksonville, Florida; Formerly Assistant Professor of Pathology, Vanderbilt University, Nashville, Tennessee, USA

Contents

Introduction

This book is intended for histopathologists who practise surgical pathology. It will also be of value to surgeons and other physicians because cooperation and understanding between surgical pathologists and clinicians is essential in the management of breast disease. As stated in the book's title, we will stress histopathological classification and, when possible, confines of histological definition. Clinical correlation and prognostical implications will be emphasized. Although many different terms are used throughout the world, there is general agreement among histopathologists concerning most of the reproducibly recognizable categories of mammary alterations. It is the recognition of this basic agreement, despite differing terminology, which led to the writing of this book. Each chapter will relate not only our own terms and their definitions, but also terms used by others for the recording of similar changes. Agreement is fostered by the avoidance of more general terms such as 'fibrocystic disease' and 'benign mammary dysplasia' which seek to include a wide variety of changes within their confines of definition. We believe that the use of terms indicating more specific alterations, although recognizing that the changes often occur together, is the only way to achieve consistency in communication and understanding.

The role of the histopathologist in breast disease is primarily one of prognostication. The usefulness of histologic evaluation of tumours and associated conditions is to predict what might happen to an individual patient. It must be remembered, however, that even in the best of circumstances this prognostic ability rests on experience gained from diagnosis of large numbers of patients, and applies to an individual patient in a probabilistic

fashion. These considerations are of particular importance to the relationship of cooperation and mutual trust which must exist between a clinical histopathologist and the responsible physician, operating surgeon, radiation oncologist and/or radiologist. The histopathologist must record anatomic changes with care and consistency, and have an understanding of what the diagnostic terms chosen to record these changes will mean to the clinician receiving them.

We have come a long way since the last century in which classification of breast cancer progressed little further than the identification of soft cancers called 'medullary' and the identification of hard cancers termed 'scirrhous'. The attempt to classify breast cancers into groups with significant prognostic and therapeutic implications is a continual process which demands careful study of large numbers of cases with extended follow-up periods. Histopathology continues to be the most reliable source of data for breast disease classification. Many investigators are searching for ultrastructural, biochemical and hormonal correlates which can, either distinct from or in concert with histopathology, enable more precise prognostication. As is so often the case in histopathology, the introduction of new clinical tools (particularly mammography) has placed new pressure on histopathologists for more precise categorization of changes within the breast which will correlate with clinical features. The realization that the breast cancer death rate has remained essentially unchanged for several decades has also necessitated better understanding of changes within the breast which may have premalignant significance. We hope that the study of these changes will lead to prevention of breast cancer development, or at

1

least increased vigilance directed toward high risk groups which could reduce the death rate. Knowledge of changes with premalignant significance identified by careful epidemiologic techniques is just beginning. It is hoped that this book will be useful in allowing consistent classification of lesions, so that such epidemiologic studies by different investigative teams will be aided by the use of similar terms for comparable lesions.

The last decade has seen a general trend toward conservatism as regards surgical therapy for breast cancer. The general standard of practice in the 1950s was to consider any doubtful lesion a cancer, and proceed with extirpative therapy in the belief that this was the best course of action for the patient. The last decade has produced a wide acceptance that less radical surgical procedures, associated with less physical and psychological trauma to the patient are followed by survival rates not appreciably different from those attained by more radical procedures. This has significantly challenged the earlier approach, and clinical practice has changed. Modified radical mastectomy and simple mastectomy, with or without lymph node dissection, has replaced the standard radical mastectomy (including removal of the pectoralis muscles) as the most common surgical practice for breast cancer. At many centres, local removal of tumours and radiotherapy are used to conserve the breast containing cancers. The surgical pathologist has shared in this trend, and has had to cease being an accomplice in the approach of 'when in doubt, cut it off'. This approach must now be considered as of historical interest only. There are recognizable conditions which are followed by malignant biologic behaviour in only a small percentage of cases, and these can no longer be recognized as cancers without at least the understanding that they represent a threat to life of minimal magnitude. The recognition of these 'minimal' lesions has produced a great pressure for precision and consistency in diagnosis of borderline or difficult lesions. Indeed, it is likely that not all breast cancers need be treated in the same manner, and the stratification of different cancers to different available treatment modalities is a current challenge. There has also been a recent tendency toward the creation of new diagnostic terms for

lesions which grossly and microscopically mimic carcinoma.

In most chapters of this book we will first present a section entitled 'Anatomic pathology' which will briefly state gross anatomical features and go on to cite histological appearances central to the diagnosis. A section on 'Differential diagnosis' will relate similar appearances representing other entities as well as borderline or variant appearances of the change discussed. A practical approach to the diagnostic reporting of cases with mixed histopathological features will often be presented in this section. A final section in each chapter will present relevant 'Clinical and prognostic features'. This last section will be brief, but reference to the literature cited at the end of each chapter will provide the reader with currently available information on clinical features. Some chapters will begin with a section entitled 'Terminology and historical development' or 'Background'. This discussion is intended to place in historic perspective more recent entities and will present the terms in widest current use.

We have attempted to cover, at least briefly, the areas of proper concern to the practising pathologist relevant to the breast. Hyperplasias and neoplasms are emphasized, and we present histological patterns in proximity to clinical correlates and prognostic implications. Invasive tumours are presented in different chapters whose titles indicate their relative importance and certainty as to status as specific or special types of breast cancer.

Many difficult and borderline diagnostic dilemmas would never arise if tissue processing were ideal. The optimal processing and staining of tissue is an absolute necessity, and no degree of experience or expertise will be able to overcome a poorly fixed or poorly prepared histological section. There will always be diagnostic dilemmas, particularly at the borderline between what is called cancer and what is not, but these difficulties will be reduced to a minimum if tissue is adequately prepared and sampled. The routine haematoxylin and eosin stained slide remains the mainstay of breast cancer diagnosis. All photographs presented here have been taken from haematoxylin and eosin stained tissue unless otherwise stated.

Our greatest debt is to the many authors of

papers and books cited in this volume. Each chapter contains the references felt to be most current and most relevant. They should be consulted if a complete understanding of the current state of the art of breast pathology is to be understood by the reader. General reference works, both books and major papers are listed following this introduction. Mastery of histopathology of the human breast can only be gained by viewing many slides and understanding the experience of others as recorded in the literature. We hope this book will serve as a guide and starting point for both.

BIBLIOGRAPHY

General

Ames F C 1984 The place of radical surgery for stages I and II breast cancer. In: Ames F C, Blumenschein G R, Montague E D (eds) Current Controversies in Breast Cancer, 1st edn. Univ Texas, Austin p 103–109

Brennan M J, McGrath C M, Rich M A (eds) 1980 Breast Cancer. New concepts in etiology and control. Academic Press, New York

Gallager E S, Leis H P Jr, Synderman R K, Urban J A (eds) 1978 The Breast. Mosby, St Louis

Grundmann E, Beck L (eds) 1978 Early Diagnosis of Breast Cancer: Methods and Results. Fischer Verlag, Stuttgart

Haagensen C D 1986 Diseases of the Breast. 3rd edn. Saunders, Philadelphia

Hayward J 1974 The conservative treatment of breast cancer. Cancer 33: 595–599

Henderson C I, Canellos P 1980 Cancer of the breast — the past decade. New Eng J Med 302: 17–30

Russel W O (Chairman) 1975 Cancer of the breast: early detection, diagnosis, therapy and end results. First cancer symposium sponsored by the Cancer Task Force and the Commission on Continuing Education. Am J Clin Path 64: 717–809

Saxen E 1979 Histopathology in cancer epidemiology. Path Annual 14 (part 1): 203–217

Urban J A 1978 Management of operable breast cancer. A surgeon's view. Cancer 42: 2066–2077

Pathology

Ahmed A 1978 Atlas of the Ultrastructure of Human Breast Diseases. Churchill Livingstone, Edinburgh

Azzopardi J G 1979 Problems in Breast Pathology. W B Saunders, London

Bassler R 1978 Pathologie der Brustdruse in Handbuch der speziellen pathologie, Bd 11 Springer, Berlin

Bassler R 1984 Mamma In: Remmele W (ed) Pathologie 3 Springer, Berlin p 305–391

Carter D 1984 Interpretation of Breast Biopsies. Raven, New York

Fisher E R 1977 Pathology of breast cancer. In: McGuire W L (ed) Breast cancer I. Advances of invasive breast cancer. Plenum, New York p 43–123

Fisher E R 1978 The pathologist's role in the diagnosis and treatment of invasive breast cancer. Surg Clin North Amer 58: 705–721

Fisher E R 1984 The impact of pathology on the biologic, diagnostic, prognostic, and therapeutic considerations in breast cancer. Surg Clin North Amer 64: 1073–1093

Fisher B, Wolmark N 1986 Conservative surgery: the American experience. Sem Oncol 13: 425–433

Hellman S, Harris J R 1987 The appropriate breast paradigm. Cancer Res 47: 339–342

Hutter R V P 1980 The influence of pathologic factors on breast cancer management. Cancer 46: 961–976

Hutter R V P 1984 Pathological parameters useful in predicting prognosis for patients with breast cancer. In: The Breast. McDivitt R W, Oberman H A, Ozzello L, Kaufman N (eds). Williams and Wilkins, Baltimore

McDivitt R W, Stewart F W, Berg J W 1968 Tumors of the breast. In: Atlas of Tumour Pathology, Second Series. Armed Forces Institute of Pathology, Washington, DC

McDivitt R W, Oberman H A, Ozzello L, Kaufman N (eds) 1984 The Breast. Williams & Wilkins, Baltimore

Millis R R 1984 Atlas of Breast Pathology. MTP Press, Lancaster

Pathology Working Group, Breast Cancer Task Force, National Cancer Institute 1973 Standardized management of breast specimens. Am J Clin Path 60: 789–798

Rilke F, Andreola S, Carbone A, Clements C, Pilotti S 1978 The importance of pathology in prognosis and management of breast cancer. Semin Oncol 5: 360–372

Rosen P P 1979 The pathological classification of human mammary carcinoma: past, present and future. Annals of Clinical and Laboratory Science 9: 144–156

Sloane J P 1985 Biopsy Pathology of the Breast. Chapman Hall, London

World Health Organization 1981 International histological classification of tumors. No. 2, 2nd ed. Histologic typing of breast tumors. WHO, Geneva

1

Anatomy

The functional components of the mature breast comprise the milk-producing lobular units and a system of branching ducts which connect them with the nipple-areolar complex (Fig. 1.1). Surrounding these functioning units are varying amounts of fat and connective tissue which make up most of the bulk of the breast. Dense connective tissue extends from the underlying pectoralis fascia to the skin of the breast (Cooper's ligaments). These 'ligaments' hold the breast upward and their lengthening is presumed responsible for drooping of the breast with advancing age.

Nipple and areola

The nipple-areolar complex (Fig. 1.2) appears from the exterior aspect as a disc of increased pigmentation. The nipple is centrally placed, surrounded by the areola, and slightly elevated above it. The tip of the nipple usually possesses 15–20 orifices which lead into the collecting ducts and which deliver milk to the exterior. These duct openings are usually filled with plugs of keratin in the non-lactating breast, and some of them may end blindly. Over the surface of the areola are small, rounded elevations, the tubercles of Montgomery. The nipple-areolar complex is free of hairs except at the periphery.

The nipple and areola are covered by stratified squamous epithelium surmounted by anucleate squames, similar to that seen in the epidermis elsewhere in the body. Abundant sebaceous glands open directly on to the surface of both the nipple and the areola. The areolar tubercles of Mont-

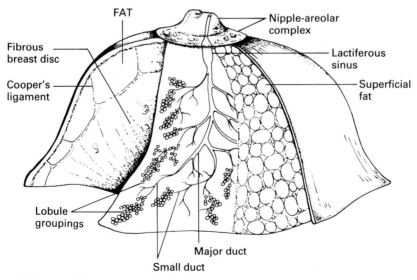

Fig. 1.1 A schematic diagram of the mature breast components in sagittal section (left) and 'window' view of duct and lobular system (centre) connecting with the nipple-areolar complex.

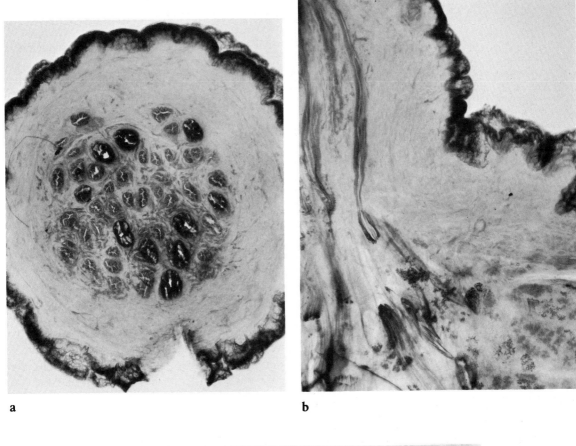

a   b

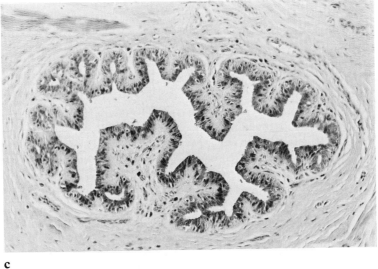

c

Fig. 1.2a–c Stereomicroscopic views of nipple slice to show ducts in central core with small outbranchings, leading into lactiferous sinus. Note lobular developments at base of nipple (**a**) transverse plane; (**b**) vertical plane; (**c**) a histological section of nipple duct in transverse plane shows grooved lining with double epithelial and myoepithelial lining (**a** × 7; **b** × 8; **c** × 150).

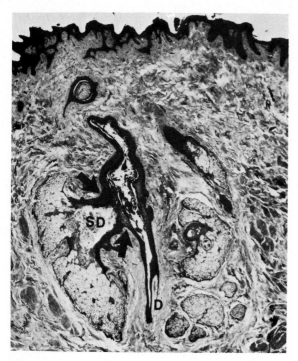

Fig. 1.3 Tubercle of Montgomery, showing sebaceous apparatus emptying through sebaceous duct (SD) into lactiferous nipple duct (D) (× 40). (Courtesy of Dr Smith.)

gomery consist of a sebaceous apparatus associated with a portion of lactiferous duct (Fig. 1.3); this duct is linked to lobular breast parenchyma located deep to the areola (Smith et al 1982). The lactiferous duct and the sebaceous gland duct either terminate adjacent to one another at the areolar epidermis or merge to empty at a common ostium (Montagna & MacPherson 1974). Some glandular units within the areola also resemble eccrine sweat glands, but those which appear as classic apocrine glands are found predominantly near the periphery of the areola (Montagna & MacPherson 1974). Connective tissues ridged with bundles of smooth muscle and elastic tissue lie deep to the epidermis of the nipple and areola. Most of these smooth muscle bundles seem to converge towards the region of the nipple.

Duct system

The breast's system of branching ducts is arranged in a segmental, roughly radial pattern; thus, different regions of the breast, both directly deep

to the nipple and extending outward from the nipple, are drained by their own collecting system whose duct opens at the nipple. This arrangement divides the breast into poorly defined segments or lobes but it is stressed that these may overlap and have no macroscopic or anatomical delineation (Fig. 1.4). Just deep to the nipple a collecting duct widens for a distance, defining an area termed the lactiferous sinus. The ducts have longitudinal ridges which appear as prominent in foldings on cross-section. This pattern of folds is particularly prominent in the region of the lactiferous sinus. The branching of the duct system is complex in that bifurcations often occur at acute angles (Fig. 1.5). Ducts within the breast may appear dilated, with areas closer to the nipple having a smaller diameter than those more distal.

The stratified squamous epithelium of the surface extends a short distance into the openings of the major ducts. The transition from this squamous epithelium to the columnar or cuboidal epithelium which characterizes the entire duct system usually occurs abruptly (Fig. 1.6). A continuous layer of luminal epithelial cells with oval nuclei perpendicular to the surface lines the lactiferous ducts. A discontinuous layer of myoepithelial cells exists between the basement membrane and the luminal epithelial cells. In haematoxylin and eosin stained tissue, the luminal epithelial cells usually have a pale eosinophilic cytoplasm and oval nuclei, whereas the myoepithelial cells possess clearer cytoplasm and rounder nuclei (Fig. 1.7).

The ducts are surrounded by a loose fibrous tissue with a capillary network richer than that seen in the surrounding connective tissue and fat beyond this area. The tissue immediately surrounding the duct is characterized by the presence of elastic fibres which end gradually in the region of the extralobular terminal duct (Fig. 1.8).

Glandular area

The terminal element of the ductal system enters a cluster of blind-ending glandular spaces which are the milk-producing units of the breast (Fig. 1.9). These final elements of the transport system within the breast are called ductules by some and terminal ducts by others. During

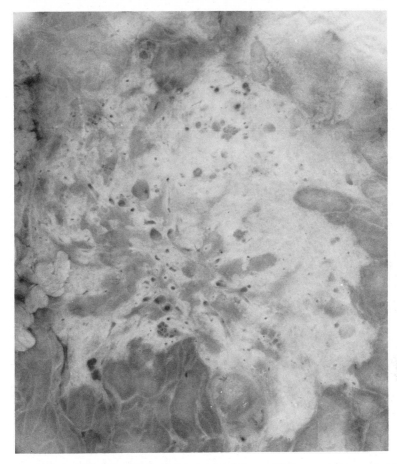

Fig. 1.4 Mature breast in coronal plane to show lack of segmented definition with fatty periphery around irregular placement of fibrous disc from below central nipple point (×1).

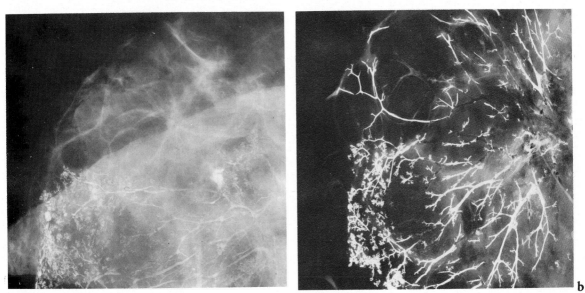

a

b

Fig. 1.5 (a) Ramification of single nipple duct system injected with radio-opaque dye leading to peripheral lobules (whole breast and skin ellipse). (b) Same breast, now sliced at 4 mm, giving clearer view of duct bifurcations and peripheral lobules (a × 0.7; b × 1). (Courtesy of S. Manton.)

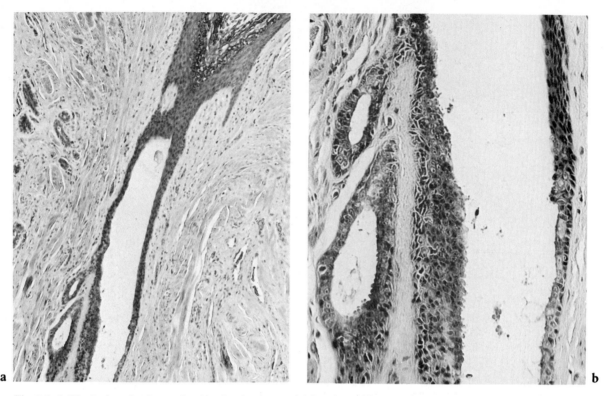

a

b

Fig. 1.6a,b Nipple duct showing surface keratin plug (upper right) and transition zone between squamous and cuboidal lining (**a** × 80; **b** × 250).

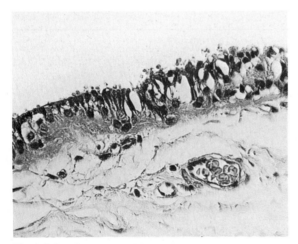

Fig. 1.7 Luminal epithelial and outer myoepithelial layers of major duct (× 500).

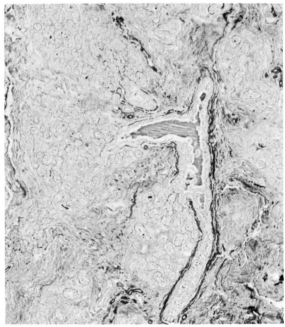

Fig. 1.8 The black elastin outline of the duct disappears as the terminal ducts enter the lobules in upper field. Miller's elastic tartrazine (× 60).

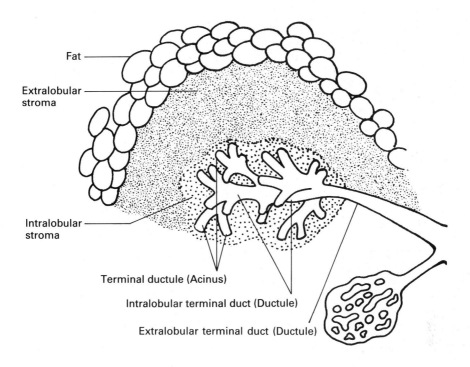

Fat

Extralobular stroma

Intralobular stroma

Terminal ductule (Acinus)

Intralobular terminal duct (Ductule)

Extralobular terminal duct (Ductule)

Fig. 1.9 A schematic diagram of mature resting lobular unit to show distinction of intralobular from extralobular stroma.

lactation, these terminal ducts develop secretory changes precisely similar to those of the acini and thus have a dual role of both transport and secretion. This situation in the breast is analogous to that seen in the lung where respiratory bronchioles both transport air distally and function in air exchange. Disagreements concerning terminology have arisen because many wish to retain the term 'acinus' for the very terminal units seen within the breast during the resting stage, while others feel that these terminal units should be called acini only in the secretory units of breasts of lactating women (McDivitt et al 1968). Either system of terminology may be seen in the literature on breast disease. For purposes of clarification, the term ductule, undefined, should be understood to mean that portion of the breast parenchymal anatomy interposed between the lobular units and the most distal bifurcation of the duct system. These terminal ducts (ductules) have no elastic around them, again demonstrating their close analogy with the acini.

The terminal ductules or acini are set within a rich and specialized stroma which defines the lobular unit (Fig. 1.9). This lobular connective tissue is usually loose, possesses many capillaries, and often contains a few lymphocytes, histiocytes, plasma cells and mast cells. This specialized connective tissue is sharply demarcated from the surrounding fat and from the more dense fibrous tissue of the structural rather than functional portion of the breast. The rounded acini have a luminal epithelium which is either cuboidal or columnar. The cells in different lobular units vary greatly in their cytoplasmic features, but the cells within an individual lobular unit are usually similar to one another. Beneath the luminal epithelium is a discontinuous layer of myoepithelial cells which tend to have smaller nuclei and clearer cytoplasm when compared to the luminal cells in haematoxylin and eosin stained section (Fig. 1.10). Between the epithelial and myoepithelial cells, occasional lymphocytes or macrophages may be seen (Stirling & Chandler 1976; Ferguson 1985).

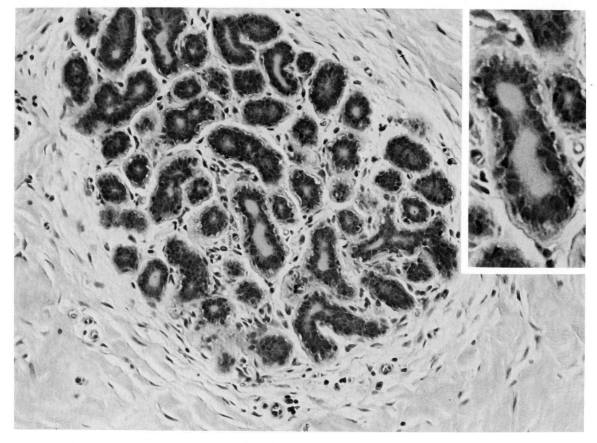

Fig. 1.10 Mature resting lobule with rounded and oblong transection of terminal ductules; luminal epithelial and outer myoepithelial layers are distinguished in the inset. (× 250; inset × 500)

REFERENCES

Ferguson D J P 1985 Intraepithelial lymphocytes and macrophages in the normal breast. Virchows Arch A 407: 369–378

McDivitt R W, Stewart F W, Berg J W 1968 Carcinoma of mammary lobules. In: Tumors of the breast. Atlas of tumor pathology, second series, fascicle 2. Armed Forces Institute of Pathology, Washington, D C, p 63–86

Montagna W, MacPherson E E 1974 Some neglected aspects of the anatomy of human breasts. J Invest Dermatol 63: 10–16

Montagna W, Yun J S 1972 The glands of Montgomery. Br J Dermatol 86: 126–133

Smith D M Jr, Peters T G, Donegan W L 1982 Montgomery's areolar tubercle. A light microscopic study. Arch Pathol Lab Med 106: 60–63

Stirling J W, Chandler J A 1976 The fine structure of the normal, resting terminal ductal-lobular unit of the female breast. Virchows Arch (A) 372: 205–226

2

Stages of breast development

Amongst her own related species, the human female is unusual in that her breasts develop without the stimulus of copulation or pregnancy. After preliminary embryological and anatomical development of the mammary bud, there are major changes during puberty. Thereafter, the breast is a 'resting' organ undergoing minor repeated stimulation associated with menstrual cycles (to be equated with maturation) whilst the fully differentiated state is obtained in pregnancy, culminating in lactation (Fig. 2.1). These physiological changes alternate until there is a major regression at the time of the menopause and after.

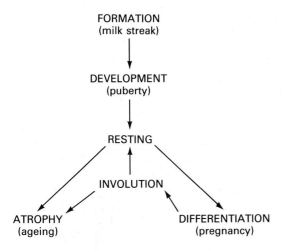

Fig. 2.1 The principal stages of development and physiological alteration in the life cycle of the breast.

The following paragraphs contain the salient features on which to build an awareness of the variable histological patterns occurring physiologically in the breast, and against which to contrast the pathological developments described in

following chapters. Detailed accounts are available in other publications (Bonser et al 1961; Bassler 1970; Vorherr 1974).

PUBERTY

Puberty occurs around the twelfth year in European and North American girls, though somewhat later in Asians and Japanese; during this period there is hormone-induced growth and maturation of the tissues of the genital organs and the breasts. With ovarian development there is first of all production of oestrogens, then progesterone with occurrence of ovulation, both hormones being stimulants of mammary parenchymal growth and acting in association with other factors such as growth hormone, thyroxine and insulin. Morphological evidence for this process in the human is not well documented but, by analogy with animal studies, these steroid hormones promote ductal elongation, reduplication and branching as well as formation of buds for development of new lobular structures. At this time also, changes take place in the volume and elasticity of the connective tissue, whilst vascularization proceeds and fat deposition occurs. This fat, which contributes the major part to breast disc protrusion, serves also as a matrix tissue for future parenchymal mammary growth. The areola and nipple likewise undergo alteration, principally in size, projection and pigmentation. Variations take place in the rate of formation and projection of the breast disc such that pubertal hyperplasia should not be confused with pathological processes; pubertal gynaecomastia is a well-recognized entity which subsides spontaneously with sexual maturation.

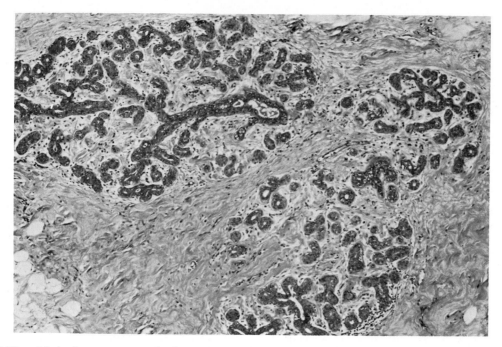

Fig. 2.2 Three lobules from a mature resting breast. Note minor but definite difference between intra- and extralobular stroma (× 60).

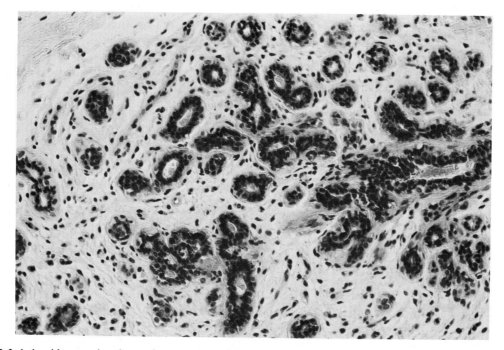

Fig. 2.3 Lobule with many ductules cut in transverse section showing two-cell layer with cuboidal luminal epithelium. Intralobular stroma is cellular and partially fibrosed and can be distinguished easily from the extralobular stroma upper left (× 225).

MATURATION

The functional unit composed of lobule and terminal duct is readily defined under the microscope (Figs 2.2–2.4) but the mode and rate of formation of such units are not clearly understood in the human. Whether development of mature 'resting' units takes place throughout reproductive life (and is accentuated in pregnancy) or only around the time of puberty and early maturation has not been established, although the former seems likely. Variation in stromal and parenchymal composition of different breasts and lack of structural uniformity within individual breasts make it very difficult to understand the morphological changes of hormone response in the 'resting' breast. Observations on the response to repeated stimuli occurring with cyclic menstruation are available, but have not received general recognition. For example, comments have been made on the altered appearance of intralobular connective tissue and of luminal secretions (Ozzello & Speer 1958), of 'basal' or myoepithelial cell

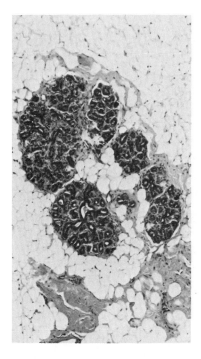

Fig. 2.4 A group of lobules lacking prominent extralobular fibrous tissue support in fat of breast at 28 years (× 60).

character and arrangement (Dieckman 1926; Ingleby 1942) and of ultrastructural features in ductular cells (Fanger & Ree 1974) in response to phases of the menstrual cycle, but agreement on their value and applicability is by no means universal. Recent interest in such changes has been stimulated by the work of McCarty and colleagues (Vogel et al 1981). These workers made a study of histological changes in normal mammary parenchyma of women with regular menstrual cycling and identified criteria for reproducible categorization into five phases, namely, early and late follicular phase, early and late luteal phase, and menstrual phase (Figs 2.5–2.9). Parenchymal cell turnover in relation to the menstrual cycles has also been examined (Anderson et al 1982) from an assessment of frequency of cell division (mitosis) and individual cell death (apoptosis) in the lobule. This disclosed a significant and separable fluctuation in these events, in phase with the menstrual cycles, with the peak of mitosis preceding by three days that of apoptosis, which was most frequent at the onset of menstruation.

Prominence of parenchymal proliferation in the late luteal phase was also noted by Longacre & Bartow (1986) in a study of breast and endometrial tissues obtained at medico-legal autopsy for accidental death of premenopausal women. This analysis provides qualitative and quantitative data concerning epithelium and stroma, supporting and expanding on those of Vogel et al (1981) and stresses that while morphological changes are variably expressed among the lobules of any one breast, a dominant morphological pattern is present. The basal cell vacuolation of the late luteal phase is again commented upon. However, in the light of negative tests for mucopolysaccharides and fat, the likelihood that this is an artefact of impaired fixation or processing should perhaps receive more emphasis. Nevertheless, the report highlighted the difference in cyclic response between breast parenchyma and endometrium. The possibility of stromal epithelial interaction in breast response was also considered. It is likely that the mysteries of the hormonal modulation of breast parenchyma will only be resolved with difficulty (McManus & Welsch 1984). The question of stem cell populations existing in breast parenchyma has never been satisfactorily resolved,

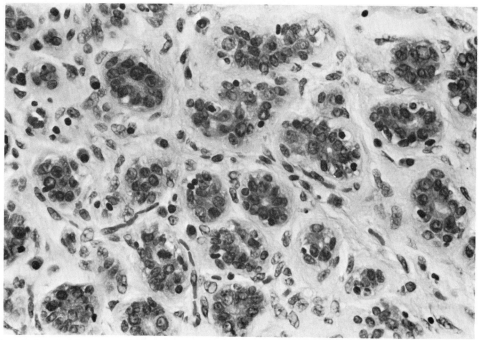

Fig. 2.5 Phase I characteristics with single dominant ductular cell type showing pale homogenous eosinophilic cytoplasm, round, centrally placed nucleus with prominent nuclei, poorly defined cell borders and little orientation to a lumen. Plasma cell infiltrates are evident (× 180). (Courtesy of Dr K. McCarty.)

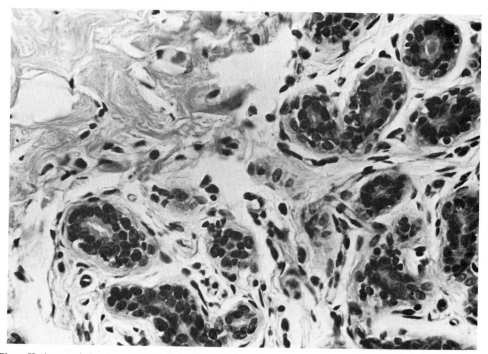

Fig. 2.6 Phase II characteristics showing stratified differentiation of ductular epithelial cell types as basophilic luminal cells with oblong darkly staining nuclei, intermediate pale cells and basal cells with transparent cytoplasm and small hyperchromatic nuclei (upper right) (× 180). (Courtesy of Dr K. McCarty.)

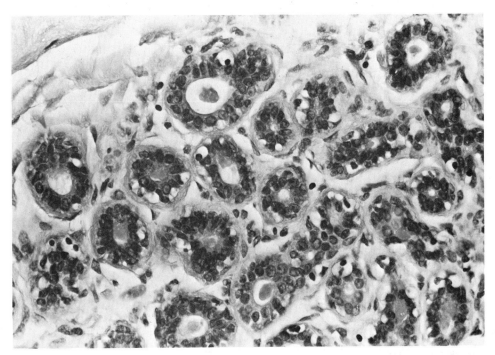

Fig. 2.7 Phase III characteristics to show ductules with three dominant cell types comprising columnar basophilic cells at the lumen, pale cells as described in the prior phase and basal myoepithelial cells with prominent vacuolation and ballooning. There is little evidence of secretion (× 180). (Courtesy of Dr K. McCarty.)

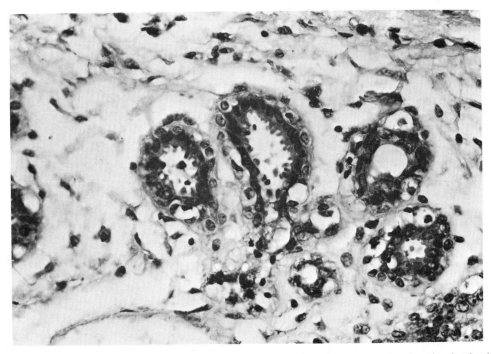

Fig. 2.8 Phase IV characteristics showing oedematous intralobular stroma around more distended ductules showing luminal epithelium with apocrine blebbing and border of basal vacuolated and pale cells (× 180). (Courtesy of Dr K. McCarty.)

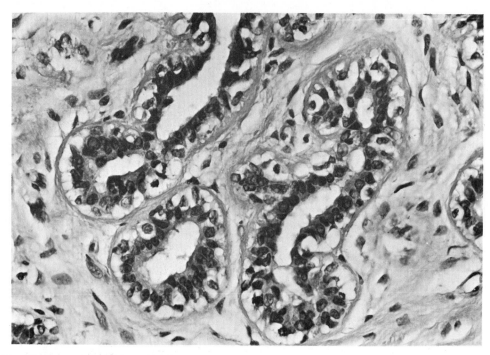

Fig. 2.9 Phase V characteristics with two dominant ductular epithelium cell types comprising luminal cells with scant basic cytoplasm and nuclei which occasionally indent into distended lumens, all supported on basal cells with ballooned transparent cytoplasm. Active secretion is not apparent (× 180). (Courtesy of Dr K. McCarty.)

but the nature of the clear cells occasionally found within epithelial layers being of lymphocyte or macrophage lineage is now evident (Ferguson 1985).

The other cells besides fibroblasts that may be found in the loose intralobular stroma include lymphocytes, plasma cells, and mast cells. The variability in the cellular constituents of the stroma at different phases of breast activity are not satisfactorily documented.

DIFFERENTIATION

Pregnancy results in a series of changes in the breast that end in the fully differentiated state of lactation. Descriptions of external early changes within the second month of pregnancy emphasize enlargement, vascularity, and pigmentation of the areola and nipple. Changes within terminal duct lobular units involve enlargement with early signs of secretory differentiation but lacking in fat. The lobular enlargement and formation of new units contribute to the term 'adenosis of pregnancy' but the generality of this alteration throughout the breast is not clearly defined. The histological appearance of events occurring in the first trimester consists of features that can be seen in non-pregnant breasts, but with scanty supra-nuclear vacuolation (Fig. 2.10), whereas by the end of the second trimester (Fig. 2.11) the appearances of secretory activity are well developed and begin to resemble the lactational state; indeed the fully differentiated secretory lobule is occasionally focally observed in the nulliparous breast (Fig. 2.12) (McFarland 1922; Tavassoli & Yeh 1987). In the third trimester (Figs 2.13 and 2.14) accumulation of fat droplets occurs within the cytoplasm of the epithelium in the lobular units which become increasingly dilated and may contain colostrum (Fig. 2.15). There is corre-sponding diminution of the interlobular connec-tive tissue to allow for expansion of these lobular units, which progress to milk synthesis following

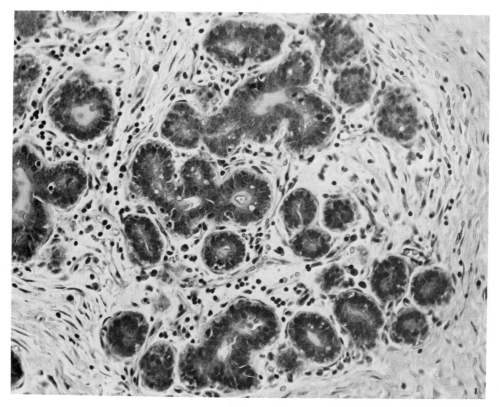

Fig. 2.10 Cellular ductules with plump luminal lining cells that show occasional supranuclear vacuolation. 17 weeks pregnant (× 250).

delivery and removal of oestrogen and progesterone inhibitory effects on prolactin influence resulting in the fully differentiated state of lactation (Figs 2.16–2.18).

INVOLUTION FOLLOWING LACTATION

The return to the 'resting' state after lactation encompasses a period of at least three months, but the degree and rate at which it occurs varies amongst individuals; abrupt cessation of nursing is said to favour more intense and rapid changes. Although tempting to invoke pressure-induced atrophy from failure of milk release, there is greater evidence for gradual demolition by auto- and heterophagic processes leading to reduction and reformation of lobular units in the 'resting' phase (Lascelles & Lee 1978). The extent to which these events are due to mechanical, vascular or hormonal factors is not known, although the reduction in prolactin levels with involution of specific anterior pituitary cells must be considered a major influence.

The topographical distribution of involutional changes within a breast is likewise poorly defined. The amount of fat and fibrous tissue will be likely to increase with each succeeding involution, but the control of these events has not been determined. No morphological correlation has been given to explain the difference in degree of involution between women grouped according to cerumenal secretory phenotype (wet or dry) commented upon by Petrakis (1977). As in menopausal involution, where the parenchymal elements, especially the lobules, undergo fibrous replacement and hyalinization, the constitutional element of body build plays a major role. It is probable that serial mammography studies will increase our understanding of these processes

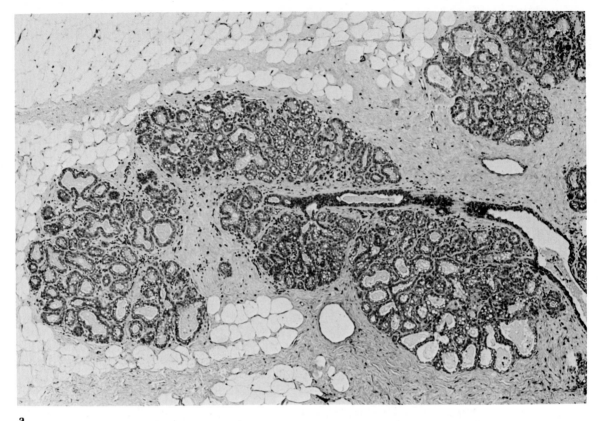

a

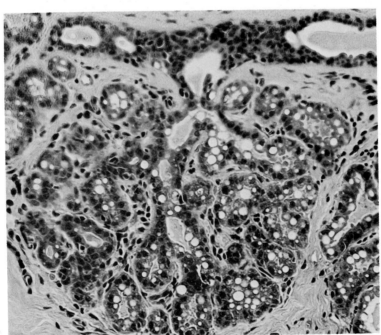

b

Fig. 2.11a, b Terminal duct and distended ductules of lobule at 22 weeks' pregnancy now showing prominent supranuclear vacuolation. Note terminal duct epithelium not participating in this change ($a \times 80$; $b \times 250$).

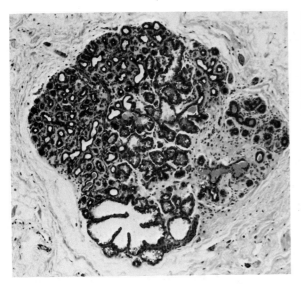

a

Fig. 2.12a, b Lobule in resting breast showing partial lactational differentiation in a 50-year-old resting breast (**a** × 60; **b** × 200).

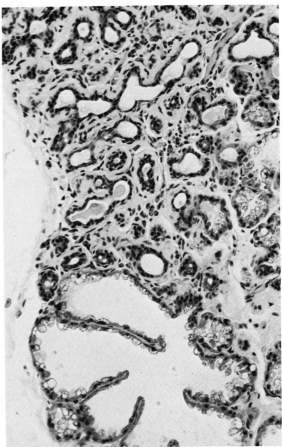

b

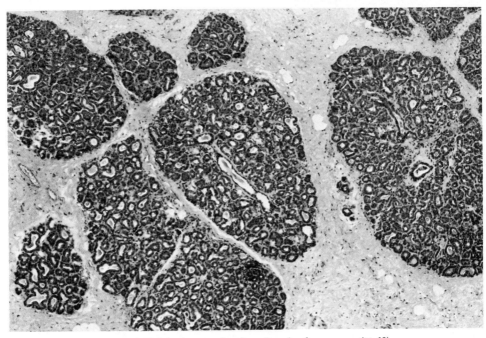

Fig. 2.13 Third trimester showing adenosis of pregnancy (× 60).

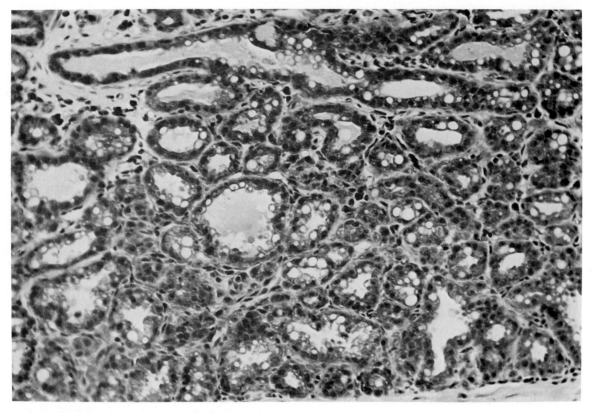

a

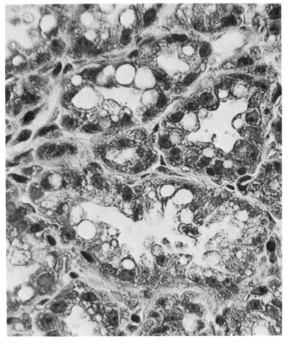

b

Fig. 2.14a, b Vacuolation of lipid droplets now prominent with greater distension of lumens and diminution of intralobular stroma (a × 250; b × 500).

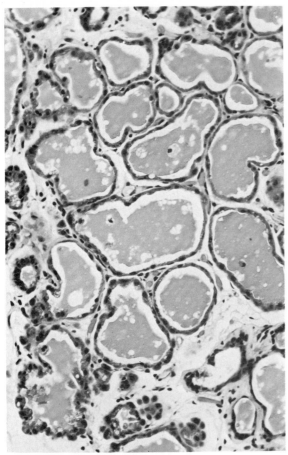

Fig. 2.15 Eosinophilic colostrum accumulated in distended acini with single epithelial lining (× 200).

Fig. 2.16 Full lactational differentiation with compact uniform glandular units and stroma surrounding the ducts which do not take part in the differentiation (× 80).

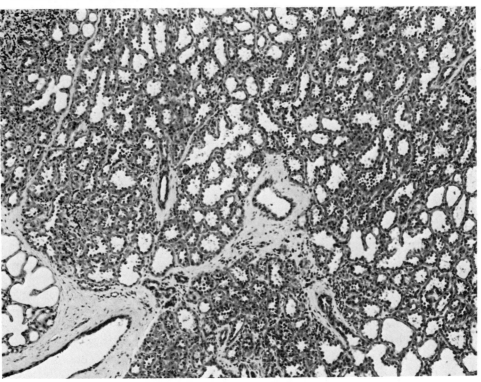

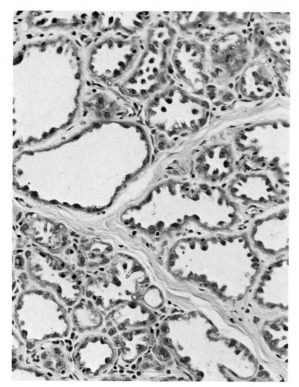

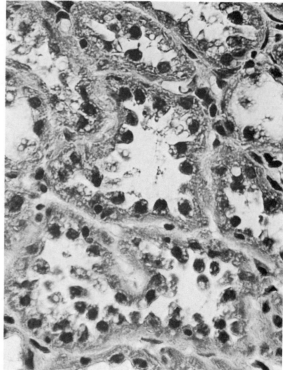

Fig. 2.17 Detail of lactational acini with 'hobnailing' of lining epithelium and prominent apocrine blebbing (× 200).

Fig. 2.18 Detail of lactational acinus to show prominence of hyperchromatic nuclei in luminal blebs (× 500).

(Wolfe et al 1980; Andersson et al 1981) but the need for carefully documented morphological evaluations of the postlactational involuting human breast remains a challenge.

INVOLUTION WITH AGE

Autopsy studies of postmenopausal involution have verified the general diminution and atrophy of parenchymal component (Prechtel 1971; Wellings et al 1975; Hutson et al 1985). Decreased parenchymal division with age has been reported (Meyer 1977) but menopausal changes in the resting breast must take account of alterations in the stromal elements such as collagen, elastic and fat, as well as parenchymal structures (Fig. 2.19). The latter may be regarded as undergoing a slowing of their turnover, with atrophy of parenchymal cells, an increase in intralobular fibrosis and a hyalinization of structures in response to

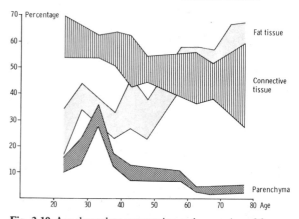

Fig. 2.19 Age-dependent progression and regression of fat, connective and glandular tissue determined from macrosections. (From Prechtel 1971.)

lack of hormone stimulation (Figs 2.20 and 2.21). Such regressive changes may be seen focally in mature resting breasts (Fig. 2.22) but are most complete in the postmenopausal breast, which shows increased fat deposition, diminished

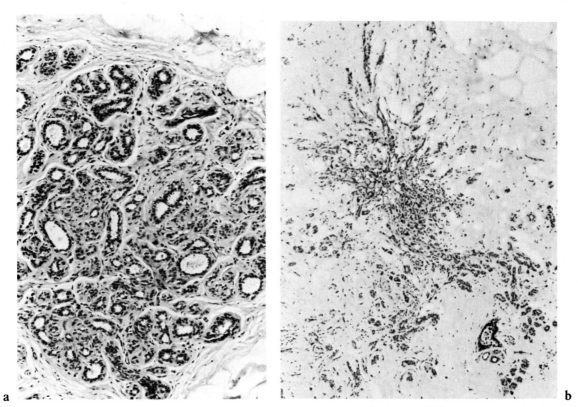

Fig. 2.20 (a) Activity of interstitial fibrosis is evident with early deformation of the lobule. (b) More extreme example with virtual disappearance of ductules but residuum of central fibrosis (**a** × 80; **b** × 60).

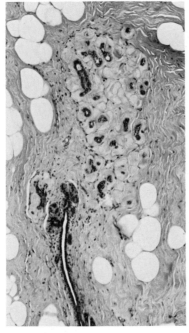

Fig. 2.21 Lobule showing prominent hyalinization by thickening of basal lamina around atrophic ductules at end of a terminal duct (× 60).

connective tissue component and persistence of simple mammary ducts with virtual disappearance of lobules (Fig. 2.23). Microcystic lobular change is frequently seen (Fig. 2.24) but the parenchymal structure may show an unusual appearance (Figs 2.25 and 2.26), termed myoid atrophy by Foote & Stewart (1945), which often has a stellate or satellite configuration. Lobules may also be seen undergoing fibrosis with some distortion (Fig. 2.27) but this should not be confused with the process described in Chapter 9 and may even show the plump, pink cells characterizing myofibroblasts (Fig. 2.28). Persistence of mature lobules within the postmenopausal breast (Fig. 2.29) must be taken as a sign of abnormality (Wellings et al 1976) with particular recognition as a risk factor for coexistent or subsequent cancer. The extent to which local steroid metabolism in the fat may contribute to these appearances has only recently become apparent, providing yet a further influence on the variability in degree and uniformity of involutional occurrence.

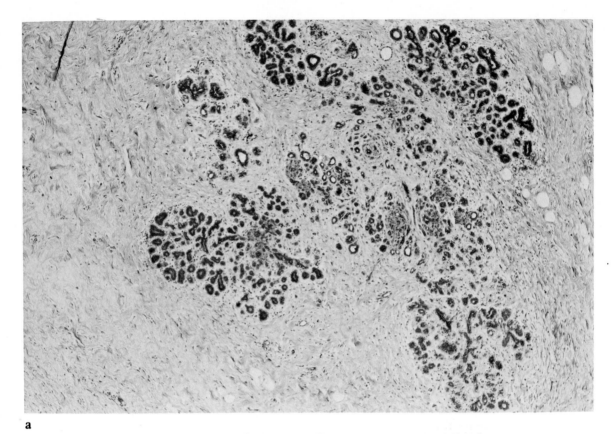

a

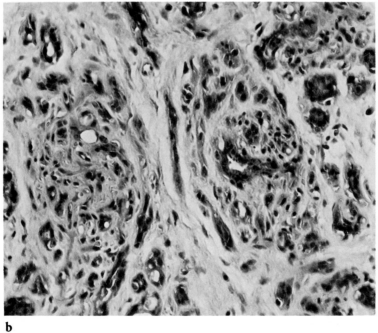

b

Fig. 2.22   (a) Resting breast of 32-year-old showing sclerosis of lobules occurring at the centre of this cluster. (b) Distinction between parenchyma and stroma may be difficult (**a** × 50; **b** × 250).

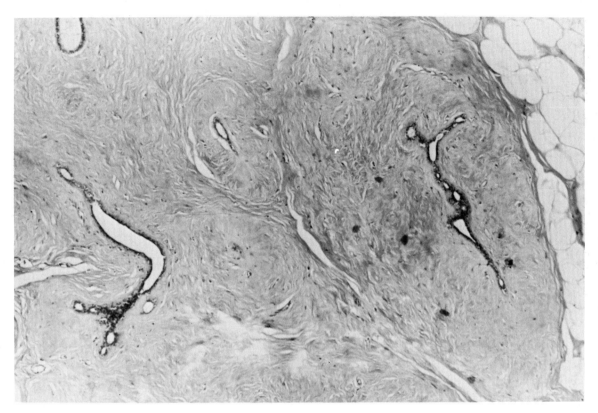

Fig. 2.23 Only ducts remain in this fibrous breast although a few microcystic end-groupings indicate the remains of lobules (× 80).

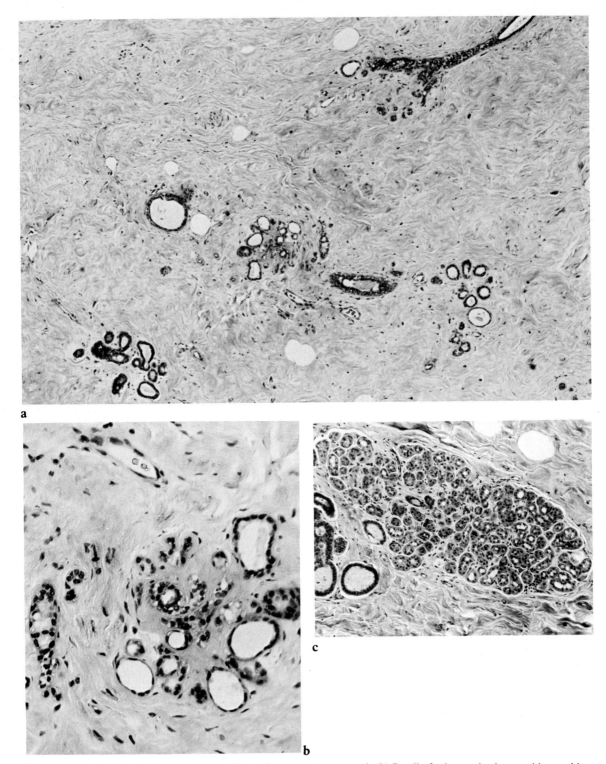

Fig. 2.24 (a) Scattered microcystic lobular atrophy at three years menopausal. (b) Detail of microcystic change with atrophic epithelium and loss of distinction between intra- and extralobular stroma. (c) Perimenopausal lobules may show persistence of luminal epithelium adjacent to microcystic change. (a × 80; b × 250; c × 100).

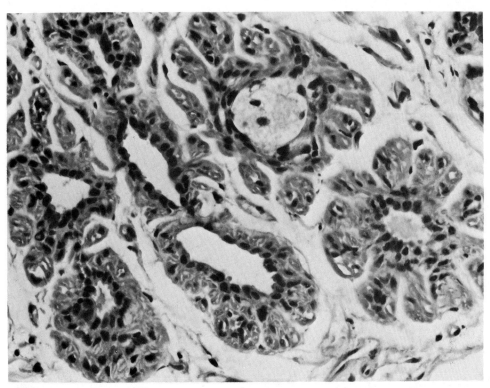

Fig. 2.25 Myoid atrophy with radial arrangement of pink myoepithelial cells around residual luminal epithelium probably representing intralobular terminal ducts (× 400).

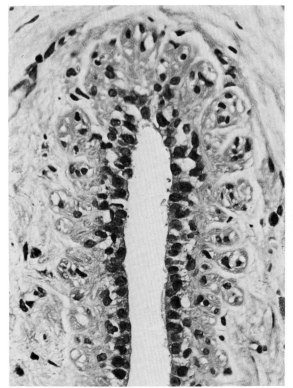

Fig. 2.26 Terminal duct cut longitudinally with surrounding mild atrophy (× 450).

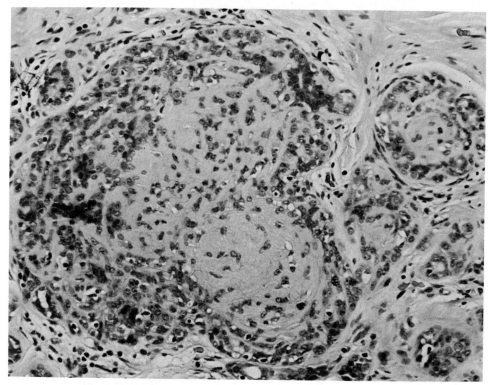

Fig. 2.27 Detail of lobular cluster undergoing hyalinization (× 250).

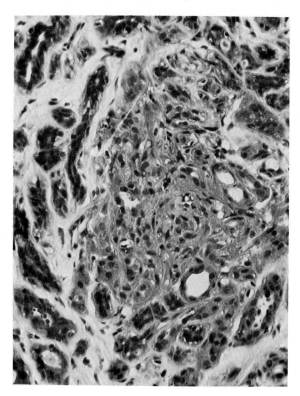

Fig. 2.28 Many of the cells in the central sclerosing area of this lobule will show the features of myofibroblasts on ultrastructure (× 250).

REFERENCES

Anderson T J, Ferguson D J P, Raab G 1982 Cell turnover in the 'resting' human breast: influence of parity, contraceptive pill, age and laterality. Br J Cancer 46: 376–382

Andersson I, Janzon J, Petersson H 1981 Radiographic patterns of mammary parenchyma. Variation with age at examination and age at first birth. Radiology 138: 59–62

Bassler R 1970 The morphology of hormone-induced structural changes in the female breast. Curr Top Pathol 53: 1–89

Bonser G M, Dossett J A, Jull J W 1961 Human and experimental breast cancer. In: The structure of the human breast. Pitman Medical, London, p 98–129

Dieckmann H 1926 Uber der Histologie der Brustdruse bei gestortens und ungestortem Menstruationsablauf. Arch Pathol Anat 256: 321–356

Fanger H, Ree H J 1974 Cyclic changes of human mammary gland epithelium in relation to the menstrual cycle — an ultrastructural study. Cancer 34: 571–585

Ferguson D J P 1985 Intraepithelial lymphocytes and macrophages in the normal breast. Virchows Arch (A) 407: 369–378

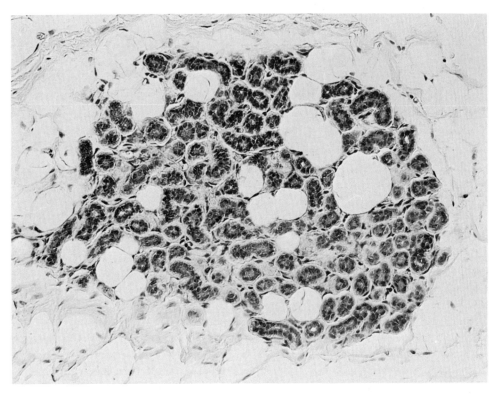

Fig. 2.29 Postmenopausal persistence of resting lobule in the fat of a 52-year-old (× 250).

Foote F N, Stewart F W 1945 Comparative studies of cancerous vs noncancerous breasts. Ann Surg 121: 6–53

Hutson S W, Cowen P N, Bird C C 1985 Morphologic studies of age related changes in normal human breast and their significance to evolution of mammary cancer. J Clin Pathol 38: 281–287

Ingleby H 1942 Normal and pathological proliferation in the breast with special reference to cystic disease. Arch Pathol 33: 573–588

Lascelles A K, Lee C S 1978 Involution of the mammary gland. In: Larson B L (ed) Lactation. A comprehensive treatise. Academic Press, New York

Longacre T A, Bartow S A 1986 A correlative morphologic study of human breast and endometrium in the menstrual cycle. Am J Surg Pathol 10: 382–393

McFarland J 1922 Residual lactation acini in the female breast: their relation to chronic cystic mastitis and malignant disease. Arch Surg 5: 1–64

McManus M J, Welsch C W 1984 The effect of estrogen, progesterone, thyroxine and human placental lactogen on DNA synthesis of human breast ductal epithelium maintained in athymic nude mice. Cancer 54: 1920–1927

Meyer J S 1977 Cell proliferation in normal human breast duct, fibroadenomas and other ductal hyperplasias measured by nuclear labelling with tritiated thymidine. Hum Pathol 8: 67–81

Ozzello L, Speer F O 1958 The mucopolysaccharides in the normal and diseased breast. Am J Pathol 34: 993–1009

Petrakis N L 1977 Breast secretory activity in non-lactating women, post partum breast involution and the epidemiology of breast cancer. Natl Cancer Inst Monogr 47: 161–164

Prechtel K 1971 Mastopathic und Altersabhangige Brustdrusen verandernagen. Fortschr Med 89: 1312–1315

Tavassoli F A, Yeh I T 1987 Lactational and clear cell changes of the breast in nonlactating nonpregnant women. Am J Clin Pathol 87: 23–29

Vogel P M, Georgiade N G, Fetter B F, Vogel F S, McCarty K S Jr 1981 The correlation of histologic changes in the human breast with the menstrual cycle. Am J Pathol 104: 23–34

Vorherr H 1974 The breast: morphology, physiology and lactation. Academic Press, New York

Wellings S R, Jensen H M, Marcum R G 1975 An atlas of subgross pathology of the human breast with special reference to possible precancerous lesions. J Natl Cancer Inst 55: 231–273

Wellings S R, Jensen H M, DeVault M R 1976 Persistent and atypical lobules in the human breast may be precancerous. Experientia 32: 1463–1465

Wolfe J N, Albert S, Belle S, Salane M 1980 Familial influence on breast parenchymal patterns. Cancer 46: 2433–2437

The male breast and gynaecomastia

GYNAECOMASTIA

Anatomical pathology

Enlargement of the male breast, known as gynae-comastia, may be unilateral or bilateral. In either instance the male breast shows variable enlargement usually presenting as a palpable subareolar cone of hyperplastic tissue that is often quite distinct from adjacent adipose tissue. However, gynaecomastia may be diffuse, merging imperceptibly with the surrounding breast tissue.

Grossly, gynaecomastic tissue is smooth, glistening and white. The histological appearance correlates with the duration of gynaecomastia, irrespective of the aetiology, as demonstrated by Nicolis et al (1971). There are two main histological patterns in gynaecomastia: the florid pattern, which is probably more commonly encountered in surgical pathology specimens, and the fibrous pattern that often characterizes senescent gynaecomastia. The florid pattern represents the early proliferative phase of the disorder, while the fibrous pattern represents a 'burned-out' or involuted state. Williams (1963) referred to this inactive phase as the quiescent fibrous type.

The florid pattern displays a proliferation of irregularly branching ducts surrounded by a loose, cellular, periductal connective tissue that has a characteristic bluish-staining quality on haematoxylin and eosin stained sections (Figs 3.1 and 3.2). The epithelial proliferation varies within the ducts. In extreme hyperplasia, the ducts are lined by delicate papillary projections (Figs 3.3 and 3.4) that may undergo focal squamous metaplasia (Gottfried 1986) (Fig. 3.5). Epithelial clusters may fragment and shed into the ductal lumen.

Although these papillations may arouse momentary concern, their benignancy is underscored by the absence of features defining atypia and in situ carcinoma (see chs 11 and 12). This papillary pattern of hyperplasia seen in gynaecomastia differs from in situ carcinoma of micropapillary carcinoma in lacking the bulbous and rigid character of the latter.

The hallmark of fibrous gynaecomastia is a dense, sparsely cellular, fibrous stroma with fewer epithelial elements than the florid type (Fig. 3.6). There is a general absence of periductal oedema and decreased or absent adipose tissue as compared to the florid type. Although the ducts show more distortion and dilatation, they are lined by a resting epithelium showing minimal hyperplasia.

Lobule formation is uncommon, occurring in less than 0.1% in a large series of gynaecomastia (Bannayan & Hajdu 1972). When lobule formation does occur, it is about three times more common in the fibrous type, while hyperplasia is more common in the florid type.

As is true in any dynamic biological system, transition or intermediate forms are encountered. Indeed, some cases of gynaecomastia demonstrate histological features of both patterns. Apocrine change (Figs 3.7 and 3.8) and epithelial hyperplasia mimicking atypical patterns (Fig. 3.9) may be encountered. The male breast may show virtually the whole spectrum of changes seen in the female breast including sclerosing adenosis (Bigotti & Kasznica 1986).

Differential diagnosis

The distinction between gynaecomastia and

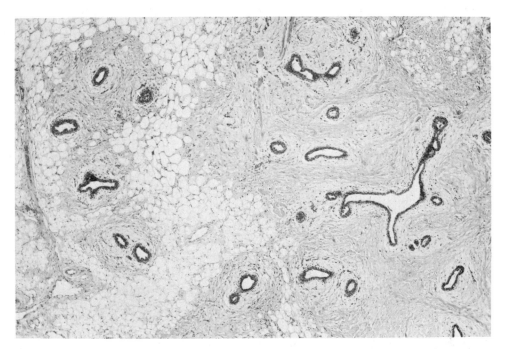

Fig. 3.1 Florid stage of gynaecomastia. Prominent epithelium is highlighted by an immediately enveloping, oedematous stroma (× 60).

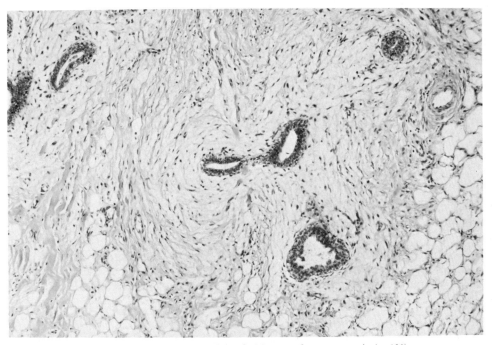

Fig. 3.2 Higher power view of the florid stage of gynaecomastia (× 120).

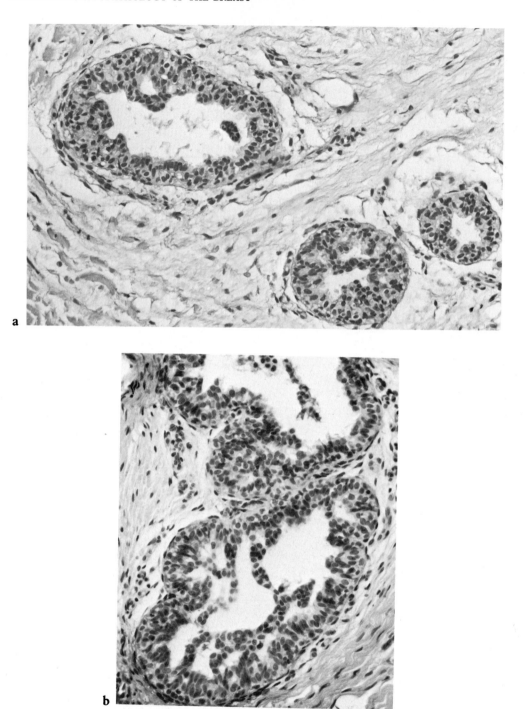

Fig. 3.3a, b Extreme degrees of epithelial hyperplasia seen in florid stage of gynaecomastia. The patterns are characteristic of this condition with slender papillae tending to taper slightly towards the ends (**a** × 180; **b** × 200).

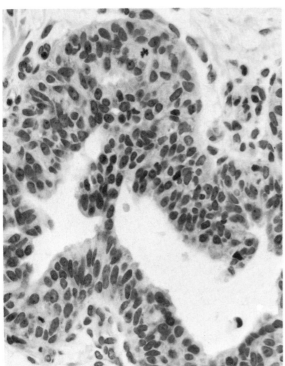

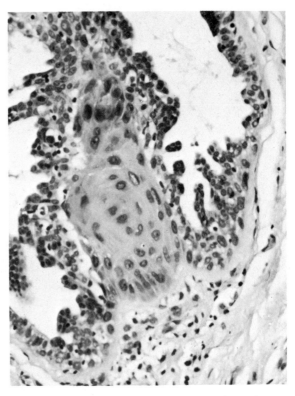

Fig. 3.4 This example of epithelial hyperplasia in florid gynaecomastia demonstrates mitoses above and at lower left (× 360).

Fig. 3.5 Squamous metaplasia is seen at mid-left in this case of gynaecomastia (× 200).

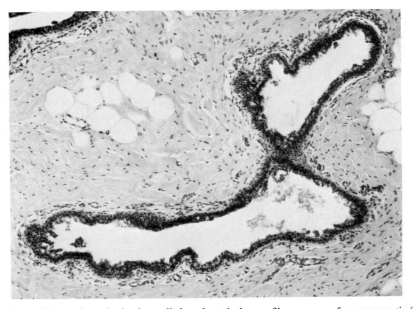

Fig. 3.6 Dense fibrous tissue is closely applied to ducts in late or fibrous stage of gynaecomastia (× 120).

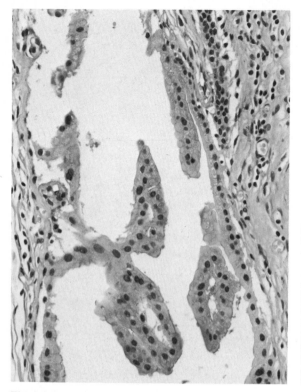

Fig. 3.7 Apocrine metaplasia is evidenced in this duct from a case of gynaecomastia by ductal lining cells with a rich endowment of granular, deeply eosinophilic cytoplasm (× 180).

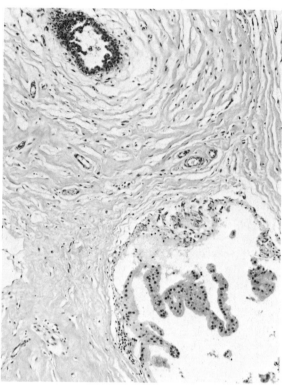

Fig. 3.8 A lesser power view from the same case as Figure 3.7 has apocrine change at lower aspect and diagnostic evidence of gynaecomastia in upper duct (× 120).

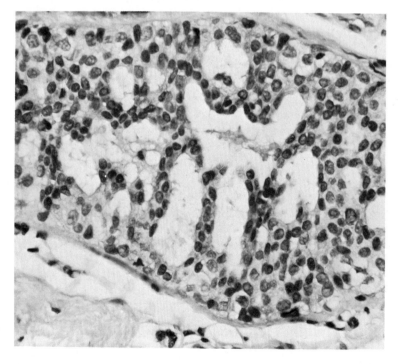

Fig. 3.9 Epithelial hyperplasia mimics atypical patterns in this case of gynaecomastia; however, irregularities of pattern and overall tendency of fronds to taper are benign features (× 360).

pseudogynaecomastia is easily made on a histological basis. The latter is seen primarily in obese individuals and consists of merely increased adipose tissue without the associated proliferation of ducts and supporting connective tissue. True lipomas may be rarely encountered in male breasts.

The fibrous type of senescent gynaecomastia may clinically mimic a carcinoma because of its firm consistency and irregular margins. However, microscopically, the sparse epithelium is rarely remotely suggestive of malignancy or atypia.

In a rare instance, one may be tempted to mistake a focus of fibrous gynaecomastia for a tubular carcinoma. One can avoid this pitfall by remembering that the hyalinized stroma causes a progressive distortion and destruction of the ducts that may create a pseudoinfiltrating appearance. Such a sclerotic focus is similar to the complex sclerosing lesions discussed in Chapter 9.

The entrapped, atrophic ducts lack the architectural and cytological features of tubular carcinoma discussed in Chapter 13.

True fibroadenomas have not been documented in the male, although gynaecomastia may be quite discrete and bear gross resemblance to a fibroadenoma.

Clinical significance and prognostic implications

Enlargement of the male breast occurs over a wide age range and may be due to multiple causes. The prevalance is highest during puberty and old age — times of greatest physiological hormonal imbalance. Pubertal gynaecomastia, usually the most frequent form of male breast enlargement, usually regresses within one to two years after its appearance. Bannayan & Hajdu (1972) have stressed that pubertal and hormonal-induced gynaecomastias tend to be bilateral, whereas idiopathic and non-hormonal drug-induced gynaecomastias are commonly unilateral. The various diseases and clinical situations associated with gynaecomastia are presented in Table 3.1 and are discussed completely along with the approach to clinical evaluation by Carlson (1980) and Niewoehner & Nuttal (1984). The relationship of gynaecomastia to the development of male breast cancer has not

Table 3.1 The diseases and clinical states associated with gynaecomastia.

1. Endogenous hormonal imbalance

2. Exogenous hormone and drug therapy

3. Neoplasms
   a. Leydig-cell tumours
   b. Germ cell tumours
   c. Hepatoma
   d. Feminizing adrenal tumours
   e. Pituitary tumours

4. Hypogonadism including Klinefelter's syndrome

5. Systemic diseases
   a. Hepatic disease
   b. Renal disease
   c. Hyperthyroidism
   d. Others

been established by a controlled epidemiological study. While gynaecomastia has been reported to exist in up to 20% of cancerous male breasts (Meyskens et al 1976), it was almost never found in the Memorial Hospital series (McDivitt et al 1968). Carcinoma arising in ducts clearly showing histological features of gynaecomastia can rarely be documented.

CARCINOMA OF THE MALE BREAST

Carcinoma of the breast is 100 times more common in women than men. Despite its low prevalence in males the histology of mammary carcinoma is strikingly similar in both sexes (Wainwright 1927). The notable exception is the rarity of lobular carcinoma in the male breast. Several reviews have explored the demographical, epidemiological, and clinical aspects of male breast cancer (Everson & Lippman 1980; Axelsson & Andersson 1983).

The earlier series of male breast cancer contained few cases of carcinoma in situ, as the disease was often advanced when first recognized. The yield of carcinoma in situ has increased with clinical detection of smaller tumours.

IN SITU CARCINOMA
Anatomical pathology

The typical male breast cancer is subareolar, as practically all arise from the major ducts. Extreme

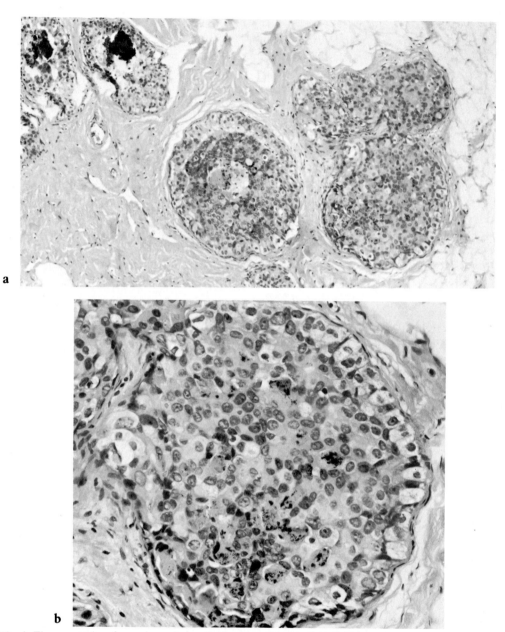

Fig. 3.10a, b These examples of comedo carcinoma in situ demonstrate well-developed examples of central necrosis with calcification at the upper left (a) and less developed central necrosis elsewhere in each figure (a × 120; b 320).

epithelial hyperplasia in the male breast is rare, but it shows the same appearance as seen in the female breast. Occasionally, borderline lesions are seen and may be difficult to distinguish from in situ carcinoma (Waldo et al 1975).

In situ ductal carcinoma may exhibit solid, comedo, cribriform or papillary patterns. The diagnostic criteria are the same as used in the

female breast.

The solid pattern contains ducts that show variable distension by pleomorphic tumour cells of high nuclear grade. Individual cell necrosis may be patchy and precede the central zonal necrosis of the well-developed comedo pattern. The comedo pattern does not generally present a diagnostic problem (Fig. 3.10).

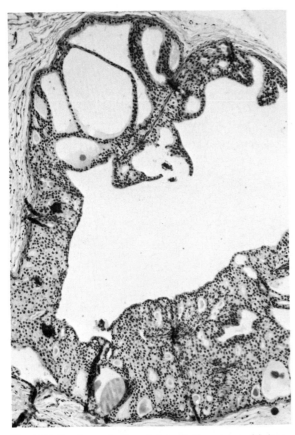

Fig. 3.11 Carcinoma in situ of the cribriform type with long, non-tapering cellular arches of classical pattern (× 90).

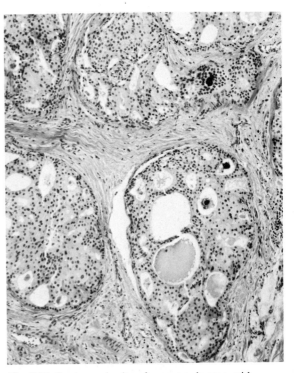

Fig. 3.12 Carcinoma in situ of non-comedo type, with cribriform features predominating. Note particularly the cribriform cell population in all spaces (× 90).

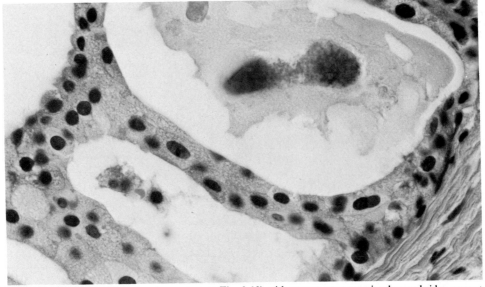

Fig. 3.13 Carcinoma in situ at high power (same case as Fig. 3.12) with narrow, non-tapering bar or bridge present centrally. Note the hyperchromatic nuclei. (× 360).

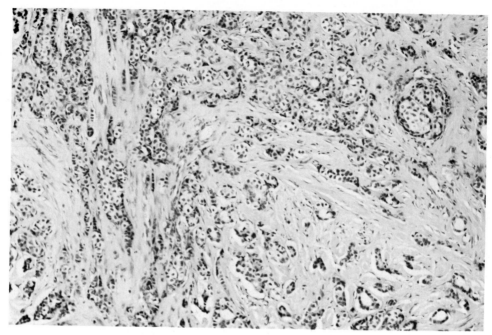

Fig. 3.14 Infiltrating carcinoma of no special type characterized by rounded groups of carcinoma cells with solid and glandular arrays (× 90).

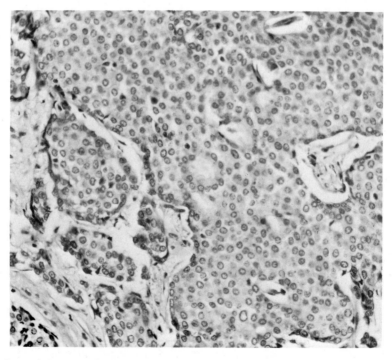

Fig. 3.15 This somewhat varied pattern of infiltrating carcinoma has large, irregularly bordered islands of quite uniform cells as well as small groups of cancer cells. Note glandular differentiation centrally (× 230).

The cribriform pattern is common. In this type the tumour produces tense, round to slightly oval structures that are a hallmark of in situ carcinoma. The cribriform spaces vary in size and may either fill the duct or grow in a circumferential fashion leaving a large central lumen (Fig. 3.11). Occasionally the neoplastic cells are small and lack obvious cytological features of malignancy. Such cells have rounded nuclei, centrally placed in pale to eosinophilic cytoplasm: yet the presence of sharply defined luminal borders in cribriform lesions should suggest malignancy. Likewise, the spaces in the cribriform pattern have sharp borders and the lumina may contain inspissated debris and psammoma bodies (Figs 3.12 and 3.13).

Apocrine carcinoma in situ of the cribriform type may have apocrine cytological features. Nuclear hyperchromasia and, often, pleomorphism, as well as architectural features of carcinoma in situ, distinguish it from benign papillary apocrine change. A micropapillary pattern of carcinoma in situ is relatively uncommon (see Ch. 12).

INVASIVE CARCINOMAS

Anatomical pathology

Male mammary carcinomas average 2.5 cm in diameter and bear striking similarity to those in the female. Most present as an irregular, scirrhous, grey to tan mass. Some show focal haemorrhage and yellow streaks correlating with necrosis. Larger tumours tend to invade the skin and pectoral muscle. There may be retraction of the nipple and atrophy of the overlying skin. Inflammatory carcinoma occurs in 2% of men in some series (Treves 1953). Paget's disease is occasionally encountered demonstrating excoriation or ulceration of the nipple and areola (Crichlow & Czernobilsky 1969; Gupta et al 1983).

Histologically, at least 75% of male breast cancers are infiltrating carcinomas of no special type. Such tumours grow as solid sheets or trabeculae (Fig. 3.14) separated by a dense collagenous stroma. The combination of tumours of no special type with other histological types is common. This is especially true with tubular carcinoma. However, tubular carcinoma should not be diagnosed unless the tumour is almost

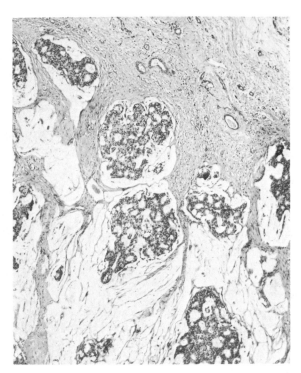

Fig. 3.16 Relatively large collections of cancer cells float in mucin pools in this example of mucinous carcinoma in a male (× 60).

purely tubular (Taxy 1975). Some more solid patterns are seen (Fig. 3.15). Pure mucinous carcinomas are rare (Fig. 3.16) and the pure patterns of invasive cribriform carcinoma (Fig. 3.17) is rarely seen in the male.

Medullary carcinoma of the male breast should be diagnosed only if the rigid criteria set forth in Chapter 13 are met. This is important since circumscribed carcinomas (Fisher et al 1975) may mimic medullary carcinoma histologically. Although medullary carcinoma comprises 4% of male breast cancers in several series (Visfeldt & Scheike 1973; Giffler & Kay 1976), the diagnosis is suspect in older series that do not show convincing photomicrographs or fail to state their diagnostic criteria. No medullary carcinomas were found among the Armed Forces Institute of Pathology series of 113 male breast cancers (Norris & Taylor 1969). Lobular carcinoma or small cell carcinoma is an uncommon occurrence in the male breast (Giffler & Kay 1976; Sanchez et al 1986). Such cases apparently arise in lobules formed during hyperoestrogenic states.

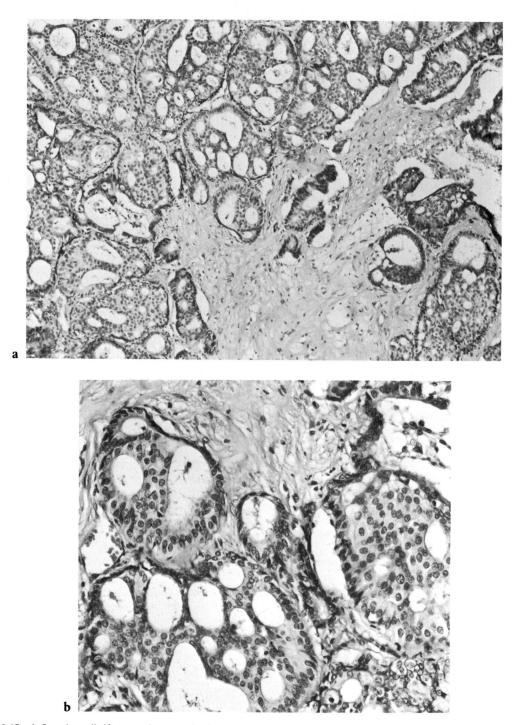

Fig. 3.17a, b Invasive cribriform carcinoma maintains the rigid arches of the companion type of non-invasive disease (**a** × 90; **b** × 230).

Differential diagnosis

The histological differential diagnosis of male breast cancer includes gynaecomastia, leukaemia, malignant lymphoma and metastatic carcinoma. It is very rare to find breast cancer arising out of gynaecomastic ducts (McDivitt et al 1968). Gynaecomastia may show atypical patterns of hyperplasia and occasional mitoses. The breast is a known site for relapse of leukaemia and lymphoma. Granulocytic leukaemia presenting as a chloroma may be identified by staining for non-specific esterase, since granulocytic tumour cells will be positive. Large cell lymphomas are usually recognized by occurrence of the disease at other sites, but electron microscopy may be needed if the breast is the only site of involvement.

Other disseminated malignancies that occasionally involve the male breast are malignant melanoma and carcinomas of the lung, kidney and prostate. Differentiation of metastatic prostate carcinoma from primary breast carcinoma is made by the demonstration of acid phosphatase in the former (Wilson & Hutchison 1976). This is the only reliable method of separating the two tumours as the cribriform and glandular patterns of most prostate cancers mimic a breast primary. Furthermore, histological separation becomes more difficult given the propensity for metastatic prostate carcinoma to have a different histological appearance than the primary tumour. In addition, oestrogen therapy may induce striking alterations in the histology of prostate carcinoma (Salyer & Salyer 1973).

Isolated reports of unusual male breast lesions have included leiomyosarcoma of the nipple (Hernandez 1978) and a phyllodes tumour in a man with gynaecomastia (Reingold & Ascher, 1970).

Clinical significance and prognostic implications

Patients with Klinefelter's syndrome have close to 20 times the risk of developing breast cancer than do normal males. About 3.7% of males with breast cancer have Klinefelter's syndrome (Cole 1976).

In the literature, there is a general impression that breast cancer in males has a worse prognosis than in females. Although a number of reasons have been cited for this, the conclusion is not entirely valid.

According to Norris & Taylor (1969) the worse prognosis is partially explained by the subareolar location of tumours and the aggressive behaviour of tumours under 3 cm diameter in males. In their series 78% of the cancers were located beneath the nipple, a site that carries a greater incidence of metastasis to internal mammary nodes. The aggressive nature of relatively small cancers in males has been thought to be a reflection of the scant substance of the male breast, thereby allowing easier spread to the lymphatics, skin and pectoral fascia. Histological grade (Visfeldt & Scheike 1973) and pathological stage (Ouriel et al 1984) influence the prognosis of male breast cancer.

The belief that men have a worse survival from breast cancer than women is also fostered by the use of crude survival statistics that favour women, i.e. because men die earlier from other causes and they develop breast cancer at a later age than women (Norris & Taylor 1969). The average five-year survival in male breast cancer is 44% in series corrected for intercurrent deaths from other causes (Moss 1964; Scheike 1974; Ribeiro 1977). The study of Ribeiro (1977) is informative as he compared survival curves of male and female patients matched for age and stage. In stage I disease he found no difference in women. The review of Everson & Lippman (1980) summarized the problem by indicating that survival may favour women only slightly, but probably without statistical assurance.

Breast cancer occurring in males closely resembles the natural history of breast cancer in women after initial treatment (Wolff & Rienis 1981; Appelqvist & Salmo 1982; Adami et al 1985).

REFERENCES

Adami H O, Holmberg L, Malker B, Ries L 1985 Long-term survival in 406 males with breast cancer. Br J Cancer 52: 99–103

Appelqvist P, Salmo M 1982 Prognosis in carcinoma of the male breast. Acta Chir Scand 148: 499–502

Axelsson J, Andersson A 1983 Cancer of the male breast. World J Surg 7: 281–287

Bannayan G A, Hajdu S I 1972 Gynecomastia: clinico-pathologic study of 351 cases. Am J Clin Pathol 57: 431–437

Bigotti G, Kasznica J 1986 Sclerosing adenosis in the breast of a man with pulmonary oat cell carcinoma. Hum Pathol 17: 861–863

Carlson H E 1980 Gynecomastia. N Engl J Med 303: 795–799

Cole, E W 1976 Klinefelter syndrome and breast cancer. Johns Hopkins Med J 138: 102–108

Crichlow R W, Czernobilsky B 1969 Paget's disease of the male breast. Cancer 24: 1033–1040

Everson R B, Lippman M E 1980 Male breast cancer. In: McGuire W L (ed) Breast cancer. 3. Advances in research and treatment, vol. 3. Plenum, New York, ch. 8, p 239–267

Fisher E R, Gregorio R M, Fischer B, Redmond C, Vellios F, Sommer S C 1975 The pathology of invasive breast cancer. A syllabus derived from findings of the national surgical adjuvant breast project (protocol no 4). Cancer 36: 1–85

Giffler R F, Kay S 1976 Small-cell carcinoma of the male mammary gland. Am J Clin Pathol 66: 715–722

Gottfried M R 1986 Extensive squamous metaplasia in gynecomastia. Arch Pathol Lab Med 110: 971–973

Gupta S, Khanna N N, Khanna S, Gupta S 1983 Paget's disease of the male breast: a clinicopathologic study and a collective review. J Surg Oncol 22: 151–156

Hernandez F J 1978 Leiomyosarcoma of male breast originating in the nipple. Am J Surg Pathol 2: 299–304

McDivitt R W, Stewart F W, Berg J W 1968 Tumors of the breast. Atlas of tumor pathology, second series, fascicle 2. Armed Forces Institute of Pathology, Washington, D C

Meyskens F L, Tormey D C, Neifeld J P 1976 Male breast cancer: a review. Cancer Treat Rev 3: 83–93

Moss N H 1964 Cancer of the male breast. Ann N Y Acad Sci 114: 937–950

Nicolis G L, Modlinger R S, Gabrilove J L 1971 A study of the histopathology of human gynecomastia. J Clin Endocrinol 32: 173–178

Niewoehner C B, Nuttal F Q 1984 Gynecomastia in a hospitalized male population. Am J Med 77: 633–638

Norris J B, Taylor H B 1969 Carcinoma of the male breast. Cancer 23: 1428–1435

Ouriel K, Lotze M T, Hinshaw J R 1984 Prognostic factors of carcinoma of the male breast. Surg Gynecol Obstet 159: 373–376

Reingold I M, Ascher G S 1970 Cystosarcoma phyllodes in a man with gynecomastia. Am J Clin Pathol 53: 852–856

Ribeiro G G 1977 Carcinoma of the male breast: A review of 200 cases. B J Surg 64: 381–383

Salyer W R, Salyer D C 1973 Metastases of prostatic carcinoma to the breast. J Urol 109: 671–675

Sanchez A G, Villanueva A G. Redondo C 1986 Lobular carcinoma of the breast in a patient with Klinefelter's syndrome. Cancer 57: 1181–1183

Scheike O 1974 Male breast cancer. Six factors influencing prognosis. Br J Surg 39: 296–303

Taxy J B 1975 Tubular carcinoma of the male breast: report of a case. Cancer 36: 462–465

Treves N 1953 Inflammatory carcinoma of the breast in the male patient. Surgery 34: 810–820

Visfeldt J, Scheike O 1973 Male breast cancer. I. Histologic typing and grading of 187 Danish cases. Cancer 32: 985–990

Wainwright J M 1927 Carcinoma of the male breast: clinical and pathologic study. Arch Surg 14: 836–859

Waldo E D, Sidhu G S, Hu A W 1975 Florid papillomatosis of the male nipple after diethylstilbesterol therapy. Arch Pathol 99: 364–366

Williams M J 1963 Gynecomastia: its incidence, recognition and host characterization in 447 autopsy cases. Am J Med 34: 103–112

Wilson S E, Hutchison W B 1976 Breast masses in males with carcinoma of the prostate. J Surg Oncol 8: 105–112

Wolff M, Rienis M S 1981 Breast cancer in the male: clinipathologic study of 40 patients and review of the literature. In: Fenoglio C M, Wolff M (eds) Progress in surgical pathology, vol III. Masson New York, p 77–109

4

Cysts and apocrine change

Anatomical Pathology

Cysts are defined by the presence of walled spaces filled with fluid. They range in size up to several centimetres in largest dimension. Cysts are rarely solitary and are usually multifocal and bilateral. Occasionally, a relatively localized area of many small cysts clustered together will produce a clinically palpable lump.

The usual large cyst has a rounded contour and a bluish colour when viewed prior to opening ('blue-domed cyst'). Cysts may contain thin, yellowish fluid, but often contain a thicker and darker fluid ranging from green-grey to brown. Colour is undoubtedly due to the accumulation of cellular and blood products within the cyst fluid. Cyst walls may be thin and delicate, but larger ones often have a thick, fibrous lining. Although the cysts are regularly unilocular, the walls may occasionally have trabeculae.

Microscopically, the cyst lining may demonstrate a wide variety of appearances. Often, the epithelium is flattened or absent (Fig. 4.1). Inflammatory cells, usually lymphocytes, plasma cells and histiocytes, are generally present adjacent

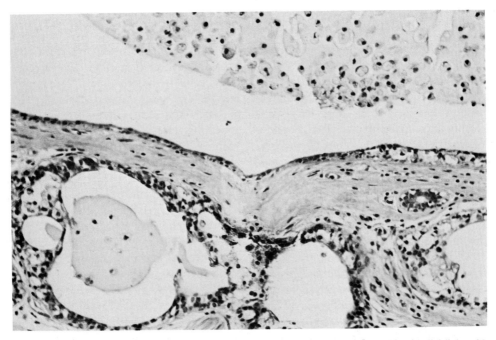

Fig. 4.1 This large cyst has an attenuated, simple, indeterminant type of cuboidal and flattened epithelial lining. Note foam cells in lumen above and similar epithelial changes in adjacent glands below. The stromal wall of the cyst has hyalinized collagen ($\times$ 225).

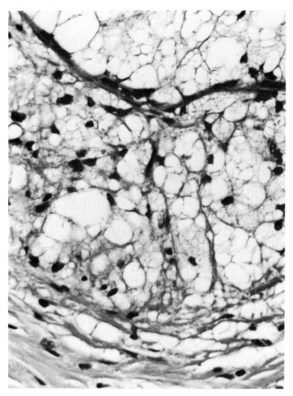

Fig. 4.2 A thinned epithelium with dark cytoplasm crosses picture at the top, separating two populations of foamy cells in a small cyst. Stroma is below (× 400).

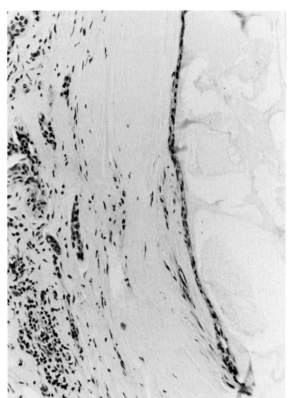

Fig. 4.3 Cystic space at right is lined by an attenuated epithelium. Note at left that similar benign epithelium is trapped in fibrous wall (× 95).

to foci where epithelium is absent. Acute inflammatory cells are unusual. Cells with multi-vacuolated or foamy cytoplasm are often seen within the cyst, along the lining and occasionally within the surrounding stroma (Fig. 4.2). Cells with this foamy appearance may be altered epithelial cells or macrophages. Granulation tissue, with its characteristic active fibroblasts and rich capillary network is often seen within the surrounding cyst wall. Dense fibrous tissue about a cyst (Fig. 4.3) is presumably related to maturation of granulation tissue into scar.

Apocrine-like alteration of breast epithelium (Ahmed 1975) is most frequently seen in the lining of cysts (apocrine change or apocrine metaplasia). This well-recognized term for large, columnar cells which resemble those of the apocrine sweat glands denotes a histological similarity to apocrine glands. The individual cells of apocrine change are large, with an abundant, granular, eosinophilic cytoplasm, and are more often columnar than

cuboidal with the nucleus typically positioned in a basal location (Fig. 4.4). The apical aspect of these cells frequently has a rounded protrusion into the cyst space ('apocrine snouts'). Large granules are often seen near the surface of these cells, appearing glassy and somewhat refractile after staining with eosin. These granules stain with Sudan black B and are PAS positive after diastase digestion (Azzopardi 1979). Although the apocrine change may present as a single layer of cells, often the groups of cells (Figs 4.5–4.7) describe papillary configurations ('papillary apocrine change', Page et al 1978). The papillary clusters of the apocrine cells most often taper and do not interconnect, but complex patterns of prolonged arcades as well as anastomosing arrays of these cells may be seen (Figs 4.8 and 4.9). Least commonly, cells with an apocrine appearance describe complex interlacing patterns with smooth or irregular arches partially filling a cystic space (Fig. 4.10). Nuclei are regularly round or oval,

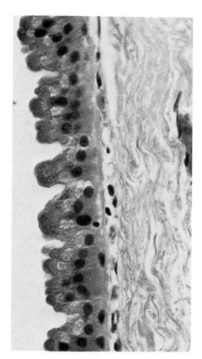

Fig. 4.4 Apocrine-like epithelium often lines cysts and is seen here in slightly heaped-up or papillary array. Note rounded apical, cyoplasmic protrusions or 'snouts' (× 450).

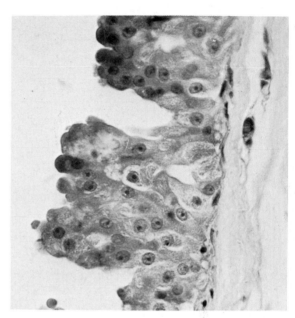

Fig. 4.5 Papillary formations of mammary apocrine epithelium occasionally have fibrovascular cores. Note prominent granularity of the apocrine cytoplasm (× 450).

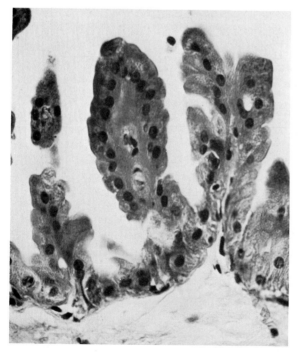

Fig. 4.6 As compared to Figure 4.5 this example of papillary apocrine change is more complex and thicker (× 450).

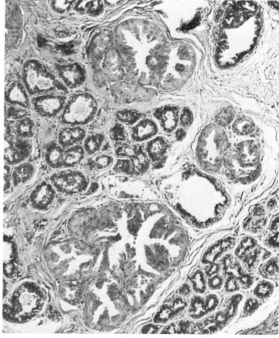

Fig. 4.7 Adjacent lobular units demostrate either columnar epithelium or apocrine change. The dilated spaces have lighter staining cells of papillary apocrine change (× 75).

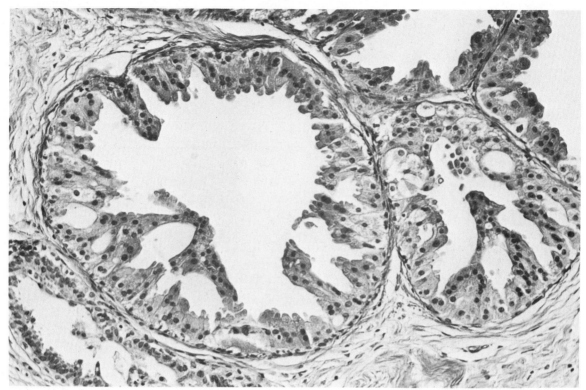

Fig. 4.8 These dilated spaces of a lobular unit demonstrate complex papillary tufts and coalescent arches occasionally seen in papillary apocrine change (× 225).

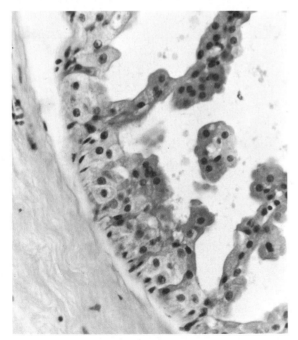

Fig. 4.9 Relatively narrow arcades or arches of apocrine cells are present. Characteristic and homogeneous apocrine cytology will avoid an atypical designation (× 300).

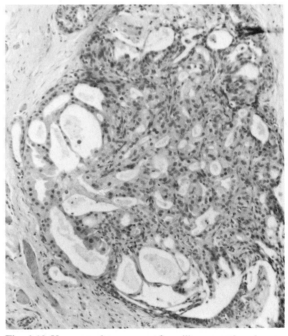

Fig. 4.10 Very complex pattern of papillary apocrine change has narrow arches and collections of apocrine cells punctuated with small, secondary spaces (× 125).

and commonly have prominent round nucleoli, particularly in the papillary configurations. Quantitative histological studies of DNA content demonstrated that some of these nuclei are tetraploid (Izuo et al 1971). The histological correlate of tetraploidy is undoubtedly the occasional enlarged nucleus (Fig. 4.11).

Many other epithelial alterations, particularly hyperplastic patterns, may coexist within or adjacent to cysts and these are discussed separately in the chapter on epithelial hyperplasia (Ch. 11).

Differential diagnosis

Slight dilatation of ductules or ducts is not recognized as cystic. Differential diagnosis from duct ectasia is discussed in that chapter (Ch. 6). Because of the difficulty of appreciating three-dimensional relationships, cystic spaces may be arbitrarily defined as having a specific diameter, usually set in the range of 1–3 mm. These small cysts may not be appreciated grossly, and this minimal definition applies to microscopic evaluation. Three-dimensional study of these microscopic cysts often demonstrates they are not closed spaces, but rather dilated terminal ductules maintaining their connection with the duct system

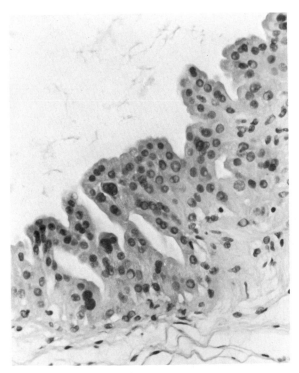

Fig. 4.11 Just to left of centre, several nuclei in this focus of papillary apocrine change have notably enlarged nuclei. This pattern of anisonucleosis has no known clinical significance (× 300).

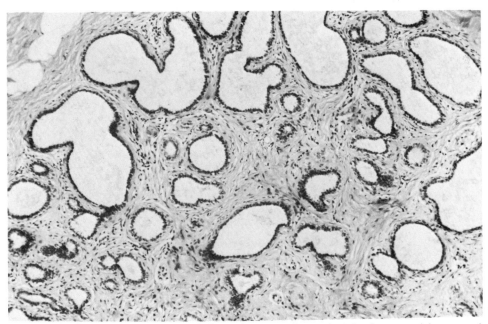

Fig. 4.12 Acini of this lobular unit have dilated and distorted as connections or branches between acini may now be seen in two dimensions (× 125).

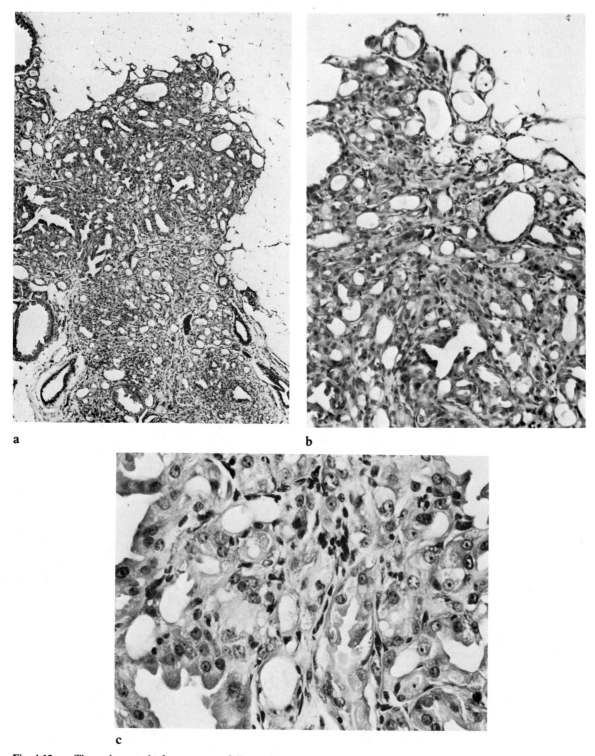

Fig. 4.13a–c These photographs from a group of distorted and enlarged lobular units contain cells with apocrine features. The vesicular, enlarged nuclei with nucleoli may lead the unwary to view these changes with suspicion (a × 75; b × 225; c × 450).

(Wellings et al 1975). In essence, cyst formation appears to be a condition of lobules in which the terminal ductules dilate and 'unfold' (Fig. 4.12) eventuating in the formation of clusters of cysts having the same spatial relationship to each other that lobular units ordinarily display (Tanaka & Oota 1970).

For purposes of practical diagnostic recording, we believe that cysts should be diagnosed if they may be reasonably assumed to have produced a local irregularity in the breast which occasioned biopsy. The use of the widely inclusive and non-specific diagnostic term 'fibrocystic change' will continue to be useful in that it indicates there is some alteration of breast tissue. It is important, however, to add to the report the presence of other changes of clinical significance, if present, and also to record specifically the information of cyst size if this may be assumed to have produced the local abnormality.

The so-called *galactocoele* is a usually palpable area of discomfort presenting during lactation and revealed to represent only dilated ductal spaces filled with milky material if biopsied (Ironside & Guthrie 1985).

Apocrine change may be seen in lobular units without the formation of cystic spaces. Because of the regular presence of large nuclei and prominent nucleoli as well as the irregular arrangement of cells (Figs 4.13 and 4.14) this change may be viewed with suspicion by the unwary. Such a change might be termed 'apocrine adenosis' and may even produce a palpable lesion (Tesluk et al 1986). Nuclear alterations in this setting of the type found in more common apocrine lesions are not accepted as atypical, nor should complex arcades be so considered. This is because the term atypical implies increased cancer risk, an implication which is unproven for apocrine cytology without advanced atypia of carcinoma in situ.

Clinical features and prognostic implications

Presentation of palpable lumps within the breast due to cyst formation is termed 'cystic disease' or 'cystic change'. Clinical presentation with cysts is unusual prior to the age of 30 and rare before the age of 25 (Haagensen 1986). Most women with cystic change present between the ages of 35 and

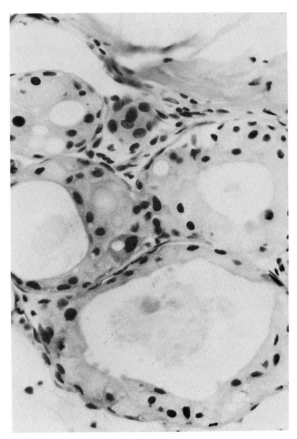

Fig. 4.14 Apocrine cytology in a lobular unit with some variation in nuclear size. This pattern is not recognized to be atypical in the sense of indicating increased cancer risk (×400).

50. Cysts are rare after the menopause. These age relationships are confirmed in autopsy studies (Frantz et al 1951; Sandison 1962).

No clinical significance may be ascribed to small cysts. No study has demonstrated an increased risk of carcinoma in these women. Although it may seem arbitrary to separate small and large cysts, the work of Haagensen (1977, 1986) has indicated that large cysts (defined essentially as cysts large enough to produce palpable masses) may be associated with an elevated risk of subsequent cancer development of two to three times. Although there continues to be acceptance by many that mammary cysts are a marker of elevated cancer risk (Editorial 1985), the studies of Page et al (1978) and Dupont & Page (1985) have not found this to be true in follow-up of over

4000 women for over 15 years. These studies separately analysed cysts and epithelial hyperplasia. Even when cysts are considered alone, not considering concurrent presence or absence of hyperplasia, they do not elevate cancer risk even if large (over 1 cm). However, the presence of cysts elevated cancer risk slightly in women already at somewhat elevated risk with a family history of breast cancer (Dupont & Page 1985). Although epithelial hyperplasia (which is related to increased cancer risk, Ch. 11) often coexists with cysts, either change may be present without the other in an individual biopsy specimen or entire breast. For this reason we feel that cysts and hyperplastic epithelial changes of various types are preferably diagnosed separately, and not presented in a 'catch-all' phrase such as 'hyperplastic cystic disease' or understood to be included together in 'fibrocystic disease' or 'fibrocystic change'. Indeed, the separate consideration of cysts from epithelial changes was well established 50 years ago (Geschickter 1939).

Apocrine change, when present in papillary formations, is more common in breasts with cancer than it is in breasts not containing cancer (Wellings et al 1975). This change, when noted microscopically at time of biopsy in a woman in the perimenopausal and postmenopausal age group, may be associated with a slight elevation of cancer risk, approximately twice that of the age-matched population without such changes (Page et al 1978). These findings have not yet been confirmed, and must be regarded as suggestive only. Papillary apocrine change when identified prior to the age of 45 was not associated with an increased risk of cancer development in that study.

In summary, neither cysts nor apocrine change may be viewed as significantly elevating cancer risk in an individual woman in the absence of other considerations (Page & Dupont 1986). It is also possible that separation of cysts into different types may produce more distinct clinical correlates. For example, Dixon et al (1985) have separated cysts into flattened (as in Fig. 4.1) and apocrine types. After initial studies correlating

histological findings with biochemical ones, they have documented strong correlation of cyst multiplicity and recurrence to the apocrine type. An apocrine lining is indicated by a relatively high potassium content in cyst fluid.

REFERENCES

Ahmed A 1975 Aprocine metaplasia in cystic hyperplastic mastopathy. Histochemical and ultrastuctural observations. J Pathol 115: 211–214

Azzopardi J G 1979 Problems in breast pathology. Saunders Philadelphia, p 57–91

Dixon J M, Scott W N, Miller W R 1985 Natural history of cystic disease: the importance of cyst type. Br J Surg 72: 190–192

Dupont W D, Page D L 1985 Risk factors for breast cancer in women with proliferative breast disease. N Engl J Med 312: 146–151

Editorial 1985 Cystic disease of the breast. Lancet 2: 253–254

Frantz V K, Pickren J W, Melcher G W, Auchincloss H Jr 1951 Incidence of chronic cystic disease in so-called normal breasts. A study based on 225 postmortem examinations. Cancer 4: 762–783

Geschickter C F 1939 The early literature of chronic cystic mastitis. Bull Inst Hist Med 2: 249–257

Haagensen C D 1977 The relationship of gross cystic disease of the breast and carcinoma. Surgery 185: 375–376

Haagensen C D 1986 Diseases of the breast, 3rd edn. Saunders Philadelphia, p 250–266

Ironside J W, Guthrie W 1985 The galactocoele: a light- and electronmicroscopic study. Histopathology 9: 457–467

Izuo M, Okagaki T, Richard R M, Lattes R 1971 DNA content in 'apocrine metaplasia' of fibrocystic disease complex and breast cancer. Cancer 27: 643–650

Page D L, Vander Zwaag R, Rogers L W, Williams L T, Walker W E, Hartmann W H 1978 Relation between component parts of fibrocystic disease complex and breast cancer. J Natl Cancer Inst 61: 1055–1063

Page D L, Dupont W D 1986 Are breast cysts a premalignant marker? Eur J Cancer Clin Oncol 22: 635–636

Sandison A T 1962 An autopsy study of the adult human breast. J Natl Cancer Inst Monogr 8: 1–145. Department of Health, Education and Welfare, Washington, D C

Tanaka Y, Oota K 1970 A stereomicroscopic study of the mastopathic human breast. II. Peripheral type of duct evolution and its relation to cystic disease. Virchows Arch (A) 349: 215–228

Tesluk H, Amott T, Goodnight J E Jr 1986 Apocrine adenoma of the breast. Arch Pathol Lab Med 110: 351–352

Wellings S R, Jensen H M, Marcum R G 1975 An atlas of subgross pathology of the human breast with special reference to possible precancerous lesions. J Natl Cancer Inst 55: 231–273

5

Adenosis

The term 'adenosis' when not further specified denotes only a condition of glandular elements. As such, the term serves to give a name indicating benignancy to histological alterations of glandular elements reminiscent of the acini or ductules normally found in the breast. When not further modified, 'adenosis' may indicate any change from enlarged lobular units to mild alterations of acini. Thus, lactational or pregnancy changes could be viewed as examples of adenosis. It is clear that adenosis is not a diagnostic term, but rather a broadly descriptive one.

Two diagnostically unified terms are discussed in detail below: sclerosing adenosis and microglandular adenosis. Another phrase that is used is 'blunt duct adenosis', but it has little diagnostic usefulness. This deficiency of utility derives from lack of clinical correlates as well as loose application of the term to various histological patterns. Most frequently 'blunt duct adenosis' has indicated slight dilatation of acini in lobular units with a prominence of luminal cells (see 'columnar alteration of lobules', Ch. 8). It has also been applied to slight increases in the number of benign cells above the acinar basement membrane mimicking lobular carcinoma in situ because of tight packing of cells (McDivitt et al 1968).

SCLEROSING ADENOSIS

Anatomical pathology

Sclerosing adenosis presents a broad spectrum from gross tumour masses to trivial microscopic alterations of lobular units which must be interpreted as physiological. This is a lobular change, involving an enlargement and distortion of lobular units, with a combination of increased numbers of acinar structures and coexistent fibrous alteration of the specialized lobular stroma while maintaining a normal two-cell population central to the enveloping basement membrane. The term was proposed by Ewing (1919) and used by Edith Dawson (1934) in order to separate it from the other common change involving increased cells which she termed 'epitheliosis'. In the latter change (see 'Epithelial hyperplasia', Ch. 11) there is an increase in cell numbers contained within the basement membrane.

The intermingling of many adjacent lobules undergoing this alteration produces gross masses which have been designated appropriately, 'adenosis tumour' (Haagensen 1971) and may be termed 'aggregate adenosis'. The tumour masses are firm and often well demarcated from the surrounding breast parenchyma, but not encapsulated. The cut surface may appear glandular as the individual lobules of 1–3 mm diameter bulge somewhat above the cut surface, appearing light-pink to brown in a background of white fibrous tissue. These tumour masses of sclerosing adenosis may approach several centimetres in diameter (averaging 2.4 cm prior to mammography, Haagensen et al 1972), but are usually only several millimetres in size and are sometimes indistinguishable from unaltered lobular units grossly.

Microscopically, the characteristic changes of sclerosing adenosis are easily identified. Enlarged lobular units, expanded because of an increased number of acini, present in whorled patterns of compressed and often elongated tubules (Figs 5.1–5.3). The individual deformed acini maintain, at least focally, a normal two-cell popu-

51

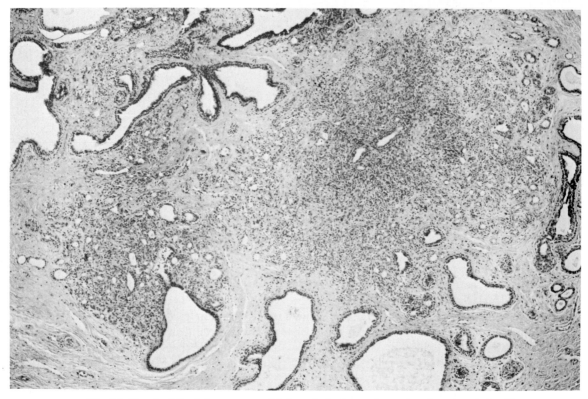

Fig. 5.1 Vaguely defined, large groups of deformed glands constitute sclerosing adenosis (× 40).

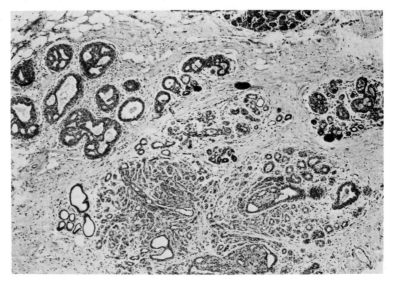

Fig. 5.2 Lobulocentric character of sclerosing adenosis is evident in lobular units at lower centre. Note that adjacent acini within each unit are similar and that unit at upper left demonstrates hyperplasia (× 50).

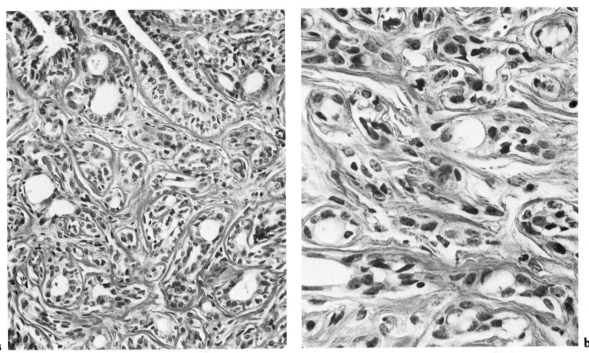

Fig. 5.3a, b Deformed glandular elements are seen in sclerosing adenosis. Note slight apparent increase in cellularity. Focally, the maintenance of a two-cell population (basal or myoepithelial and luminal) is inapparent (**a** × 225, **b** × 450).

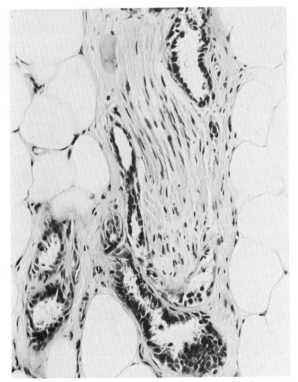

Fig. 5.4 Peripheral nerve within the breast with benign perineural glands near a focus of sclerosing adenosis (× 200).

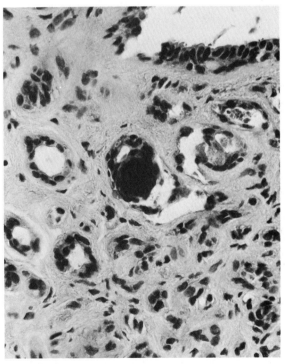

Fig. 5.5 Within a dense stroma, these deformed and miniaturized acini are also often compacted, lacking lumina. Note solitary, dark calcification just above centre (× 350).

lation surrounded by a cellular and active-appearing stroma. There may be extreme disorder and distortion, but the lobular, 'organoid' character is readily apparent under the scanning lens (Fig. 5.1).

The proliferative and expansive nature of this change is demonstrated by the extension of these benign glands into perineural spaces (Fig. 5.4) (Taylor & Norris 1967; Davies 1973; Gould et al 1975). This phenomenon is reported in 2% of cases with sclerosing adenosis (Taylor & Norris 1967), although some cases presented by them would probably be currently accepted as complex sclerosing lesions (see Ch. 9).

Calcifications may be found in the glandular spaces of sclerosing adenosis (Fig. 5.5). These calcifications are often found in areas having collapsed spaces with inapparent lumina and small nuclei with little cytoplasm.

Differential diagnosis

Grossly evident examples of sclerosing adenosis may mimic the appearance of carcinoma by physical examination and mammography as well as gross examination in the surgical pathology laboratory. There are irregular but smooth, finely nodular contours to the outer edges of these lesions. They may contain sufficient calcification to be viewed by mammography (MacErlean & Nathan 1972). Although firm in consistency, these lesions are not as hard as carcinomas with extensive sclerosis, nor as soft as medullary carcinomas.

Although the many small spaces of sclerosing adenosis may superficially mimic carcinoma microscopically, the maintenance of a lobular architecture ('lobulocentricity') as determined by low power evaluation allows sclerosing adenosis to be identified as the benign lesion that it is. The differential diagnosis of this lesion from carcinoma is made primarily at low power microscopic examination. Since that information is not ordinarily available with the small amount of material obtained by needle core biopsy, the possibility that closely clustered glands may be sclerosing adenosis and not invasive carcinoma should be kept in mind when dealing with material obtained in this way.

Adjacent glandular spaces in sclerosing adenosis often have similar shapes and tend to have parallel orientation. The maintenance of regular basement membrane about each glandular space, and the presentation of a two-cell layer within it, are the hallmarks of sclerosing adenosis. The central area of each lobule involved by sclerosing adenosis tends to be most cellular, whereas the special type of invasive carcinoma known as tubular carcinoma, which most resembles sclerosing adenosis, often has a fibrotic and elastotic centre which is poorly cellular (see Ch. 13).

Elastosis is unusual in sclerosing adenosis and, when present, is sparse. When large areas of elastosis and epithelial proliferation are present, the lesion would be considered a radial scar or complex sclerosing lesion (CSL, Ch. 9). The differential diagnosis of CSL from sclerosing adenosis presents little difficulty as the complexity of the CSL lesion involves the loss of lobular orientation and is usually the result of involvement with several separated and altered lobular elements oriented toward a central scar. Sclerosed lobules, often qualifying for the designation 'sclerosing adenosis' may be seen adjacent to a CSL. Although sclerosing adenosis may extend into fat, as may normal lobules, the maintenance of the lobular pattern identifies the lesion as benign.

Enlarged, non-deformed lobular units are often seen as an incidental histological finding. Although these lobules have been termed 'adenosis' by some pathologists, we feel there is no practical use for this diagnostic term because it has no clinical significance.

The proliferating units of sclerosing adenosis may extend focally into perineural spaces and this does not indicate the lesion is malignant if other features of sclerosing adenosis are present. The benign glands may also extend into the wall of vessels (Eusebi & Azzopardi 1976), although it may be extremely difficult to differentiate between vessels and ducts containing irregular connective tissue positive with elastic stains.

One of the most difficult differential diagnostic problems in all of breast pathology is seen when the epithelial cells in a focus of sclerosing adenosis resemble the rounded and evenly demarcated cells of atypical lobular hyperplasia (Fechner 1981). If

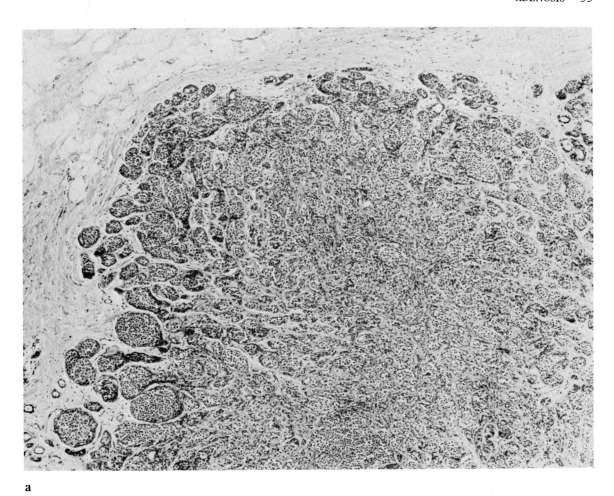

a

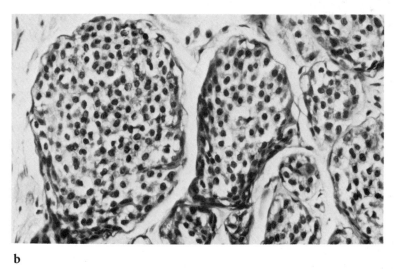

b

Fig. 5.6a, b Large focus with increased numbers of acini. Centrally, dense fibrous tissue separates somewhat deformed acini. Peripherally, the acini are greatly distended and filled with cells characteristic of LCIS (**a** × 50; **b** × 350).

the involved spaces appear expanded and filled, atypical lobular hyperplasia may be diagnosed (Ch. 12). The diagnosis of lobular carcinoma in situ, however, should be approached with caution in the setting of sclerosed lobules (Fig. 5.6), the pathologist being alerted to search carefully through all tissue available to determine if more characteristic changes are present.

The cells within the spaces of a lesion of sclerosing adenosis may demonstrate apocrine change (Fig. 5.7), but this is regarded as a benign lesion despite the frequent presence of large nuclei and nucleoli as discussed in the chapter on cysts and apocrine change (Ch. 4).

Sclerosing adenosis should not be diagnosed unless the lesion can be distinguished from a physiological sclerosis of lobules and is a well-developed example of this change. In general, we require that involved, sclerotic lobules be enlarged to at least twice the size of nearby lobules before the altered lobules are given the diagnosis of sclerosing adenosis. In older and occasionally young women, lobules may be seen in which the acini are somewhat deformed, but contain small, apparently inactive and even atrophic cells with a stroma containing predominantly collagen and few fibroblasts. Such deformed lobules are not diagnosed as sclerosing adenosis by us. Also not recognized as fully developed examples of sclerosing adenosis are lobules which are partially involved (Fig. 5.8). Epithelial cells in deformed and enlarged lobules may become spindled (Fig. 5.9). Although the significance of this last change is unknown, it is regarded as benign without premalignant significance (see Ch. 2).

Clinical features and prognostic implications

Sclerosing adenosis is confined for the most part to the child-bearing and perimenopausal years. Marked examples of this phenomenon are seen primarily between the ages of 30 and 45 (Haagensen 1971). Sclerosing adenosis has no proven premalignant implications, despite the single report of a slight predictability of increased cancer risk (Dupont & Page 1985). A consensus statement has placed sclerosing adenosis in the no-risk category (Hutter et al 1986). The importance of sclerosing adenosis to clinical medicine is its gross and microscopic resemblance to carcinoma.

It is quite probable that aggregate masses of sclerosing adenosis may recede following menopause. Haagensen et al (1972) presented a case with biopsied sclerosing adenosis and an extensive mass lesion. The involved area was not totally excised because an entire quadrant was involved, and the remaining region of induration disappeared after menopause.

MICROGLANDULAR ADENOSIS

Background and terminology

Noted briefly in McDivitt et al (1968), microglandular adenosis has recently achieved more formal recognition with the publication of three series of cases (Clement & Azzopardi 1983; Rosen 1983; Tavassoli & Norris 1983).

Microglandular adenosis (MGA) recognizes a rare histological pattern of increased numbers of acinar-like elements which are not lobulocentric.

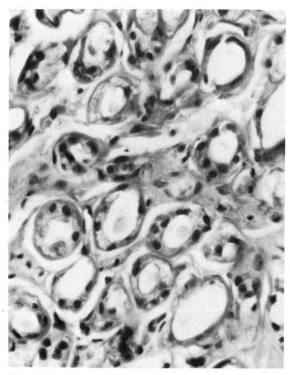

Fig. 5.7 A portion of a focus of sclerosing adenosis contains variable sized glands and cells with prominent nuclei and dark, finely granular cytoplasm resembling apocrine change (× 400).

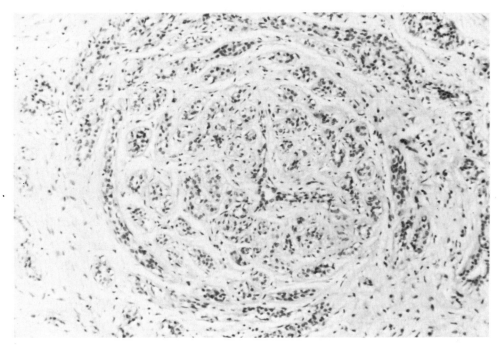

Fig. 5.8 Only the periphery of this lobular unit has elongated, deformed glands. Sclerosing adenosis is suggested, but not present in fully developed form (× 200).

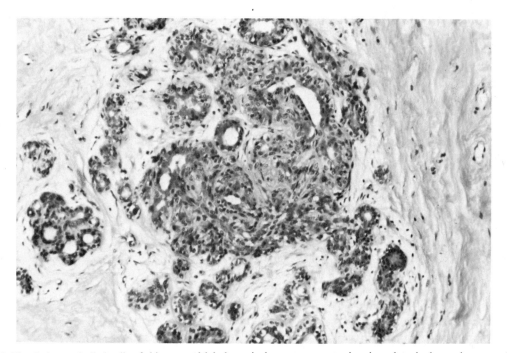

Fig. 5.9 The darker, spindled cells of this unusual lobular unit do not represent sclerosing adenosis, but rather an undefined alteration (× 200).

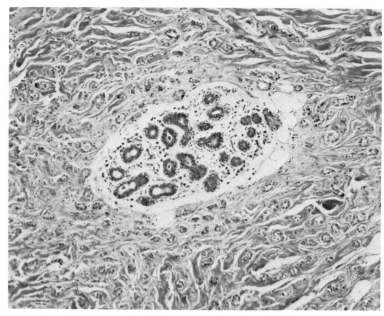

Fig. 5.10 The lack of lobulocentricity of microglandular adenosis (MGA) is well shown as glandular elements infiltrate diffusely around a normal lobular unit (× 125). (Courtesy of H.J. Norris, Washington, DC.)

Anatomical pathology

Palpable mass lesions of several centimetres may be produced which may be fairly sharply demarcated, though irregularly so, from surrounding tissue. Other examples are difficult to differentiate grossly from surrounding tissue. When characteristic, the histological features are clearly separable from similar mammary alterations. One sees a haphazard increase in round, gland-like cellular aggregates with no discernible lobular or organoid orientation extending through stroma and fat (Figs 5.10 and 5.11). Usually the glands have a central space containing hyaline and eosinophilic material (Fig. 5.12). This is often PAS positive, but may also stain with mucicarmine and Alcian blue (Tavassoli & Norris 1983). The lining cell cytoplasm is frequently clear and apparently glycogen containing as PAS positivity may be removed by diastase. There is no nuclear pleomorphism or atypia. A second, basal population of myoepithelial cells is absent. The stroma is either dense fibrous with few evident fibroblasts or is absent, leaving the glands haphazardly placed within otherwise usual loose connective tissue or fat with no alteration of immediately adjacent tissue.

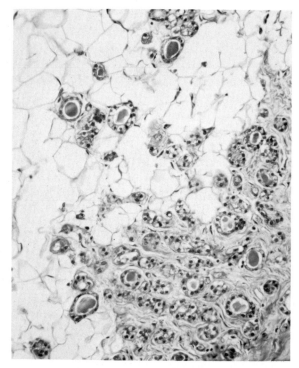

Fig. 5.11 Haphazard arrangement of glandular elements extend into fat in this example of MGA (× 150). (Courtesy of H.J. Norris, Washington, DC.)

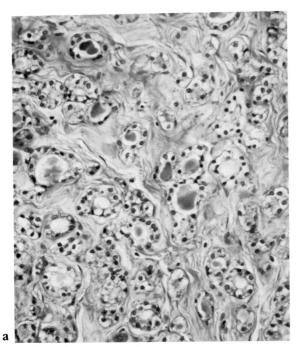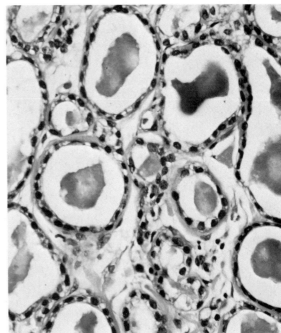

a   b

Fig. 5.12a, b Irregular arrangement of a single layer of clear cells, frequently with central colloid-like material are the histological hallmarks of the glandular elements in MGA (**a** × 200; **b** × 400). (Courtesy of H.J. Norris, Washington, DC.)

Similar glandular changes may be seen as recognizably lobulocentric (Figs 5.13–5.15) and thus not diagnosable as MGA.

Differential diagnosis

The major consideration in differential diagnosis is tubular carcinoma (Table 5.1). A similar condition with myoepithelial cells has been described (Kiaer et al 1984; Eusebi et al 1987).

Clinical features and prognosis

Small examples of this histological appearance may be found, and are of unknown clinical significance. Most reported examples have presented as palpable masses, a presentation which is the only known clinical importance as lack of recurrence of further breast disease is the norm for reported women. Rosen (1983) supported the benignancy of this condition and noted the subsequent development of carcinoma in two women with MGA. Each of these had hyperplastic foci within MGA at initial biopsy, and are, thus, different from uncomplicated MGA. One of these two cases was

separately reported by Kiaer et al (1984), and probably represents a different condition altogether as there were multiple recurrences over several years and myoepithelial cells were present in the benign tumour. Rosen (1983) also noted atypical proliferation in one case, interpreted as DCIS, and the coexistence of in situ lobular carcinoma in another case. Rosenblum et al (1986)

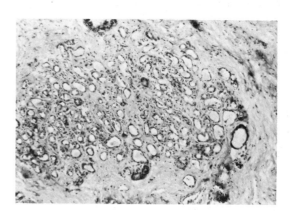

Fig. 5.13 Lobulocentric collection of dilated acini resembles microglandular adenosis, but containment into a rounded, local area (lobulocentric) means that only an altered lobule is present (× 50).

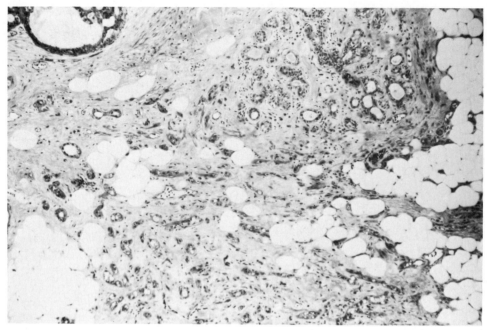

Fig. 5.14 Unusual alteration of glandular elements which could be characterized as a form of adenosis. Miniaturized and collapsed acini are interspersed through fibrous tissue maintaining a vague clustering pattern, although they are almost haphazard (× 125).

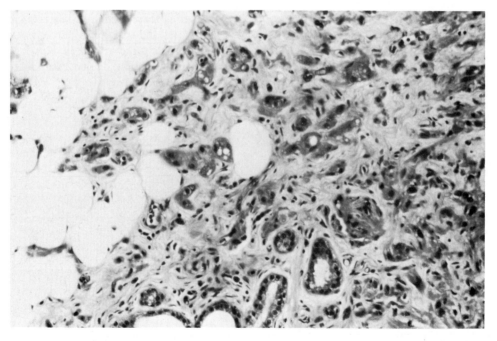

Fig. 5.15 Higher power of Figure 5.14 demonstrates collapsed acini with dark cytoplasm probably representing enhanced myoid differentiation of myoepithelial cells in this unusual example of adenosis. Small nuclei and gradual transition to more opened glands should avoid overdiagnosis of malignancy (× 250).

Table 5.1 Histological criteria for microglandular adenosis and tubular carcinoma

	Microglandular adenosis	Tubular carcinoma
Focality	Unifocal or multifocal	Unifocal*
Lobular	+ or −	−
Glandular size and shape	Small, round, uniform	Slightly irregular with oval or angular and elongated shapes
Lumina	Open or closed	Open
Secretion	Often prominent and usually eosinophilic	Often absent and sometimes basophilic
Apical snouts	−	+
Cellular pleomorphism	Absent	Mild
Cribriform patterns	−	+
Periglandular reticulin	Complete	Incomplete
Fibrous stroma	Absent or hyalinized	Cellular and frequently elastotic
Local in situ carcinoma or atypical ductal hyperplasia	−	Two-thirds or more

* This does not refer to separate lesions in different areas of the breast, but rather to the usual lack of interspersed mammary elements within a tumour mass (modified from Clement & Azzopardi 1983).

have added to the sparse literature on MGA with a presentation of seven patients who developed patterns of infiltrative carcinoma in the background of MGA. These authors hypothesize that MGA may, on occasion, serve as the substrate for the development of mammary carcinoma. Obviously, careful histological sampling is indicated.

REFERENCES

Clement P B & Azzopardi J G 1983 Microglandular adenosis of the breast — a lesion simulating tubular carcinoma. Histopathology 7: 169–180

Davies J D 1973 Neural invasion in benign mammary dysplasia. J Pathol 109: 225–231

Dawson E K 1934 A histological study of the normal mammal in relation to tumour growth. Early development to maturity. Edinb Med J 41: 653–681

Dupont W D, Page D L 1985 Risk factors for breast cancer in women with proliferative breast disease. N Engl J Med 312: 146–151

Eusebi V, Azzopardi J G 1976 Breast disease. J. Pathol 118: 9–16

Eusebi V, Casadei G P, Bussolati G, Azzopardi J G Adenomyoepithelioma of the breast with a distinctive type of apocrine adenosis. Histopathology 11: 305–315

Ewing J 1919 Neoplastic disease. Saunders, Philadelphia, p 473

Fechner R E 1981 Lobular carcinoma in situ in sclerosing adenosis. Am J Surg Pathol 5: 233–239

Gould V E, Rogers D R, Sommers S C 1975 Epithelial-nerve intermingling in benign breast lesions. Arch Pathol 99: 596–598

Haagensen C D 1971 Diseases of the breast, 2nd edn. Saunders, Philadelphia, p 177–184

Haagensen C D, Lane N, Lattes R 1972 Neoplastic proliferation of the epithelium of the mammary lobules: adenosis, lobular neoplasia and small cell carcinoma. Surg Clin North Am 52: 497–524

Hutter R V P et al 1986 Consensus meeting. Is 'fibrocystic disease' of the breast precancerous? Arch Pathol Lab Med 110:171

Kiaer H, Neilsen B, Paulsen S, Sorensen I M, Dyreborg U, Blichert-Toft M 1984 Adenomyoepithelial adenosis and low-grade malignant adenomyoepithelioma of the breast. Virchows Arch (A) 405: 55–67

McDivitt R W, Stewart F W, Berg J W 1968 Tumors of the breast, Atlas of tumor pathology, second series, fascicle 2. Armed Forces Institute of Pathology, Washington, D C, p 74–75, 91

MacErlean D P, Nathan B E 1972 Calcification in sclerosing adenosis simulating malignant breast calcification. Br J Radiol 45: 944–945

Rosen P P 1983 Microglandular adenosis: a benign lesion simulating invasive mammary carcinoma. Am J Surg Pathol 7(2): 137–144

Rosenblum M K, Purrazella R, Rosen P P 1986 Is microglandular adenosis a precancerous disease? A study of carcinoma arising therein. Am J Surg Pathol 10: 237–245

Tavassoli F A, Norris H J 1983 Microglandular adenosis of the breast: a clinicopathologic study of 11 cases with ultrastructural observations. Am J Surg Pathol 7: 731–737

Taylor H B, Norris H J 1967 Epithelial invasion of nerves in benign diseases of the breast. Cancer 20: 2245–2249

6

Miscellaneous non-neoplastic conditions

Background

Several of the conditions presented in this chapter are poorly understood. This is particularly true for 'duct ectasia', 'fibrous mastopathy', and 'idiopathic granulomatous mastitis'. The greatest medical significance of these conditions lies in their clinical mimicry of invasive carcinoma when seen in late stages or extreme degrees. They are grouped together here as they have in common an inflammatory component or are associated with pronounced stromal changes.

DUCT ECTASIA

Duct ectasia is a disease complex involving the larger and intermediate ducts of the breast. In common with other types of benign breast disease it may clinically mimic carcinoma in its more severe forms. In its milder manifestations of dilated ducts with inspissated secretions it is commonly seen as an incidental histological finding (Sandison 1962). In fact, post-mortem studies have indicated that it is present in almost half the women older than 60 (Frantz et al 1951). Various anatomical features of this condition have led to proposals of several diagnostic terms. Each term highlights a prominent feature, but the descriptions indicate that there are many features in common. The frequent presence of dilated ducts filled with a pasty material led to the term 'duct ectasia' (Haagensen 1951) which is the one in current general use (Haagensen 1986). This term should be maintained until a pathogenetically or aetiologically related phrase may be suggested to replace it. Periductal inflammation is a histological hallmark of this condition (Azzopardi

1979). It is now generally believed that the process begins with such a change, being seen more commonly in the younger age group (Dixon et al 1983), and proceeds by destruction of the elastic network to ectasia and periductal fibrosis. Pasty intraductal debris suggested the diagnostic phrase, comedomastitis (Tice et al 1984) analogizing the condition to comedo CIS (Ch. 12). Less often, the inflammatory changes result in scar which may obliterate the ducts. Finally, 'obliterative mastitis' and 'plasma cell mastitis' are terms which have been applied to the late stages of this spectrum.

Duct ectasia is most often recognized clinically by the presence of palpable, dilated ducts filled with grumous material. Focal lesions with scar formation may be seen. Duct ectasia tends to present centrally, in the area adjacent to the areola but may be distant from it, and is ordinarily confined to a few duct systems in a segmental fashion. In late stages of the process, nipple inversion may be seen (Rees et al 1977). Histologically, the diagnostic phase is recognized when the dilated ducts are seen to contain amorphous debris, frequently foam cells, and occasionally spiculated, crystalline-like material (Figs 6.1 and 6.2). Epithelial cell proliferation is conspicuous by its absence as the epithelial cells often appear attenuated, deformed and flattened (Figs 6.2 and 6.3). Inflammatory cells are frequently interspersed among the epithelial cells as are foam cells and occasionally the epithelium is ulcerated or absent. Foam cells may contain pigment and are often seen in periductal stroma (Davies 1974). Chronic inflammatory cell infiltrate, frequently with many plasma cells, is usually present in marked degree about the duct, along with increased fibrous tissue which may present as

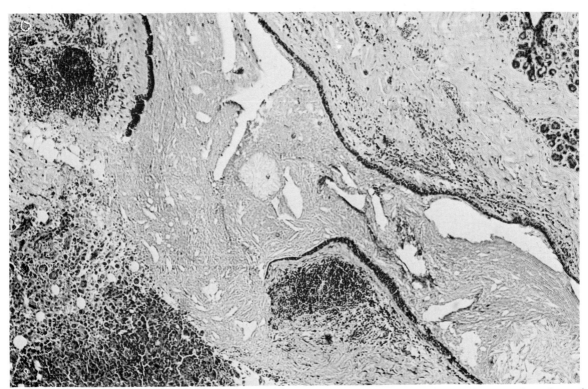

Fig. 6.1 Grumous material in dilated duct affected by duct ectasia with cholesterol clefts apparent within, as well as release of ductal contents into stroma at left with dense inflammatory reactions (× 40).

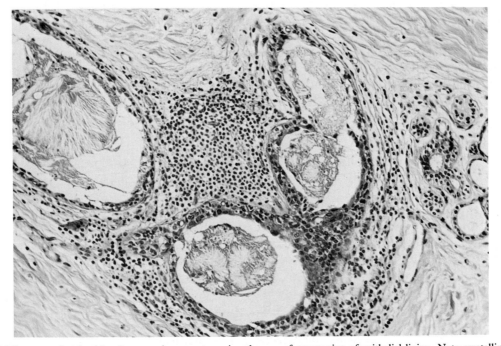

Fig. 6.2 The spaces involved by duct ectasia present varying degrees of attenuation of epithelial lining. Note crystalline arrays of contained material, dense lymphocytic and plasmacytic infiltrate and unaffected lobular unit at right (× 200).

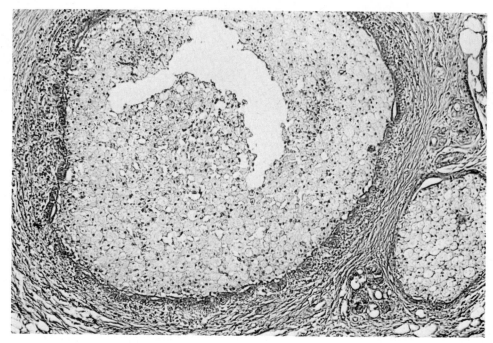

Fig. 6.3 Large duct affected by duct ectasia which is filled with foam cells. Periductal fibrosis is evident (× 40).

dense hyaline scar (Davies 1973). The periductal inflammation may be intense and, with histiocytic giant cells, appear granulomatous (Figs. 6.4 and 6.5). Rounded foci of many cholesterol crystals surrounded by giant cells may be found (Wilhelmus et al 1982). Apocrine change of the involved epithelium is rare. Calcification may be seen in the periductal and obliterative fibrous tissue or within the inspissated luminal contents. Although dilatation of the ducts characterizes most examples of this entity, well-developed cases may demonstrate obliteration of ducts with disappearance of ductal lumina, leaving irregularly rounded masses of fibrous and elastic tissue with varying amounts of inflammation (Davies 1975).

It is important to differentiate duct ectasia, which is a ductal disease, from cysts, which are a lobular disease. Important points of distinction are: duct ectasia is frequently seen in linear formation with an elastica that is sometimes focally increased and has irregular ductal dilatation with inspissated granular eosinophilic contents frequently with foamy cells. On the other hand, cysts lack elastica and are round or oval, with empty lumens or a content of homogenous pale material sometimes including foam cells, and often have an apocrine lining.

Clinically, nipple discharge may be seen in about 25% of women with duct ectasia, and local pain is common, with no discernible relationship to menstrual cycle (Preece et al 1976). Extreme examples may produce mass lesions with or without local surface deformity. It is likely that clinical presentation of fistulae or sinuses in the region of the areola is usually related to duct ectasia (Abramson 1969). Nipple retraction and inversion may be produced with or without mass formation. Mammographically, linear calcifications along the ducts in duct ectasia may resemble the pattern seen with the calcification of intraductal carcinoma of comedo type. Gross examination of a biopsy with duct ectasia also resembles the comedo type of intraductal carcinoma as dilated spaces are distended with pultaceous material. There is no demonstrated relationship to cancer risk, and also no proof that there is an association with parity or history of breast feeding (Dixon et al 1983).

Granulomatous mastitis

Granulomatous mastitis may be merely an unusual manifestation of the spectrum of duct ectasia, but it may occur without duct dilatation (Kessler &

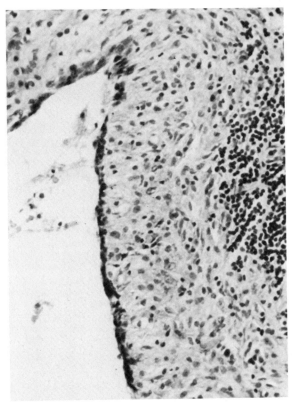

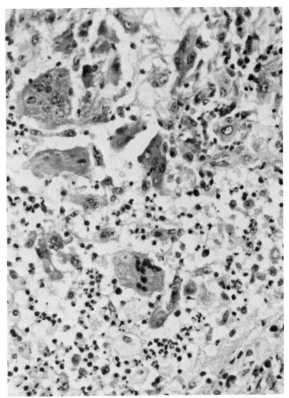

Fig. 6.4 The flattened epithelium of this ectatic duct is immediately surrounded by a histiocytic infiltrate with dense foci of lymphocytes at right (× 225).

Fig. 6.5 Intense and mixed type of inflammation adjacent to duct involved by duct ectasia or 'periductal mastitis'. Both polymorphonuclear leucocytes and histiocytic giant cells are evident (× 225).

Wolloch 1972). On the one hand there are cases with lobulocentric lesions frequently associated with recent pregnancy or high prolactin (Going et al 1987) which have a strong tendency for post-surgical recurrence or failure to heal. Improved awareness of this situation will help identify the cause and perhaps lead to better management with chemotherapy. At the other extreme, granulomatous inflammation may, rarely, be the declaration of a systemic disorder such as Wegener's granulomatosis (Douglas et al 1976; Deininger 1985). Probably the word 'idiopathic' should be added when appropriate so that the necessity of considering a specific, primarily infectious, aetiology will not be overlooked. Idiopathic granulomatous mastitis may respond to corticosteroid therapy (DeHertogh et al 1980), but specific granulomatous infections such as tuberculosis do present in the breast, even if very uncommonly (Ikard & Perkins 1977; Wapnir et al 1985) and

therefore must be carefully ruled out. In general, infectious granulomatous mastitis will be more destructive of tissue and less evidently confined to regions of ducts than idiopathic granulomatous mastitis or duct ectasia. The variety of infectious and non-infectious granulomatous mammary conditions are listed by Symmers & McKeown (1984). Recognition of a granulomatous inflammation at time of frozen section should indicate the need for culture studies to identify possible infectious aetiology. Sarcoidosis may be associated with granulomas in the breast and is another diagnostic consideration when granulomas are found in breast (Fitzgibbons et al 1985; Banik et al 1986). In sarcoidosis the associated features of duct ectasia should be absent.

Although not granulomatous, it is relevant to state here that giant cell arteritis may present in the breasts (Thaell & Saue 1983; Stephenson & Underwood 1986).

FIBROUS MASTOPATHY

Fibrous mastopathy as a diagnostic term and conceptual entity stands on shaky ground. It is a last refuge for the histopathologist who wishes to apply some diagnostic term to an individual biopsy occasioned by a clinically palpable mass. Haagensen (1986) presented this condition as a clinical entity and proposed the term 'fibrous disease of the breast'. Vassar & Culling (1959) have proposed the term 'fibrosis of the breast', and Puente & Potel (1974) prefer 'fibrous tumour', while Rivera-Pomar et al (1980) prefer 'focal fibrous disease of the breast'. Our preference, for no impelling good reason, is the term 'fibrous mastopathy' introduced by Minkowitz et al (1973).

Fibrous mastopathy presents as a poorly defined, indurated area consisting of predominantly fibrous tissue. Histologically, there is no significant inflammation, the broad areas of fibrous tissue extending between separated parenchymal elements which are most often characterized by miniaturization and apparent atrophy of both ducts and lobules (Fig. 6.6). The loose specialized connective tissue of lobular units is often continuous with or replaced by the increased interlobular fibrous tissue. Fibrous mastopathy does not produce deformity of surrounding structures, but it does produce a palpable lump in the breast necessitating biopsy. In essence, there may be a need for a diagnostic term to relay to the clinician that an area of induration or mass lesion palpated clinically is explained by a focal area of increased fibrous tissue in the breast. Yet histopathologists should be aware that such stromal changes and parenchymal atrophy may well be qualitatively within normal limits of changes discussed in Chapter 2 as senile involution. Note, however, that many cases with this histology, presenting as a clinical mass, are in young women. Furthermore, the great majority of such cases are in premenopausal women. Of particular interest is the series of 12 women aged between 25 and 40 with diabetic complications, arthropathy and fibrosis of the breast (Soler & Khardori 1984) where autoimmunity and altered collagen metabolism were invoked as causative. We have seen similar cases (Fig. 6.7) but questions of interpretation and pathogenesis remain unresolved.

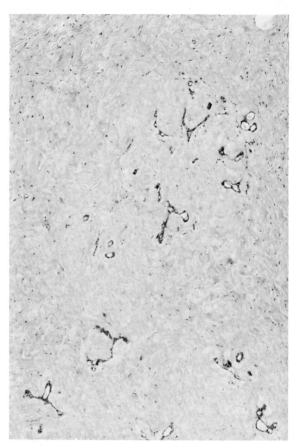

Fig. 6.6 A pronounced example in the poorly defined spectrum of change called fibrous mastopathy. Note the miniaturization of lobular units, and dense fibrous tissue in which specialized lobular and interlobular portions may no longer be differentiated (× 40).

Aggressive fibromatosis of the breast (see also Ch. 18) has been described in about 20 cases (Rosen et al 1978; Bogomoletz et al 1981) posing some difficulties in distinction from invasive carcinoma. Whilst some of the cases were associated with general abnormalities of connective tissue such as Gardner's syndrome, problems have occurred with incomplete removal (Zayid & Dihmis 1969).

FAT NECROSIS

Fat necrosis presents as a firm and rather regularly defined mass lesion which has an indurated appearance often with pale oily, cystic areas on sectioning the excised lump. Histologically, there

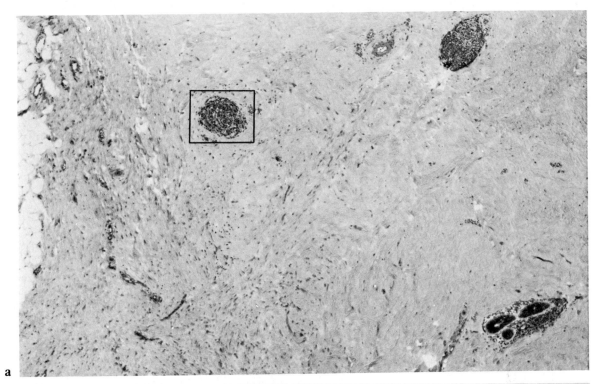

a

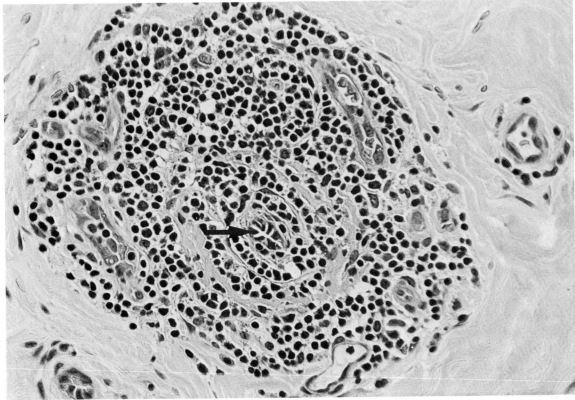

b

Fig. 6.7 (**a**) Fibrous breast tissue of second biopsy from 31-year-old diabetic with arthropathy showing only scanty parenchyma in lower right, but two lymphocyte aggregates in lower field. (**b**) Detail of left-hand lymphocytic aggregate outlined in (**a**) with vascular structures but no definitive parenchyma except possible central atrophic residuum (**a** × 50; **b** × 500).

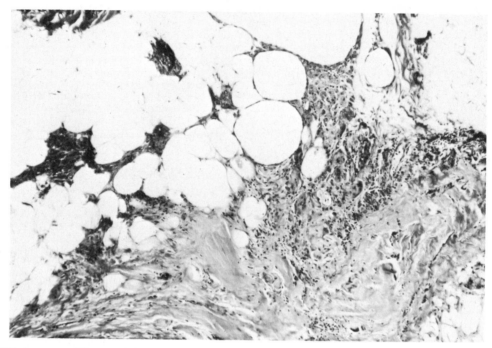

Fig. 6.8 This late stage of fat necrosis has characteristic 'fatty cysts' at upper left appearing as enlarged fat spaces. Histiocytes and lymphocytes are at the border between fat and dense fibrous scar (× 50).

is disruption of the regular pattern of lipocytes with formation of lipid-filled spaces surrounded by histiocytes with foamy cytoplasm and frequent foreign body giant cell formation. Such histological changes may be seen alone occasioning a diagnosis of fat necrosis, but are also found commonly in association with duct ectasia and of course are seen in mild form in relation to recent biopsy sites. Inflammatory infiltrates most often of a chronic character are seen in varying amounts as is fibrous scarring (Fig. 6.8), and some examples may become fixed to overlying skin.

Local trauma is accepted as the usual cause of fat necrosis, and this entity constituted about one in 200 excised breast lesions in the pre-mammography era (Meyer et al 1978). The mammographic appearance in late stages is quite characteristic (Orson & Cigtay 1983).

RECURRING SUBAREOLAR ABSCESS

Recurring subareolar abscess presents as an area of abscess and sinus formation in the subareolar area, often associated with plugging of the major ducts with keratin debris and/or advanced examples of duct ectasia (see above). Fistulous tracts from ducts to skin are relatively common. Histologically, the varied appearance of cellulitis, active abscess formation and resolving inflammatory changes are seen. This is, of course, also the appearance of any abscess which might occur within the breast. A pathogenetic relationship between duct ectasia and these conditions is strongly suggested (Sandison & Walker 1962; Abramson 1969).

AMYLOID

Amyloid masses may present within the breast, although the event is extremely rare. The knowledge of this condition is mostly useful in helping to avoid misinterpretation of other hyaline masses in the breast as amyloid. Specifically, some have misinterpreted the elastic material so commonly found in complex sclerosing lesions and cancers as amyloid because they stain with Congo red, the stain most used and useful for demonstrating amyloid materials. Use of the alkaline Congo red

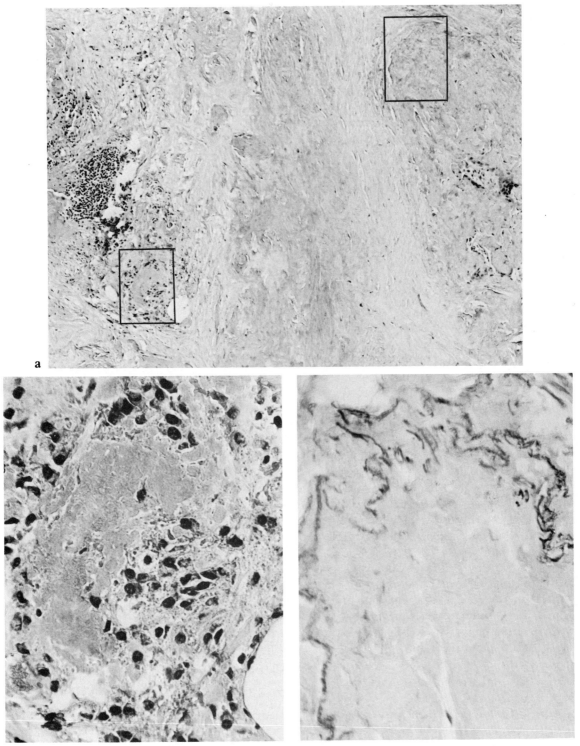

Fig. 6.9 (a) The breast mass exhibits hyalinized fibrous tissue with scanty focal cellular aggregation (b) Detail of lower left cellular aggregate around deeply eosinophilic amorphous material which polarized apple green after alkaline Congo red. (c) Detail of upper right ovoid with similar eosinophilic composition probably representing obliterated duct as judged by elastic stain (a × 80; bc × 500).

method which blocks staining of collagen (Glenner & Page 1976) will aid in avoiding this error. Most of the reported cases of amyloid in the breast presented with palpable masses (Fernandez & Hernandez 1973; Lipper & Kahn 1978) and are probably examples of localized amyloid deposition related to plasmacellular infiltration, as is the case for other examples of localized amyloid deposition (Glenner 1980; Fujihara & Glenner 1981). These cases are characterized by clumps of hyaline, eosinophilic material associated with a plasma-cellular infiltrate and occasional histiocytic giant cells (Fig. 6.9). Systemic amyloidosis may also demonstrate amyloid in breast (Cetti et al 1983; O'Connor et al 1984) which may present palpable masses (Sadeghee & Moore 1974).

COUMARIN NECROSIS

Tissue necrosis is a rare complication of anticoa-gulation therapy with coumarin, and is mentioned here because of its propensity to occur in the breast. Several days after initiation of the drug, pain, swelling, and petechiae appear. Blistering precedes the final appearance of necrosis with black, dry surface. Histologically viable areas are scattered between foci of necrosis and haemor-rhage. Thrombosis of small veins and inflamma-tion in vascular walls complete the microscopic picture which is quite different from isolated fat necrosis (Nudelman & Kempson 1966). Despite the seeming severity of the process, it may heal spontaneously after a shallow tissue slough (Mason 1970).

It is currently believed that initiation of coumarin treatment may precipitate a hyper-coagulable state by reducing levels of protein C (which exerts anticoagulant effects) before the levels of prothrombin, Factor IX, and Factor X fall (Clouse & Comp 1986).

REFERENCES

Abramson D J 1969 Mammary duct ectasia, mammillary fistula and subareolar sinuses. Ann surg 169: 217–226

Azzopardi J G 1979 Problems in breast pathology. Saunders, Philadelphia, p 72–91

Banik S, Bishop P W, Ormerod L P, O'Brien T E B 1986 Sarcoidosis of the breast. J Clin Pathol 39: 446–448

Bogomoletz W V, Boulinger E, Simatos A 1981 Infiltrative fibromatosis of the breast. J Clin Pathol 34: 30–34

Cetti R, Reuther K, Hansen J P H, Schiodt T 1983 Amyloid tumor of the breast. Dan Med Bull 30: 34–35

Clouse L H, Comp P C 1986 The regulation of hemostasis: the protein C system. N Engl J Med 314: 1298–1304.

Davies J D 1973 Hyperelastosis, obliteration and fibrous plaques in major ducts of the human breast. J Pathol 110: 13–26

Davies J D 1974 Pigmented periductal cells (ochrocytes) in mammary dysplasias: their nature and significance. J Pathol 114: 205–216

Davies J D 1975 Inflammatory damage to ducts in mammary dysplasia: a cause of duct obliteration. J Pathol 117: 47–54

DeHertogh D A, Rossof A H, Harris A A, Economou S G 1980 Prednisone management of granulomatous mastitis. N Engl J Med 303: 799–800

Deininger H K 1985 Wegener's granulomatosis of the breast. Radiology 154: 59–60

Dixon J M, Anderson T J, Lumsden A B, Elton R A, Roberts M M, Forrest A P M 1983 Mammary duct ectasia. Br J Surg 70: 601–603

Douglas A C, Anderson T J, MacDonald M, Simpson J G G 1976 Midline and Wegener's Granulomatosis. Ann N Y Acad Sci 278: 618–635

Fernandez B B, Hernandez F J 1973 Amyloid tumor of the breast. Arch Pathol 95: 102–105

Fitzgibbons P L, Smiley D F, Kern W H 1985 Sarcoidosis presenting initially as breast mass: report of two cases. Hum Pathol 16: 851–852

Frantz V K, Pickren J W, Melcher G W, Auchincloss H 1951 Incidence of chronic cystic disease in so-called 'normal breasts', a study based on 225 postmortem examinations. Cancer 4: 762–783

Fujihara S, Glenner G G 1981 Primary localized amyloidosis of the genitourinary tract: immunohistochemical study on eleven cases. Lab Invest 44: 55–60

Glenner G G 1980 Amyloid deposits and amyloidosis: the beta-fibrilloses. N Engl J Med 302: 1283–1292, 1333–1343

Glenner G G, Page D L 1976 Amyloid amyloidosis and amyloidogenesis. Int Rev Exp Pathol 15: 1–92

Going J J, Anderson T J, Wilkinson S, Chetty U 1987 Granulomatous lobular mastitis. J Clin Pathol 40: 535–540

Haagensen C D 1951 Mammary-duct ectasia: a disease that may simulate carcinoma. Cancer 4: 749–761

Haagensen C D 1986 Diseases of the breast, 3rd edn. Saunders, Philadelphia, p 125–135, 357–368

Ikard R W, Perkins D 1977 Mammary tuberculosis: a rare modern disease. South Med J 70: 208–212

Kessler E, Wolloch Y 1972 Granulomatous mastitis: a lesion clinically simulating carcinoma. Am J Clin Pathol 58: 642–646

Lipper S, Kahn L B 1978 Amyloid tumor: a clinicopathologic study of four cases. Am J Surg Pathol 2: 141–415

Mason J R 1970 Haemorrhage-induced breast gangrene. Br J Surg 57: 700–702

Meyer J E, Silverman P, Gandbhir L 1978 Fat necrosis of the breast. Arch Surg 113: 801–805

Minkowitz S, Hedayati H, Hiller S, Gardner B 1973 Fibrous mastopathy: a clinical histopathologic study. Cancer 32: 913–916

Nudelman H L, Kempson R L 1966 Necrosis of the breast: a rare complication of anticoagulant therapy. Am J Surg 111: 728–733

O'Connor C R, Rubinow A, Cohen A S 1984 Primary (AL) amyloidosis as a cause of breast masses. Am J Med 77: 981–986

Orson L W, Cigtay O S 1983 Fat necrosis of the breast: characteristic xeromammographic appearance. Radiology 146: 35–38

Preece P E, Hughes L E, Mansel R E, Baum M, Bolton P M, Gravelle I H 1976 Clinical syndromes of mastalgia. Lancet 2: 670–673

Puente J L, Potel J 1974 Fibrous tumor of the breast. Arch Surg 109: 391–394

Rees B I, Gravelle I H, Hughes L E 1977 Nipple retraction in duct ectasia. Br J Surg 64: 577–580

Rivera-Pomar J M, Vilanova J R, Burgos-Bretones J J, Arocena G 1980 Focal fibrous disease of breast: a common entity in young women. Virchows Arch (A) 386: 59–64

Rosen Y, Papasozomenos S C, Gardner B 1978 Fibromatosis of the breast. Cancer 41: 1409–1415

Sadeghee S A, Moore S W 1974 Rheumatoid arthritis, bilateral amyloid tumors of the breast and multiple cutaneous amyloid nodules. Am J Clin Pathol 62: 472–476

Sandison A T 1962 An autopsy study of the adult human breast: with special reference to proliferative epithelial changes of importance in the pathology of the breast. Nat Cancer Inst Monogr 8: 1–145

Sandison A T, Walker J C 1962 Inflammatory mastitis, mammary duct ectasia, and mammillary fistula. Br J Surg 50: 57–64

Soler N G, Khardori R 1984 Fibrous disease of the breast, thyroiditis and cheiroarthropathy in type I diabetes mellitus. Lancet 1: 193–194

Stephenson T J, Underwood J C E 1986 Giant cell arteritis: an unusual cause of palpable masses in the breast. Br J Surg 73: 105

Symmers W St C, McKeown K C 1984 Tuberculosis of the breast. Br Med J 289: 48–49

Thaell J F, Saue G L 1983 Giant cell arteritis involving the breasts. J Rheumatol 10: 329–331

Tice G I, Dockerty M B, Harrington S W 1984 Comedomastitis: a clinical and pathologic study of data in 172 cases. Surg Gynecol Obstet 87: 525–540

Vassar P S, Culling C F A 1959 Fibrosis of the breast. Arch Pathol 67: 128–133

Wapnir I L, Pallan T M, Gaudino J, Stahl W M 1985 Latent mammary tuberculosis: a case report. Surgery 98: 976–978

Wilhelmus J L, Schrodt G R, Mahaffey L M 1982 Cholesterol granulomas of the breast: a lesion which clinically mimics carcinoma. Am J Clin Pathol 77: 592–597

Zayid I, Dihmis C 1969 Familial multicentric fibromatosis-desmoids. Cancer 24: 786–795

Fibroadenoma and related lesions

Terminology

Fibroadenoma (adenofibroma) is a benign tumour of fibrous and epithelial elements. The adjectives intracanalicular and pericanalicular have been applied to fibroadenomas but are of no practical or prognostic importance. They refer to different arrangements of the fibrous tissue and the epithelium, and serve only to acknowledge that fibroadenomas have different patterns.

The adjectives 'giant' and 'juvenile' *are* of importance because they have been inconsistently used. For instance, giant fibroadenoma has often been used interchangeably with the semantically abominable term 'benign cystosarcoma phyllodes'. The distinction between giant fibroadenoma and benign phyllodes tumour rests solely on the histological features of the stroma, and the diagnosis is completely independent of size. A giant fibroadenoma is merely a fibroadenoma that has attained an immense size. There is no official minimal limit, but the term should probably be reserved for tumours greater than 8–10 cm in size. McDonald & Harrington (1950) suggested 500 g as a minimum weight. The World Health Organization has used the term 'cellular intracanalicular fibroadenoma' for giant fibroadenoma (Scarff & Torloni 1968). This term serves the important purpose of recognizing that the giant fibroadenoma is indeed a fibroadenoma and not a cystosarcoma. The term is not ideal, however, because all giant fibroadenomas do not have an intracanalicular configuration.

Juvenile fibroadenoma is a diagnostic term that is predominantly predicated on clinical grounds (Ashikari et al 1971; Oberman 1979). Because of their size, all juvenile fibroadenomas are also giant fibroadenomas by definition. The term juvenile fibroadenoma is used when the tumour (1) occurs in an adolescent, (2) grows rapidly, (3) reaches a size that is often two to four times the size of the opposite breast, (4) stretches the skin and (5) displaces the nipple. The juvenile fibroadenoma is not a specific histological entity. It has a *trend* to fewer lobules, larger ducts, and a more cellular stroma than the typical fibroadenoma. These trends are explainable by the clinical features. Since juvenile fibroadenomas often occur shortly after menarche, the entire breast, as well as the fibroadenoma, is at a stage of minimal lobular development. The trend towards an increased cellularity of stroma correlates with the fact that juvenile fibroadenomas are rapidly growing lesions that are often excised only a few months after the initial appearance. Nonetheless, juvenile fibroadenomas can have a sparsely cellular, hyalinized stroma throughout the lesion that completely belies its rapid growth. Moreover, there are large numbers of well-defined lobules in many juvenile fibroadenomas just as seen in ordinary fibroadenomas (Wuslin 1960). Finally, there is sometimes an intracanalicular pattern of stromal proliferation that is identical to the usual fibroadenoma.

Anatomical pathology

The gross appearance of the typical fibroadenoma is usually diagnostic. It is a sharply circumscribed spherical or discoid mass (Fig. 7.1). The cut surface is white, although sometimes there are small, light-brown areas when there is epithelial hyperplasia or large lobules. The cut surface glistens and is occasionally slightly myxoid. Small

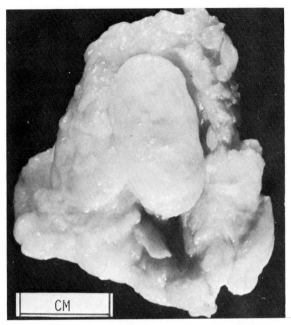

Fig. 7.1 Fibroadenoma from 72-year-old woman. Tumour was excised with surrounding margin of breast which falls away due to sharp circumscription of lesion. Microscopically, this was mostly hyalinized connective tissue with atrophic epithelium. Gross appearance of fibroadenoma is the same regardless of age.

clefts are often evident, and they may be accentuated by bending the cut surface. Most lesions are firm but not hard, although a few are soft if the stroma is myxomatous. In the elderly, fibroadenomas are often extremely firm due to sparse stromal cellularity, lack of epithelium and/or calcification. Dense fibrosis and calcification are sometimes found in tumours of young women as well. Juvenile fibroadenomas are firm, tan, pink, or grey and have a nodular cut surface (Fig. 7.2). They are either surrounded with a thin capsule or abut directly on surrounding tissue.

Microscopically, fibrous tissue comprises most of a fibroadenoma. The stroma can compress ducts so that they are reduced to slits with a curvilinear configuration (the intracanalicular pattern). In other areas the ducts maintain their patency because the stroma grows circumferentially around the ducts (the pericanalicular pattern). A single tumour can have both patterns. The stroma can be quite cellular with readily identifiable mitoses and there may be a modest degree of pleomorphism (Fig. 7.3). Other foci are sparsely cellular areas and can have broad zones of hyalinized collagen. The stroma is sometimes loose and myxomatous, and the cells in these foci are more stellate. The quality of the stroma can vary markedly even within the same lesion.

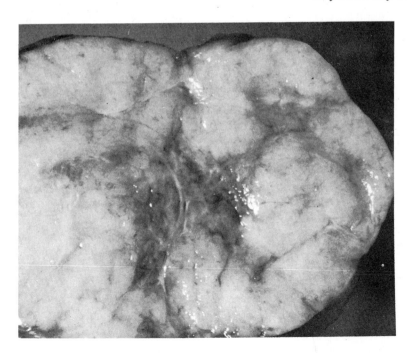

Fig. 7.2 Giant fibroadenoma measures 8 × 8 × 13 cm. Patient was an 18-year-old girl with a history of rapid breast enlargement with thinning of the overlying skin. Based on these clinical features, this lesion can also be designated as a juvenile fibroadenoma.

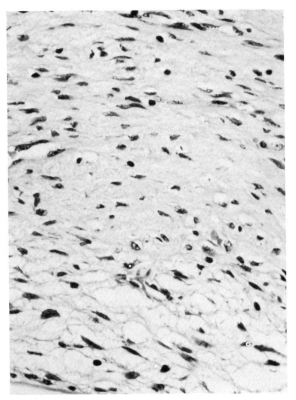

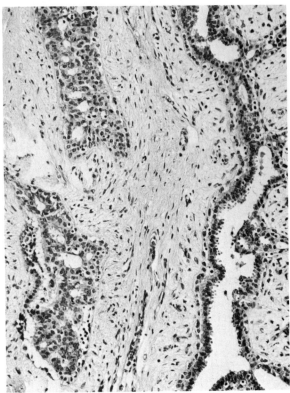

Fig. 7.3 Fibroadenoma from 31-year-old woman. Stroma was fairly uniform with cells and abundant collagen (upper) as well as looser stroma with cells having larger nuclei (lower). This degree of variation is frequent. The lack of bizarre cells and high mitotic activity separates it from cystosarcoma phyllodes (× 225).

Fig. 7.4 Prominent epithelial lining in a fibroadenoma may show complex patterns when cut tangentially or in cross-section (left half). Nuclei are active but bland. A myoepithelial layer is discernible in much of the duct in right half of field. Apocrine snouts are evident in the epithelial cells (× 150).

Rarely, fibroadenomas contain fat either in small foci or in very large areas. The small areas are probably fat that is entrapped since fibroadenomas grow, at least in part, by accretion of neighbouring breast tissue. A second possibility is metaplasia of fibroblasts into adipocytes. This seems a likely explanation for the rare lesion that has a huge quantity of fat within what otherwise appears to be a fibroadenoma (Oberman et al 1969). Osseous metaplasia has rarely been seen in fibroadenomas (Spagnola & Shilkin 1983).

Smooth muscle is an extremely rare component of fibroadenomas (Goodman & Taxy 1981). Some tumours have been so dominated by smooth muscle that Riddell & Davies (1973) called the lesions muscular hamartomas. It should be mentioned that the term muscular hamartoma has been used for masses that are predominantly smooth muscle but lack the epithelial architecture of fibroadenomas (Huntrakoon & Lin 1984).

The epithelium has diverse appearances. Normal lobules are frequent and, indeed, the smallest fibroadenoma can be traced to an origin in the lobules (Wellings et al 1975). Lobules are especially evident near the edge of fibroadenomas and may in part represent lobules incorporated into the tumour as it expands. Often the lobules immediately adjacent to a fibroadenoma have increased stroma between the ductules as if they were mini-fibroadenomas. Lobules may undergo the same changes that occur in lobules elsewhere in the breast, e.g. apocrine metaplasia, sclerosing adenosis, or blunt duct adenosis. Azzopardi (1979) found sclerosing adenosis in 6% of fibroadenomas, usually in tumours from older patients. He found apocrine metaplasia in 14%. Squamous metaplasia, with or without keratinization, is very rare (Salm 1957).

Large extralobular ducts are often numerous and usually have a double layer of epithelium and myoepithelium. The normal architecture is especially discernible with the pericanalicular growth pattern. In the intracanalicular lesions the epithelium is often stretched and the myoepithelial layer is not easily seen. Sometimes there is stratification of the epithelium and occasionally small papillary excrescences that are four to six cells in thickness. Tangential sectioning of these hyperplastic foci can produce complex patterns that may be worrisome (Fig. 7.4). The cells have plump nuclei, but atypia is not present. Mitoses are sometimes numerous, but abnormal forms do not occur.

Fibroadenomas removed from pregnant or lactating women can have acinar hyperplasia of the lobules and evidence of secretion identical to that seen in the normal lactating breast (Fig. 7.5). Secretory change has also been seen in fibroadenomas from patients taking oral contraceptives, including women who have never been pregnant (Fechner 1970). Fibroadenomas from oral contraceptive users do not have epithelial atypia (LiVolsi et al 1979), nor are there differences in cell proliferation rates (Meyer 1977).

About 0.5% of fibroadenomas are partially or completely infarcted. The inflammatory and fibrous reaction to the infarct can destroy the sharp circumscription of the fibroadenoma and fix the lesion in the breast tissue. The apparent infiltration of fat mimics carcinoma, and a frozen section from the infarcted area can be difficult to interpret because of the blurring of the characteristic fibroadenomatous architecture. The diagnosis of carcinoma may be entertained. This error can be avoided by not diagnosing carcinoma on 'ghosts' of necrotic epithelium. Other blocks must be sectioned to search for viable tissue or the frozen section diagnosis must be deferred.

The juvenile fibroadenoma can have any of the above features of the usual fibroadenoma. The major differences, when they occur, are a hypercellular stroma and hyperplastic epithelium. The stroma is sometimes accentuated around the ducts, and it usually grows in a pericanalicular pattern. Atypical nuclei are not present and few

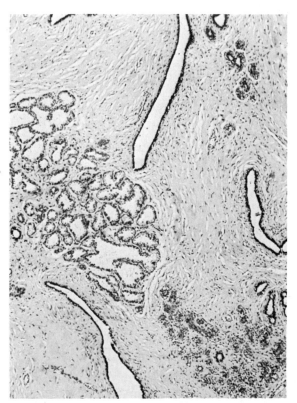

Fig. 7.5 Fibroadenoma from pregnant woman shows lactational change in one lobule. The lobule at bottom right remains inactive ($\times$ 75).

mitoses are seen despite the usual clinical history of a rapidly enlarging lesion. The epithelium is hyperplastic with cells forming a rather disorganized layer three to seven cells in thickness. Apocrine snouts are commonly evident. Small papillary excrescences may form, and the overall image is quite similar to gynaecomastia (Fig. 7.6). Some juvenile fibroadenomas are completely devoid of well-formed lobules whereas others have many. In addition, Oberman (1979) has pointed out that there are often caricatures of lobules in which clusters of small ducts are widely separated by stroma (Fig. 7.7).

Differential diagnosis

Fibroadenomas can have the entire spectrum of epithelial alterations discussed in other chapters. In effect, one can mentally isolate the epithelial changes in fibroadenoma and apply the same criteria that would be used if the changes were

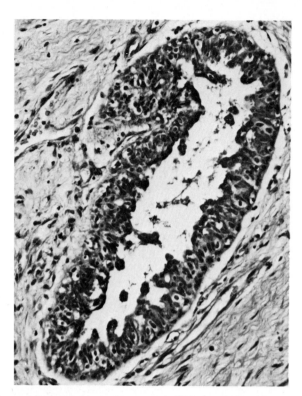

Fig. 7.6 Some ducts in juvenile fibroadenoma have stratification of epithelium with small papillary tufts mimicking gynaecomastia. Same case as Figure 7.2 (× 200).

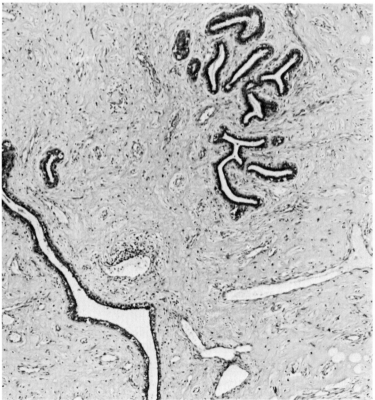

Fig. 7.7 Microscopic appearance of juvenile fibroadenoma seen in Figure 7.2 shows sparsely cellular stroma despite history of rapid growth. A caricature of a lobule is seen at upper right (× 75).

seen outside a fibroadenoma. Thus, lobular carcinoma in situ in a fibroadenoma is diagnosed utilizing the same criteria that one would use for a lobule situated in an otherwise normal breast. Similarly, sclerosing adenosis has the same features whether found within the confines of a fibroadenoma or elsewhere in the breast. These secondary changes can be acknowledged in the report, e.g. 'fibroadenoma with foci of sclerosing adenosis'.

The only entity that combines the epithelial and fibrous proliferations into a pattern resembling fibroadenoma is cystosarcoma phyllodes (or phyllodes tumour). Cystosarcoma may have sparsely cellular hyalinized areas or myxoid areas, and one must focus on the most cellular foci in order to make the diagnosis. The cystosarcoma with numerous bizzare nuclei and mitoses exceeding 5/10 hpf poses no problem. It is the lesion with fairly uniform, plump nuclei and low mitotic rates that requires the greatest judgement. If one encounters hypercellular stroma with 'active' nuclei, the mitotic rate can be used to advantage. Different criteria of mitotic counts have been used but we feel that a lesion with less than 3 mitoses/10 hpf does not warrant the diagnosis of cystosarcoma. It is prudent, however, in hypercellular lesions to acknowledge the difficulty in sharply distinguishing between some low grade cystosarcomas and fibroadenoma. This may influence the surgeon to follow the patient more closely. Should the lesion recur, wide local excision rather than enucleation could be carried out. Parenthetically, I never use the term 'benign cystosarcoma phyllodes' for a giant fibroadenoma even if it has a very cellular, myxoid stroma. The report on such a tumour, however, may include a note stating that some pathologists would prefer the term 'benign cystosarcoma phyllodes' for such a lesion. As long as the clinical implications are clear to all parties, no harm should come from the diagnosis of benign cystosarcoma phyllodes. In any case, use of the terms cystosarcoma or phyllodes tumour should always be modified and clarified by 'benign', 'borderline', or 'malignant' (see Ch. 20).

The term *sclerosing lobular hyperplasia* has been used for masses that have some minute foci resembling fibroadenoma, but otherwise consist of numerous lobules in a fibrous stroma. Conversely, about half of fibroadenomas have adjacent foci of sclerosing lobular hyperplasia. The ages of patients with sclerosing lobular hyperplasia parallel fibroadenomas. The hyperplasia is a mass ranging from 1–5 cm that seems to have a predilection for blacks (Kovi et al 1984).

Another condition that can superficially resemble fibroadenoma is fibromatosis (Ali et al 1979) (see Ch. 6). It can surround ducts and lobules so that they are incorporated into a fibrous mass several centimetres wide. Fibromatosis has a much more cellular stroma than fibroadenoma, but more importantly it has an infiltrating margin. Small tongues of fibrous tissue extend between fat cells at the advancing edge of the process. Fibroadenomas, while usually unencapsulated, have a microscopically smooth margin.

As mentioned previously, the juvenile fibroadenoma histologically overlaps the ordinary fibroadenoma although the juvenile tumour has some trends that are different. Juvenile fibroadenoma is also confused sometimes with virginal hypertrophy (adolescent hypertrophy or adolescent macromastia) because there is complete histological overlap of the two conditions. Virginal hypertrophy has a *trend* towards fewer lobules than normal breasts, often has a hyperplastic change in the epithelium as seen in juvenile fibroadenomas, and has abundant fibrous tissue ranging from cellular to hyalinized areas. The differentiation between virginal hypertrophy and juvenile fibroadenoma cannot be made on histological examination. It requires knowledge of the clinical setting. The juvenile fibroadenoma is usually a unilateral lesion resulting in displacement of the nipple. The skin is often stretched, cyanotic, and has distended veins. Conversely, virginal hypertrophy is bilateral, does not displace the nipple, and lacks the cutaneous and venous alterations seen in the patient with juvenile fibroadenoma (Hines & Geurkink 1965). Moreover, at the time of surgery, the entire breast is uniformly involved in virginal hypertrophy whereas a space is easily established between the capsule of juvenile fibroadenoma and the uninvolved breast tissue. In fact, one juvenile fibroadenoma had a distinct vascular pedicle feeding it (Jordal & Sorenson 1961).

Clinical features and prognostic implications

The prevalence of fibroadenomas can be gauged from the autopsy study by Frantz et al (1951) who found fibroadenomas in 8% of women less than 40 years of age and in 10% of women beyond 40 years. Clinically, of course, there is a peak between 20 and 30 years of age, but fibro-adenomas occur into the eighth decade. A case of recurrent fibroadenomas was reported in an infant but the exact features of the lesion were not given (Raine et al 1979). Fibroadenomas may be detected for the first time in postmenopausal women as the breast becomes pendulous and the lesion more accessible to palpation. Atrophy of the breast surrounding a fibroadenoma may also make it more readily palpable. Microscopically, many fibroadenomas removed beyond menopause are hyalinized and frequently calcified, giving the impression of an origin in the remote past. Nonetheless, some lesions from postmenopausal women appear as 'active' and as cellular as tumours in young women. This does not correlate with a history of oestrogen usage.

Blacks are more prone to develop fibroaden-omas than whites, have an age distribution shifted slightly towards a younger age, are more apt to have reoccurrence (metachromous multiplicity) and are especially susceptible to the formation of giant fibroadenomas (Funderburk et al 1972; Nigro & Organ 1976; Organ & Organ 1983). Another racial difference was also noted by Nambiar & Kannan Kutty (1974) who found that giant fibroadenomas were more common in Chinese than Indians.

Fibroadenomas that are allowed to grow after initial detection double in size within approximately six to 12 months and usually cease growing when they reach 2–3 cm in diameter (Haagensen 1986a). The tumour is nearly always painless, and it can be moved around within the breast. Between 10% and 20% of fibroadenomas are multiple when they are first seen. They may all be concentrated within one quadrant of the breast or in several quadrants. Approximately 3% of patients have at least one fibroadenoma in each breast although the duration that they have been present may differ (Oliver & Major 1934). The frequency of reoccurrence is about 5%. This term is used deliberately to recognize that it is a new lesion and not a recurrence of an incompletely removed tumour. There is a tendency for the reoc-currence to be in the same breast as the original lesion, but some patients have their subsequent lesions in the opposite breast or bilaterally. Oliver & Major (1934) noted that patients who initially had bilateral synchronous tumours did not seem to be at greater risk for reoccurrence.

One clinical subgroup of women has multiple, usually bilateral, fibroadenomas that occur in successive waves. The additional tumours appear from a few months to a few years after the previous surgery. Oberman (1979) noted that all patients in this clinical group were black. Histo-logically, the fibroadenomas are not distinctive. The simultaneous occurrence of multiple bilateral fibroadenomas and adenomas in identical twins suggests a genetic predisposition (Morris & Kelly 1982). Multiple sisters in other families have also been affected (Naraynsingh & Raju 1985).

Approximately 5–10% of the fibroadenomas that occur in teenagers are the juvenile fibro-adenomas. They grow rapidly so that the breast may double in size within a month (Jordal & Sorenson 1961). A few have occurred before menarche. In contrast to women with typical fibroadenomas, the patient with juvenile fibro-adenoma is not prone to reoccurrence.

Approximately 1 of 200 fibroadenomas is partially or totally infarcted (Wilkinson & Green 1964; Majmudar & Rosales-Quintana 1975). About half of the women have pain or tenderness and most are pregnant or lactating. Vascular occlusion is rarely demonstrable, although Newman & Kahn (1973) found thrombosed medium-sized arteries in two of their five cases. The inflammatory reaction to the altered fibroadenoma can produce a fixed mass accompanied by lymphadenopathy, and this clinical identity with cancer has led to mastectomy (Delarue & Redon 1949). Pambakian & Tighe (1971) have pointed out the danger of mistaking an infarcted fibroadenoma for cancer on frozen section.

By 1985, approximately 100 cases of either non-invasive or invasive carcinoma arising in fibro-adenomas had been reported (Fondo et al 1979; Pick & Iossifides 1984; Ozzello & Gump 1985). Approximately 50% of the tumours have been lobular carcinoma in situ, 35% have been infiltrating carcinoma, and 15% have been intraductal carcinoma. In one series, carcinoma was found in 2 of 73 fibroadenomas removed from women between the ages of 40 and 60 (Deschenes et al 1985). Roughly 40% of patients have had carcinoma in the surrounding breast tissue as well as in the fibroadenoma.

Carcinomas arising in fibroadenomas do not seem to differ in their biological potential from the same type of carcinoma arising de novo. For example, some patients with lobular carcinoma in situ in a fibroadenoma have been long-term survivors without further therapy whereas other patients have subsequently developed invasive cancers in either the ipsilateral or contralateral breast (Ozzello & Gump 1985). Such variable behaviour parallels that seen for lobular carcinoma in situ occurring outside of the fibroadenomas (see Ch. 12).

Traditionally, the risk for *subsequent* carcinoma in patients with typical fibroadenomas has not been considered to be higher than the general population. Nonetheless, there are some recent data that suggest that there may be an increased risk. Kodlin et al (1977) followed 849 women with fibroadenomas who had a mean age of 31 when they were first diagnosed. Sixteen patients developed carcinoma during the follow-up period whereas the expected number was 2.3. This increased risk was of a similar magnitude as patients with fibrocystic disease in that study. Moskowitz et al (1980) calculated that the risk of cancer was increased threefold in women with fibroadenomas. It is important to realize that the patients of Moskowitz et al (1980) were a selected group who voluntarily entered a breast cancer detection centre, and most of the women were peri- or postmenopausal.

HAMARTOMA

Terminology

In 1971, Arrigoni et al (1971) used the term hamartoma for a clinically discrete nodule comprised of lobules set in a fibrofatty stroma. Linell et al (1979) pointed out that the term hamartoma is inaccurate because the nodule does not show the architectural derangement that is the usual definition of hamartoma. Regardless of the acceptability of the term, it has been used consistently in three studies (Arrigoni et al 1971; Hessler et al 1979; Linell et al 1979).

Anatomical pathology

Lesions vary from 1–17 cm in diameter, but most are in the 2–4 cm range. The gross appearance of a hamartoma often resembles a fibroadenoma because it is sharply circumscribed and firm. The clefts of fibroadenoma are missing, however, occasionally a few cysts are present that measure up to a few millimetres. The cut surface often has a mottled yellow appearance because of the presence of fat. The fat may be inconspicuous or it may make up more than half of the cut surface.

Microscopically, numerous lobules are present (Fig. 7.8). They may be discrete or they may

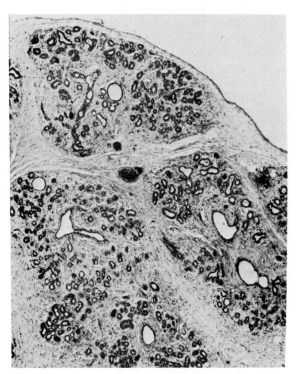

Fig. 7.8 Low power of hamartoma from 30-year-old woman shows sharply delimited margin. The mass consists of lobules with an increase of both intralobular fibrous tissue and dense interlobular fibrous tissue. The overgrowth of stroma such as seen in fibroadenoma is lacking. Mass measured 2 × 2 × 4 cm, had been present for two years, and 'popped out' of the breast at surgery (× 60).

merge into one another. Most of the lobules are normal although occasionally there is apocrine metaplasia or duct ectasia. It is the widely ectatic duct that results in the grossly visible cyst. Neither epithelial hyperplasia nor carcinoma in situ have been described. The fibrous stroma is sparsely cellular. Islands of fat are usually present and are haphazardly intermixed with the fibrous zones that contain the lobules. Although sharply delimited, a distinct fibrous capsule is not often found.

Differential diagnosis

The only consideration in the differential diagnosis is the fibroadenoma. Fibroadenomas and hamartomas share the features of gross circumscription and the presence of lobules. The lobules in a fibroadenoma are irregularly distributed and comprise a minority of the lesion. On the other hand, the lobules in the hamartoma are a major component of the nodule except in the fatty areas. The stroma of a fibroadenoma is usually more cellular than the stroma of a hamartoma. Finally, most hamartomas have at least small areas of fat whereas this is rare in fibroadenomas.

Clinical features and prognostic implications

Hamartomas have been found in women from 15–88 years old. The majority are beyond the age of 35 and the mean age in three series was 40, 43, and 45 years respectively (Arrigoni et al 1971; Hessler et al 1979; Linell et al 1979). There has been no recurrence of the lesion, although long range follow-up data are lacking. There is no association with other breast diseases. Some patients have been nulliparous indicating that the lesion is not necessarily a residuum of a breast altered by lactation.

It is possible that hamartomas may be seen with increasing frequency because they are easily detectable on mammograms. Hessler et al (1979) found hamartomas in 16 of 10 000 consecutive mammograms, and half of the lesions reported by Linell et al (1979) were detected by mammogram. It is unclear what number of these lesions were also clinically palpable.

TUBULAR ADENOMA AND LACTATING ADENOMA

Terminology

Only recently has the existence of a true mammary adenoma been firmly established. Persaud et al (1968) emphasized the rarity of this tumour by accepting only two cases from the literature prior to 1968. Most cases that had been called adenoma were really fibroadenomas that had a greater lobular component than usual. Hertel et al (1976) defined tubular adenoma as a circumscribed mass composed of closely packed ductules with minimal supporting stroma.

The existence of lactating adenoma as a clearcut entity is questionable. The term can be used for a lesion composed of closely packed ductules showing secretory activity. Small areas of tubular adenoma can be found in fibroadenomas (O'Hara & Page 1985). These adenomatous areas may be the source of some lactating adenomas. However, it seems unlikely that all lactating adenomas arise from pre-existing fibroadenomas. Fibroadenomas removed during pregnancy or lactation may have secretory activity and an accentuated lobular proliferation, but many, if not all, maintain their fibrous component (LeGal 1961) (Fig. 7.5). It is much more likely that most lactating adenomas arise in a pre-existing tubular adenoma and therefore represent a physiological response of the adenoma to pregnancy. Other so-called lactating adenomas may only be areas of lobular proliferation that stand out from the remainder of the breast as a manifestation of the physiological variability that is so characteristic of the breast. We cannot deny the possibility that some lactating adenomas are true adenomas that arise de novo during pregnancy, but doubt that it is a provable hypothesis.

Anatomical pathology

Tubular adenoma is a sharply circumscribed nodule ranging between 0.8 and 4 cm in diameter with most between 1.5 and 3.0 cm. The cut surface is tan and may have a fine nodularity (Moross et al 1983).

Microscopically, the tubular adenoma is sharply demarcated but does not always have a fibrous

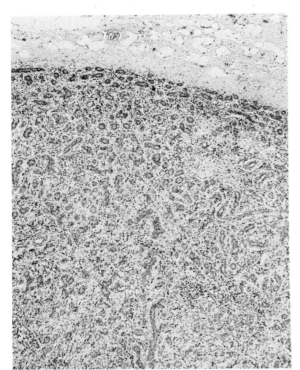

Fig. 7.9 Tubular adenoma is sharply circumscribed but not distinctly encapsulated. Tumour was 2 cm mass from a nulliparous 24-year-old woman (× 60).

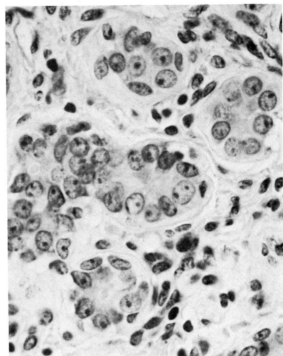

Fig. 7.10 The ductules of tubular adenomas are lined by a single layer of epithelium with an occasional myoepithelial cell. Stroma is delicate and scant (× 800).

capsule (Fig. 7.9). The epithelium consists of uniform tubular structures (30–50 microns in diameter) lined by a single layer of epithelial cells. Attenuated myoepithelial cells are seen and the individual ductule is indistinguishable from a normal lobular ductule (Fig. 7.10). Mitoses are occasionally encountered but nuclear atypia is absent.

Lactating adenomas vary from 1–4 cm in diameter and are tan or slightly yellow. They are sharply delimited but tend to be softer than the tubular adenoma and exude a milky substance when transected. A lobulated appearance is prominent on cut surface (Fig. 7.11).

Lactating adenomas form true acini with the alveolar pattern of a lactating breast (Fig. 7.12). The cells have large nuclei and abundant vacuolated cytoplasm. Hertel et al (1976) noted that the lactating adenomas removed during the first six months of pregnancy had more stroma whereas those removed later had scant stroma between the ductules as the lactational change became fully developed.

Adenomas may become infarcted, especially during pregnancy or lactation (Rickert & Rajan 1974). The caveat regarding the cautious interpretation of degenerating epithelium applies to adenomas as well as fibroadenomas (vide supra).

Differential diagnosis

The only lesions that enter into the differential diagnosis are fibroadenomas and tubular carcinoma. There may be fibrous septa in either a tubular adenoma or lactating adenoma, but the fibrous tissue is sparsely cellular. It rims groups of lobules, does not distort them, and does not appear to be an active participant in the lesion. All of these features contrast with fibroadenoma.

Tubular carcinoma is readily distinguished by gross and microscopic criteria. Grossly, tubular carcinoma has the appearance of an ordinary infiltrating carcinoma with a white, cut surface and a stellate configuration mingling with fat at its margin. Microscopically, the individual tubules

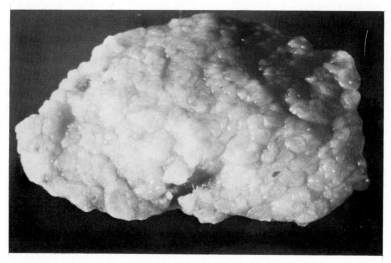

Fig. 7.11 A 2 × 3 cm lactating adenoma removed during the fifth month of pregnancy. Nodule is sharply circumscribed and lobular on cut surface.

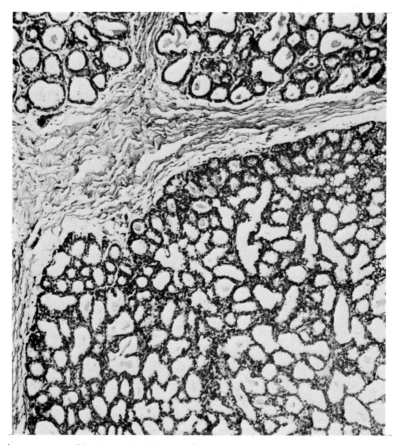

Fig. 7.12 Microscopic appearance of lesion seen in Figure 7.11 shows closely packed acini with evidence of secretion (× 75).

are lined by a single layer of cuboidal epithelium and lack a myoepithelial layer. Tubular carcinoma produces a desmoplastic response that surrounds virtually every tubule. This is quite different from the delicate and minimal stroma of adenoma.

Clinical features and prognostic implications

Patients with tubular adenomas have been between 16 and 40 years of age with most of them in their 20s. Occasionally there is a history of oral contraceptive usage, but there is no evidence of a causal effect. A few patients have had an ordinary fibroadenoma either in the same breast or in the opposite breast and, rarely, an adenoma abuts a fibroadenoma (Hertel et al 1976). Recurrence of adenomas has not been a problem.

Infarcts of the breast may occur during pregnancy or lactation and result in discrete masses (Hasson & Pope 1961). It is often arbitrary as to whether one views these as infarcted adenomas or as a localized infarct of a group of physiologically hyperplastic lobules. The distinction is unimportant and most cases are best diagnosed simply as 'infarct of the breast'. The diagnosis of infarcted adenoma can be made only if there is partial infarction so that one sees evidence of the pre-existing adenoma.

With two exceptions adenomas of the breast have not been associated with malignancy. Hill & Miller (1954) reported a case in which an adenoma was microscopically involved with carcinoma in a 34-year-old woman. She had widespread metastatic carcinoma, and no mastectomy was performed. It is likely that the adenoma was secondarily involved by the malignancy. One other case is not sufficiently documented to be certain of the relationship (Case 1977).

ADENOLIPOMA

Terminology

Adenolipoma consists of a sharply circumscribed nodule of fat that has normal lobules and ducts interspersed. Spalding of Guy's Hospital coined the term in 1945 (Spalding 1945). He pointed out that the epithelial tissue was evenly distributed throughout the tumour, and he felt that this

reflected a coordinated growth of both the epithelial elements and the fat. Moreover, there was little or no remnant of intralobular connective tissue in the lobules, and the fat cells usually came right up to the edge of the epithelium. The lesion has also been referred to as lipomatosis and 'mature breast fat with glandular tissue' (Allen 1981).

Anatomical pathology

Adenolipomas range from 2–20 cm in diameter. They are sharply delineated and have a thin capsule identical to an ordinary lipoma. A few strands of white tissue may be seen on cut surface that correspond to the breast parenchyma (Fig. 7.13).

Microscopically, the fat is cytologically normal. The lobules and ducts are fairly evenly distributed throughout the tumour. The larger ducts have a delicate fibrous coat. Most of the lobules, however, are set in the fat without any fibrous stroma (Fig. 7.14).

Differential diagnosis

Ordinary lipomas of the breast outnumber adenolipomas almost 10 to 1 (Haagensen 1986b). By definition, the lipoma will have no epithelial elements within it. Liposarcoma is an infiltrative lesion that can surround and isolate epithelial elements. Liposarcoma, however, will be much more cellular and the cells will have the nuclear abnormalities of malignant lipoblasts.

Clinical features and prognostic implications

Adenolipomas may occur at any age including teenagers. The mean age of the 22 patients reported by Haagensen (1986b) was 42 years. Many patients have had the mass for several years. Brebner et al (1976) diagnosed four adenolipomas in 5000 mammograms at the Johannesburg General Hospital in South Africa. They noted that the adenolipomas were not seen on ordinary mammograms but did appear on xerographs, presumably due to the 'edge enhancement' phenomenon inherent in the xerographic process. Adenolipomas have been seen on ordinary

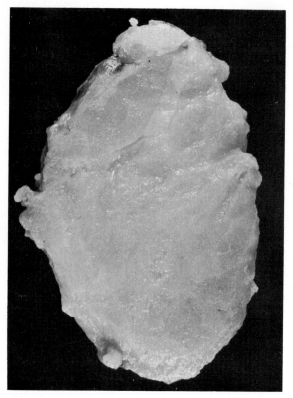

Fig. 7.13 Adenolipoma is a circumscribed nodule of fat with a few white strands of connective tissue running through it. Approximately actual size.

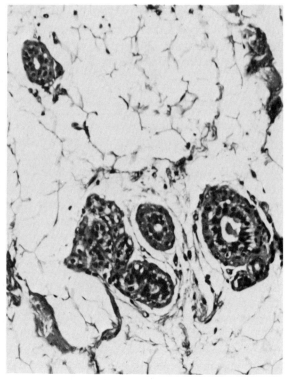

Fig. 7.14 Adenolipoma has ductules without stroma. The fat is immediately adjacent to the myoepithelial layer (× 150).

mammograms in other series (Dyreborg & Starklint 1975). Lobular carcinoma in situ has been reported within one adenolipoma (Mendiola et al 1982), but there does not appear to be any special predilection of adenolipomas to develop epithelial abnormalities.

REFERENCES

Ali M, Fayemi A O, Braun E V, Remy R 1979 Fibromatosis of the breast. Am J Surg Pathol 3: 501–505

Allen P W 1981 Tumors and proliferations of adipose tissue. A clinicopathologic approach. Masson, New York, p 78–79

Arrigoni M G, Dockerty M B, Judd E S 1971 The identification and treatment of mammary hamartoma. Surg Gynecol Obstet 133: 577–582

Ashikari R, Farrow J H, O'Hara J 1971 Fibroadenomas in the breast of juveniles. Surg Gynecol Obstet 132: 259–262

Azzopardi J G 1979 Problems in breast pathology. Saunders, Philadelphia, p 29–56

Brebner D M, Cosmann B, Shapiro J 1976 Lipomata of the breast diagnosed by film and xeromammography. S Afr Med J 50: 685–688

Case T C 1977 Adenocarcinoma of breast. Arising in adenoma. N Y State J Med 77: 2122–2123

Delarue J, Redon H 1949 Les infarctus des fibro-adénomes mammaires: probléme clinique et pathogénique. Sem Hop Paris 25: 2991–2996

Deschenes L, Jacob S, Fabia J, Christen S 1985 Beware of breast fibroadenomas in middle-aged women. Can J Surg 28: 372–374

Dyreborg U, Starklint H 1975 Adenolipoma mammae. Acta Radiol (Diagn) (Stockh) 16: 362–366

Fechner R E 1970 Fibroadenomas in patients receiving oral contraceptives. Am J Clin Pathol 53: 857–864

Fondo E Y, Rosen P P, Fracchia A A, Urban J A 1979 The problem of carcinoma developing in a fibroadenoma. Recent experience at Memorial Hospital. Cancer 43: 563–567

Frantz V K, Pickren J W, Melcher G W, Auchincloss H Jr 1951 Incidence of chronic cystic disease in so-called 'normal breasts'. A study based on 225 postmortem examinations. Cancer 4: 762–783

Funderburk W W, Rosero E, Leffall L D 1972 Breast lesions in blacks. Surg Gynecol Obstet 135: 58–60

Goodman Z D, Taxy J B 1981 Fibroadenomas of the breast with prominent smooth muscle. Am J Surg Pathol 5: 99–101

Haagensen C D 1986a Diseases of the breast, 3rd edn. Saunders, Philadelphia, p 268

Haagensen C D 1986b Diseases of the breast, 3rd edn. Saunders, Philadelphia, p 335–336

Hasson J, Pope C H 1961 Mammary infarcts associated with pregnancy presenting as breast tumors. Surgery 49: 313–316

Hertel B G, Zaloudek C, Kempson R L 1976 Breast adenomas. Cancer 37: 2891–2905

Hessler C, Schnyder P, Ozzello L 1979 Hamartoma of the breast: diagnostic observation of 16 cases. Radiology 126: 95–98

Hill R P, Miller F N Jr 1954 Adenomas of the breast. With case report of carcinomatous transformation in an adenoma. Cancer 7: 318–324

Hines J R, Geurkink R E 1965 Giant breast tumors in the adolescent. Am J Surg 109: 810–813

Huntrakoon M, Lin F 1984 Muscular hamartoma of the breast. An electron microscopic study. Virchows Arch (A) 403: 306–321

Jordal K, Sorenson B 1961 Giant fibroadenoma of the breast. Report of two cases, one treated with mammoplasty. Acta Chir Scand 122: 147–151

Kodlin D, Winger E E, Morgenstern N L, Chen U 1977 Chronic mastopathy and breast cancer. A follow-up study. Cancer 39: 2603–2607

Kovi J, Chu H B, Leffall L D Jr 1984 Sclerosing lobular hyperplasia manifesting as a palpable mass of the breast in young black women. Hum Pathol 15: 336–340

LeGal Y 1961 Adenomas of the breast — relationship of adenofibroma to pregnancy and lactation. Am Surg 27: 14–22

Linell F, Östberg G, Söderström J, Andersson I, Hildell J, Ljungqvist U 1979 Breast hamartomas. An important entity in mammary pathology. Virchows Arch (A) 383: 253–264

LiVolsi V A, Stadel B V, Kelsey J L, Holford T R 1979 Fibroadenoma in oral contraceptive users. A histopathologic evaluation of epithelial atypia. Cancer 44: 1778–1781

McDonald J R, Harrington S W 1950 Giant fibroadenoma of the breast — 'cystosarcoma phyllodes'. Ann Surg 131: 243–251

Majmudar B, Rosales-Quintana S 1975 Infarction of breast fibroadenomas during pregnancy. J A M A 231: 963–964

Mendiola H, Henrik-Nielson R, Dyreborg U et al 1982 Lobular carcinoma-in situ occurring in adenolipoma of the breast. Report of a case. Acta Radiol (Diagn) (Stockh) 23: 503–505

Meyer J S 1977 Cell proliferation in normal human breast ducts, fibroadenomas, and other ductal hyperplasias measured by nuclear labeling with tritiated thymidine. Effects of menstrual phase, age, and oral contraceptive hormones. Hum Pathol 8: 67–81

Moross T, Lang A P, Mahoney L 1983 Tubular adenoma of breast. Arch Pathol Lab Med 107: 84–86

Morris J A, Kelly J F 1982 Multiple bilateral breast adenomas in identical adolescent negro twins. Histopathology 6: 539–547

Moskowitz M, Gartside P, Wirman J A, McLaughlin C 1980 Proliferative disorders of the breast as risk factors for breast cancer in a self-selected screened population: pathologic markers. Radiology 134: 289–291

Nambiar R, Kannan Kutty M 1974 Giant fibroadenoma (cystosarcoma phyllodes) in adolescent females — a clinicopathological study. Br J Surg 61: 113–117

Naraynsingh V, Raju G C 1985 Familial bilateral multiple fibroadenomas of the breast. Postgrad Med J 61: 439–440

Newman J, Kahn L B 1973 Infarction of fibroadenoma of the breast. Br J Surg 60: 738–740

Nigro D M, Organ C H, Jr 1976 Fibroadenoma of the female breasts. Some epidemiological surprises. Postgrad Med 59: 113–117

Oberman H A 1979 Breast lesions in the adolescent female. Ann Pathol 14: 175–201

Oberman H A, Hosanchuk J S, Finger J E 1969 Periductal stromal tumors of breast with adipose metaplasia. Arch Surg 98: 384–387

O'Hara M F, Page D L 1985 Adenomas of the breast and ectopic breast under lactational influences. Hum Pathol 16: 707–712

Oliver R L, Major R C 1934 Cyclomastopathy; a physio-pathologic conception of some benign breast tumors with an analysis of four hundred cases. Am J Cancer 21: 1–85

Organ C H Jr, Organ B C 1983 Fibroadenoma of the female breast: a critical clinical assessment. J Natl Med Assoc 75: 701–704

Ozzello L, Gump F E 1985 The management of patients with carcinomas in fibroadenomatous tumors of the breast. Surg Gynecol Obstet 160: 99–104

Pambakian H, Tighe J R 1971 Mammary infarction Brit J Surg 58: 601–602

Persaud V, Talerman A, Jordan R P 1968 Pure adenoma of the breast. Arch Pathol 86: 481–483

Pick P W, Iossifides I A 1984 Occurrence of breast carcinoma within a fibroadenoma. A review. Arch Pathol Lab Med 108: 590–594

Raine P A M, Noblett H R, Houghton-Allen B W, Campbell P E 1979 Breast fibroadenoma and cardiac anomaly associated with EMG (Beckwith-Wiedemann) syndrome. J Pediatr 94: 633–634

Rickert R R, Rajan S 1974 Localized breast infarcts associated with pregnancy. Arch Pathol 97: 159–162

Riddell R H, Davies J D 1973 Muscular hamartomas of the breast. J Pathol 111: 209–211

Salm R 1957 Epidermoid metaplasia in mammary fibroadenoma with formation of keratin cysts. J Pathol Bacteriol 74: 221–222

Scarff R W, Torloni H 1968 Histological typing of breast tumours. World Health Organization, Geneva

Spagnolo D V, Shilkin K B 1983 Breast neoplasms containing bone and cartilage. Virchows Arch (A) 400: 287–295

Spalding J E 1945 Adenolipoma and lipoma of the breast. Guy's Hosp Rep 94: 80–84

Wellings S R, Jensen H M, Marcum R G 1975 An atlas of subgross pathology of the human breast with special reference to possible precancerous lesions. J Natl Cancer Inst 55: 231–273

Wilkinson L, Green W O Jr 1964 Infarction of the breast lesion during pregnancy and lactation. Cancer 17: 1567–1572

Wuslin J M 1960 Large breast tumours in adolescent females. Ann Surg 152: 151–154

8

Columnar alteration of lobules

Devotion of a chapter to this solitary alteration is done because this area has been characterized by terminological confusion. Columnar alteration of lobules is not of intrinsic clinical importance except in an attempt to be complete in describing the total histopathological, content of the human breast. These altered lobules have been termed 'hyperplastic terminal groupings' (Gallager 1976), 'columnar metaplasia' (Bonser et al 1961), 'atypical lobules type A' of minimal severity (Wellings et al 1975), and 'blunt duct adenosis' (Foote & Stewart 1945; Azzopardi 1979; Ch. 5). Most of these terms have also included lesions demonstrating an increased number of cells within acinar spaces — the most common and non-worrisome type of epithelial hyperplasia.

Anatomical pathology

Grossly, these altered lobular units are not appreciated by the naked eye. The lobular units demonstrating columnar alteration are enlarged and are also prominent under the scanning lens of the microscope (Fig. 8.1) because the glandular spaces are dilated with prominent, enlarged luminal cells. There may be secreted material in the acinar spaces. The epithelial cells are tall and columnar, usually with pink, apocrine-like cyto-

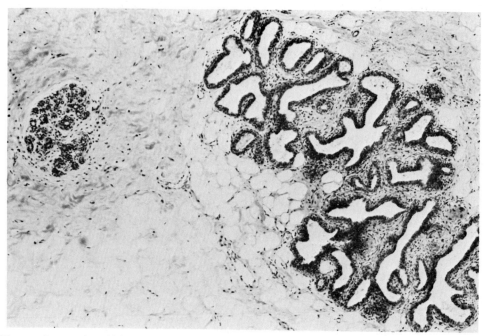

Fig. 8.1 The prominent, enlarged lobular unit at right is an example of columnar alteration of lobules. The miniaturized lobular unit at left resembles the majority of units found in this biopsy ($\times$ 60).

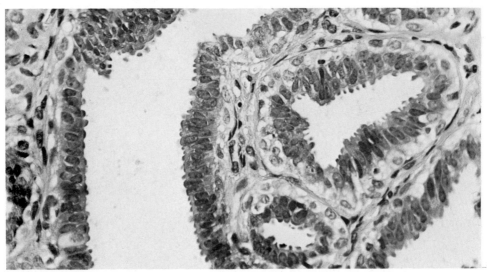

Fig. 8.2 The elongated, columnar appearance of luminal cells is apparent along with the apical, rounded protrusions (× 400).

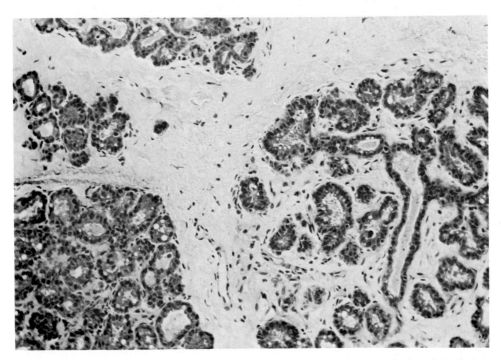

Fig. 8.3 Suggestion of secretory change (as evidenced by occasional clear vacuoles) is present in these foci of columnar alterations (× 20).

plasm and often with apical cytoplasmic blebs or 'snouts' (Fig. 8.2). Nuclei are somewhat enlarged, but are not atypical. The basal cells adjacent to the basement membrane are often prominent and usually form a complete layer about the acinar space. Cytological features suggesting pregnancy alterations (Hamperl 1975) are occasionally seen in similarly altered lobules (Fig. 8.3) and apocrine change may be seen in foci acceptable as examples of this change.

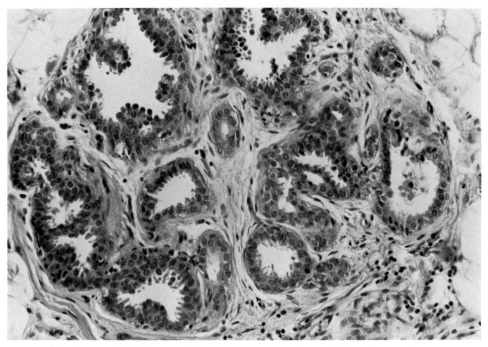

Fig. 8.4 Columnar alteration dominates in this lobular unit. However, a few acini are uninvolved and, focally, there are hillocks of increased cell number indicating mild hyperplasia of usual type (× 250).

Differential diagnosis

Columnar alteration is frequently present in lobules demonstrating mild and moderate degrees of epithelial hyperplasia of no special type (Fig. 8.4). It is almost as if the cellular prominence of columnar alteration were a background to hyperplasia. This was recognized by Wellings et al (1975) in the series of atypical lobules type A in which the first category recognized columnar alteration and the remainder of the series (2–4) recognized hyperplastic lesions of usual type. The change can seem alarming when these lobules are found in a breast which is mostly atrophic, particularly when they are placed in fat or have slight deformity of the acini resembling infiltration. The lobules demonstrating secretory or lactational changes (Ch. 2) may have a similar appearance to that of columnar alteration.

Clinical significance

There is no defined clinical usefulness to this diagnosis, although such altered lobules are more commonly found in women with breast cancer than in women without cancer (Wellings et al 1975). This may only signify that they are a sign of epithelial stimulation or activity as opposed to atrophy. They have no proven or suggested premalignant significance when identified at biopsy.

REFERENCES

Azzopardi J G 1979 Problems in breast pathology. Saunders, Philadelphia, p 25–32
Bonser G M, Dossett J A, Jull W 1961 Human and experimental breast cancer. Pitman Medical, London, p 336–347
Foote F W, Stewart F W 1945 Comparative studies of cancerous versus noncancerous breast. I. Basic morphologic characteristics. Ann Surg 121: 6–53
Gallager H S 1976 Sources of uncertainty in interpretation of breast biopsies. Breast 2: 12–15
Hamperl H 1975 Sekretionserscheinungen in der mastopathischen Brustdruse. Beitrage zur pathologischen Histological der Mamma. X. Virchows Arch (Cell Pathol) 18: 73–81
Wellings S R, Jensen H M, Marcum R G 1975 An atlas of subgross pathology of the human breast with special reference to possible precancerous lesions. J Natl Cancer Inst 55: 231–273

9

Radial scars and complex sclerosing lesions

Terminology and historical development

The breast changes which are encompassed by the terms heading this chapter have been recognized at different times in different countries. Not unnaturally this has given rise to a multitude of descriptive names that has contributed to a certain amount of confusion and dispute over the nature and significance of the lesions. Table 9.1 summarizes these various names along with the

Table 9.1 Lesion nomenclature.

Term	Reference
Rosette-like lesions	Semb (1928)
Sclerosing papillary proliferation	Fenoglio & Lattes (1974)
Radial scar	Hamperl (1975)
Complex compound, heteromorphic lesions	Wellings et al (1975)
Scleroelastic lesions	Eusebi et al (1976)
Benign sclerosing ductal proliferation	Tremblay et al (1977)
Infiltrating epitheliosis	Azzopardi (1979)
Non-encapsulated sclerosing lesion	Fisher et al (1979)
Radial scar	Linell et al (1980)
Indurative mastopathy (a benign sclerosing lesion with elastosis)	Ricket et al (1981)
Proliferation centre of Aschoff	D'Amore et al (1985)

authors promoting them. Whilst the essential feature is a central sclerosis and varying degrees of epithelial proliferation, apocrine and cystic change as well as papilloma formation, it is the gross and microscopic mimicry of cancer which has rendered these lesions most important to diagnostic histopathology. Liability to detection by mammography, despite a usual inability to produce a clinically palpable mass, explains their recent emergence as an important entity with the more widespread application of breast screening programmes.

A discussion of the relative merits of each term applied to this entity is not appropriate here but rather we recommend the usefulness of employing two of them: radial scar is best used for the smaller lesions up to a centimetre, whilst the diagnostic phrase 'complex sclerosing lesion' is appropriate for the larger ones. Radial scar is the translation of Hamperl's (1975) *strahlige Narben* and has some historical prerogative, although this may be disputed by the French (D'Amore et al 1985). Further, it has the merit of simplicity without the likelihood of confusion with the image of cancer in the minds of physicians receiving the diagnosis — as might arise with some of the alternatives. The utility of radial scar becomes less as the lesion enlarges, however, and in view of the evident complexity of structures upon subgross stereomicroscopy (Wellings et al 1975) this feature is also worthy of mention in the name. Since central sclerosis is the other hallmark the combination of these two features in 'complex sclerosing lesion' appears apt. Furthermore, the two terms have a practical merit offering a choice to distinguish between lesions of microscopic dimension and frequently incidental finding, from those accounting for severe gross alterations. Some flexibility in the application of either term must be accepted.

For readers interested in a more detailed debate over terminological preference we refer them to a recently published discussion on the topic (Andersen et al 1986). This article is of necessity somewhat wide-ranging and lengthy, but provides

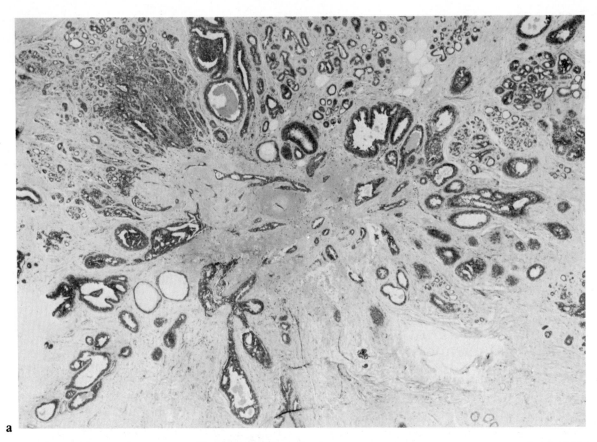

a

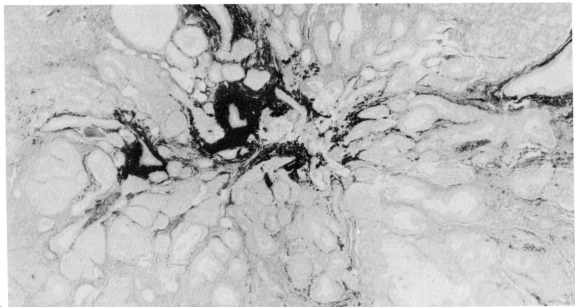

b

Fig. 9.1 (a) Mature radial scar with scleroelastic and atrophic centre, but hyperplastic peripheral region of parenchyma. (b) Abundant interstitial and periductal elastic tissue in deeper level at centre of lesion in (a) (a × 40; b elastic tartrazine × 40). (Courtesy of Editor, J Pathol.)

a useful appraisal of the development of patho-logical awareness in the collective existence of such sclerosing lesions. Uncertainty still persists about their precise histogenesis and malignant potential, but their importance to the pathologist lies in the recognition that they are distinctive lesions which can be discriminated from cancers.

Whilst there may be selected instances when any of the previously proposed terms (Table 9.1) may be useful in describing a specific lesion that prominently displays the features noted in the particular designation, the terms recommended here are in agreement with comments emerging from international discussion (Andersen et al 1986). The choice offered by the two alternatives, radial scar/complex sclerosing lesion, provides the latitude for separation by degree which answers some of the criticism contained in that discussion.

Anatomical pathology

The naked-eye appearance of many of the small lesions from 1–9 mm is often unremarkable, as only with the hand lens is the radiality evident around a central white area of fibrosis flecked with creamy elastic streaks. For such *radial scars* (RS), origination at the point of terminal duct branching from a more major stem is likely. The microscopic features will be determined by the stage of devel-opment or maturation since it is now realized that the classical appearance of central sclerosis with prominent elastosis and radial corona of paren-chymal structures (Fig. 9.1) represents the well-developed stage. The characteristic tell-tale is the arrangement of parenchyma around a fibrosing spindle rather in the manner of a central purse-string having been pulled. Lesions at an earlier stage show noticeable spindle cells and chronic inflammatory cells around the central parenchymal components which are less distorted (Fig. 9.2). The association of hyperplastic and cystic changes in parenchyma becomes more evident as the lesion matures, and apocrine blebbing is detectable in the epithelium lining many of the central and peripheral structures. Thus both maturity and plane of section will influence the patterns observed on microscopy, which may be predomi-nantly parenchymal (Fig. 9.3) or stromal (Fig. 9.4). Elastosis becomes a central feature with

conspicuous interstitial accumulations in addition to the thick bands around atrophic ducts. Within the central elastosis the randomly distributed, non-organoid arrangement of the tubules is characteristic, as is the double layering of epithe-lium and myoepithelium in these mature centres (Fig. 9.5). Appreciation of the cell types at the parenchymal borders may be less easy with earlier lesions when myofibroblasts are prominent by ultrastructural definition (Battersby & Anderson 1985). Tubular structures are not always present in the central core (Fig. 9.6), but when they are a basal membrane is identifiable indicating persist-ence of normal structural integrity characteristic of the benign process.

From an analysis of the quantitative and qualitative features of over 100 examples of radial scars from cases with and without cancer, it is apparent that frequency of scars is similar in both and is heavily dependent on the diligence of tissue scrutiny (Andersen & Battersby 1985). Bilaterality was also noted, but in those cases where mastec-tomies were available for comparison, there was an individuality of distribution and maturity of lesions in each breast. A sclerosing process formed part of the associated pathology in over 40% of the benign cases and in 15% there was coexistence of small and large lesions, the latter more appropri-ately fitting the description complex sclerosing lesions.

The *complex sclerosing lesion* (CSL) measures upwards from 10 mm and has all the same charac-teristics of the radial scar but in greater scale. A stellate or sometimes nodular appearance is usually seen around the firm, fibrous centre that is frequently puckered (Fig. 9.7). The latter appearance is probably a consequence of the varying consistency of the different elements in these lesions. Occasionally several closely adjacent small lesions will form what grossly appears to be a single mass. Flecks of creamy-yellow elastic tissue are recognized, aiding the mimicry of an invasive carcinoma, even to the extent of exhi-biting an intensified yellowed colour in the surrounding fat.

All the histological features of the radial scar are again seen in these larger lesions but the involved elements show a greater disturbance of structure with papilloma formation, apocrine change and

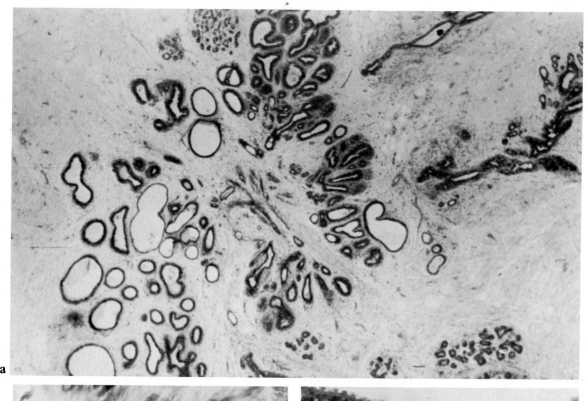

a

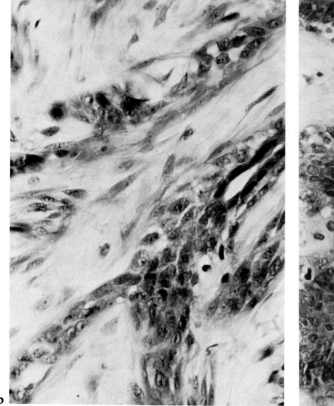

b

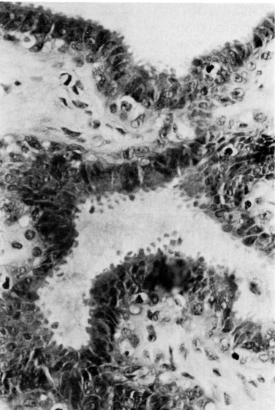

c

Fig. 9.2 (*opposite page*) (**a**) Early radial scar showing cellular centre with microcystic and hyperplastic peripheral parenchyma. (**b**) Central region of (**a**) at higher magnification to show stromal spindle cells between and merging with central parenchymal units. (**c**) Peripheral parenchyma of (**a**) to show prominent apical snouts of hyperplastic epithelium (**a** × 40; **b**, **c** × 400). (Courtesy of Editor, J. Pathol.)

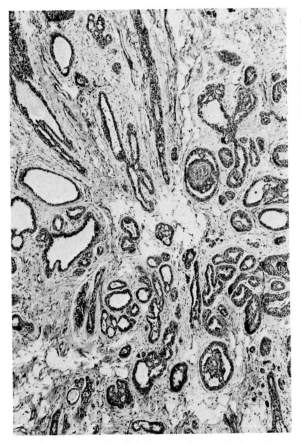

Fig. 9.3 Radial arrangement of parenchyma lacking central scleroelastosis due to plane of section (× 55).

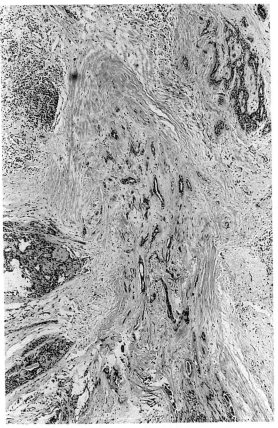

Fig. 9.4 Prominent parenchymal distortion at centre with sclerosis involving the radii; note associated chronic inflammatory infiltrate (× 60).

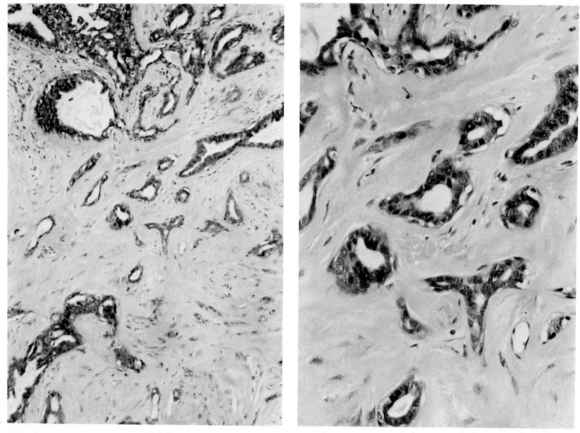

Fig. 9.5 (a) Haphazard non-organoid arrangement of parenchyma at centre of mature radial scar. (b) High magnification of (a) illustrates tubules with epithelial and myoepithelial layers (a × 100; b × 250). (Courtesy of Editor, J Pathol.)

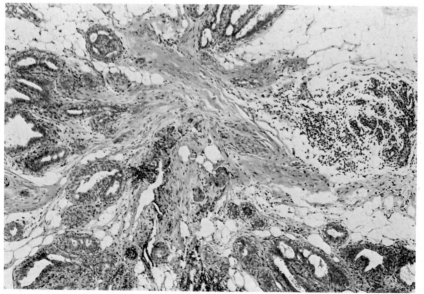

Fig. 9.6 Radial arrangement of parenchyma around fibrosis lacking tubular elements but with persistence of chronic inflammation; deeper levels may show elastosis (× 60).

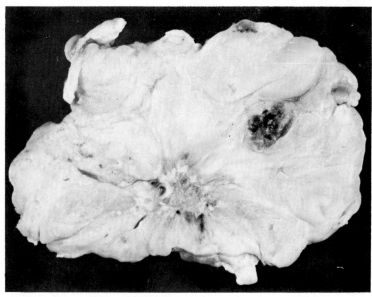

Fig. 9.7 Macroscopic appearances of complex sclerosing lesion (CSL) have marked puckering and mimicry of carcinoma (× 1).

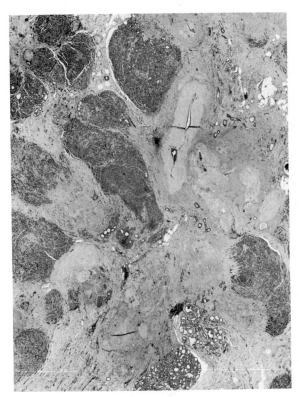

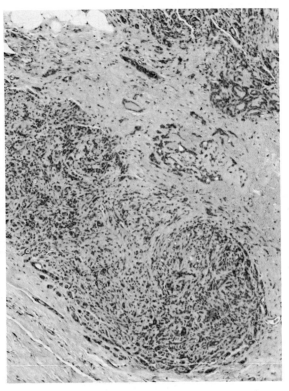

Fig. 9.8 Multiple foci of sclerosing adenosis around central fibroelastosis characterize this CSL (× 15).

Fig. 9.9 Organoid arrangement of sclerosing adenosis from bottom left of Figure 9.8 (× 60).

sclerosing adenosis (Figs 9.8 and 9.9). As in the case of radial scars, the epithelial proliferation will need to be assessed for any atypical pattern with care taken not to misinterpret entrapment in sclerosing border for infiltration (Figs 9.10 and 9.11). Sometimes the central or peripheral region of the lesions will be intensely hyaline, and rarely the lesion may consist entirely of elastic tissue (Figs 9.12–9.14).

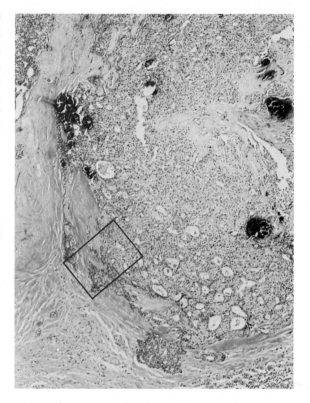

Fig. 9.10 CSL containing many foci of microcalcification has several areas of pseudoinfiltration at edge ($\times$ 60).

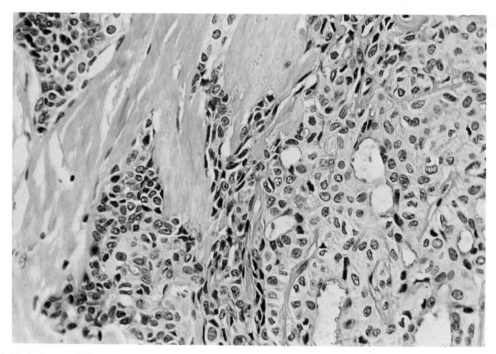

Fig. 9.11 Marked area of Figure 9.10 shows pyknotic nuclei caught up in fibrosis and associated with hypercellular regions lacking features of carcinoma ($\times$ 400).

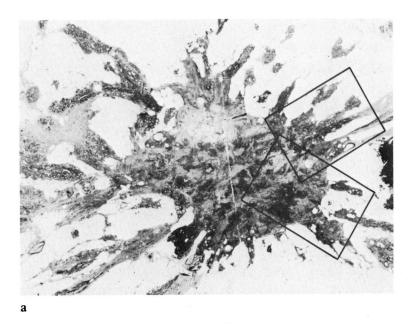

a

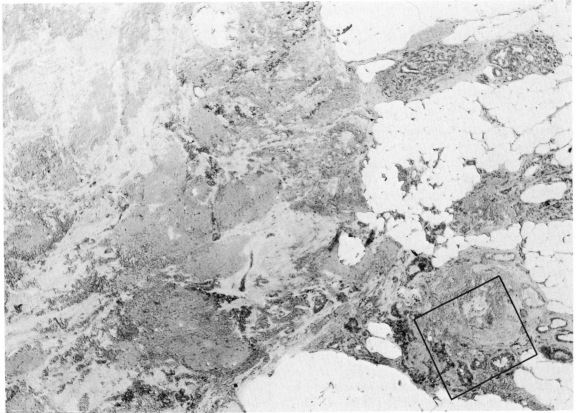

b

Fig. 9.12a, b This occult lesion was mammographically malignant and considered so at naked-eye examination of sliced tissue. Microscopy revealed only elastosis and peripheral sclerosing parenchyma. (a) Complete lesion; (b) marked area on right of (a) showing abundant elastosis (left) and sclerosing parenchyma (right) (a × 10; b × 50).

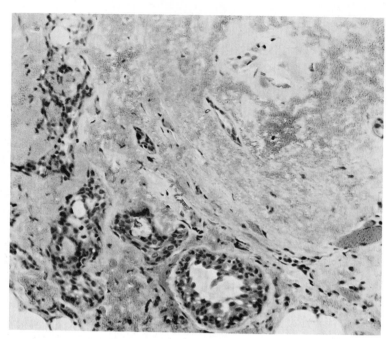

Fig. 9.13 Magnification of marked area of Figure 9.12b shows confluent elastosis, representing obliterated duct, with adjacent disorganized pyknotic parenchyma lacking malignant or atypical features (× 200).

Differential diagnosis

The diagnosis of a breast sclerosing lesion is not of necessity an exclusive one. Figure 9.15 depicts the interrelationship of these various sclerosing changes within the organ, such that the dominant pattern will give the appropriate terminology for diagnosis, without excluding the existence of the other features. As discussed in the sections on carcinoma in situ, epithelial hyperplasia, papilloma and papillary carcinoma, any existing epithelial proliferation association with RS/CSL must be separately considered and diagnosed (Figs 9.16 and 9.17). Since the entrapped epithelial elements in the central fibrous core of such a lesion resemble infiltrating carcinoma, the most important diagnostic consideration is invasive cancer, particularly tubular carcinoma. Although foci of sclerosing adenosis are commonly present within or adjacent to such major sclerosing lesions, this differential diagnosis presents little challenge as sclerosing adenosis is a change confined to recognizable lobular units.

The most important histological features sepa-

rating tubular carcinoma from the lesions of this chapter are the presence in tubular carcinoma of rounded, glandular epithelial elements which infiltrate into the adjacent fat and which are lined by a single cell layer. These defined features of tubular carcinoma must be absent in order to diagnose a radial scar/complex sclerosing lesion. In contrast to the histological characteristics of tubular carcinoma, the entrapped epithelial elements of RS/CSL are irregular in shape and usually have a two-cell epithelial layer. Furthermore, the connective tissue surrounding the infiltrating elements of a tubular cancer is often loose or myxoid, whereas that of an RS/CSL is distinctly sclerotic.

Two additional items that aid in the differentiation of an RS/CSL from a tubular carcinoma are (1) the presence of basement membrane material around the epithelial nests in question, and (2) the occurrence of epithelial hyperplasia in association with the primary lesion. The isolated groups of cells found in the RS/CSL usually, but not always, have basement membrane material around them

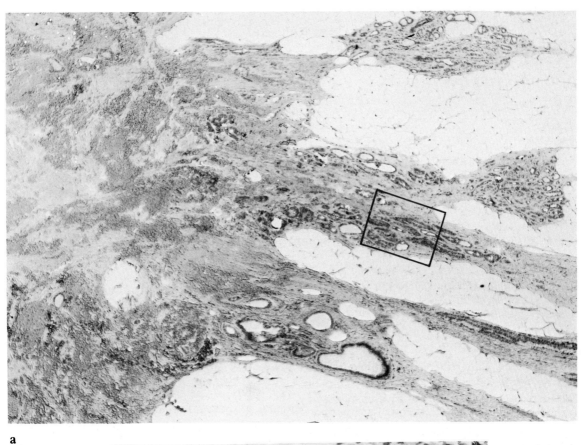

a

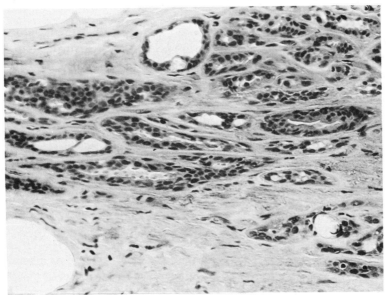

b

Fig. 9.14 (a) Magnification of left marked area of Figure 9.12a with amorphous elastosis (left) and focal sclerosing parenchyma (right). (b) Marked area of (a) to show organoid arrangement of units that often have a two-cell epithelial layer (a × 50; b × 250).

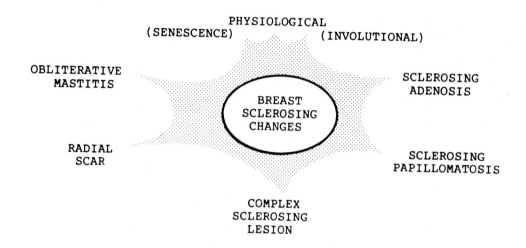

Fig. 9.15 Schematic relationship of breast sclerosing changes, progressing from physiological round to complex lesions to illustrate linkage of processes that are not exclusive of each other.

when examined with either a reticulum or PAS stain, or with antibodies for specific collagen types. Because some of the invasive elements of a tubular carcinoma may also demonstrate this characteristic, the feature is not an absolute criterion for separating these two entities. However, the RS/CSL undoubtedly demonstrates basement membrane material around a greater percentage of entrapped epithelial elements than tubular carcinoma. Because benign hyperplastic epithelial change occurs more frequently in association with the RS/CSLs than with tubular carcinomas, the identification of this feature also aids in the differential diagnosis. This epithelial hyperplasia is found usually at the periphery of the central fibrous core of an RS/CSL. Concomitant epithelial proliferation in preformed ductular structures in tubular carcinomas is usually a cribriform or micropapillary carcinoma in situ. Since both RS/CSLs and tubular carcinomas possess uniform bland nuclei microscopically and since both lesions show a stellate configuration grossly, these two features provide little aid in the differential diagnosis. Considering the excellent prognosis of tubular carcinoma, particularly when small, the doubtful lesions should be considered benign.

Prognostic and clinical features

The ability of the radial scar/complex sclerosing lesion to mimic carcinoma on mammographic examination, as well as on gross examination, constitutes its most relevant clinical feature. Currently no evidence exists to suggest that these lesions are premalignant (Andersen & Gram 1984); however, if carcinoma in situ is present within an RS/CSL, the prognostic implications of carcinoma in situ, either lobular or ductal type, would pertain. It should be stressed that the stromal cellular processes in the benign lesions under consideration in this chapter are shared with the sclerosing regions of many cancers of breast and other sites (Seemayer et al 1979; Lagace et al 1985). But this only indicates a common cellular process that is coexistent and not causal. The possibility that the epithelial elements of some radial scar/complex sclerosing lesions represent an early stage in the evolution of a tubular or other type of mammary carcinoma, as suggested by Fisher et al (1979) and Linell et al (1980), remains to be proven. No further clear evidence has emerged to support this concept and reservations continue to be expressed over the likelihood of progression to and risk association

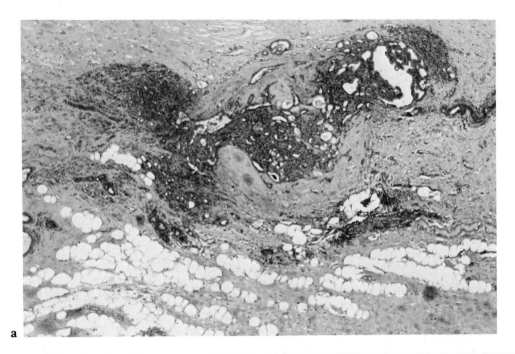

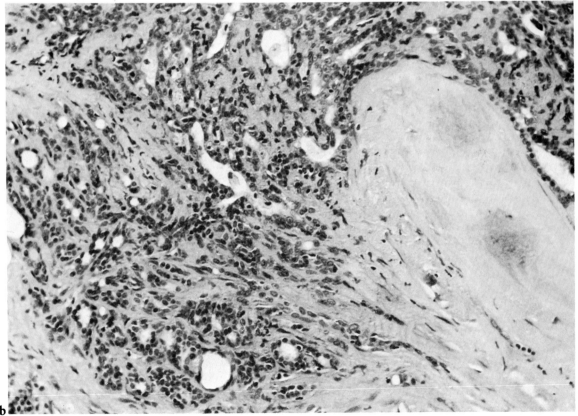

Fig. 9.16 (a) Small CSL with features of sclerosing papillomatosis and sclerosing adenosis. (b) Obliterated duct and surrounding sclerosing adenosis (**a** × 50; **b** × 250).

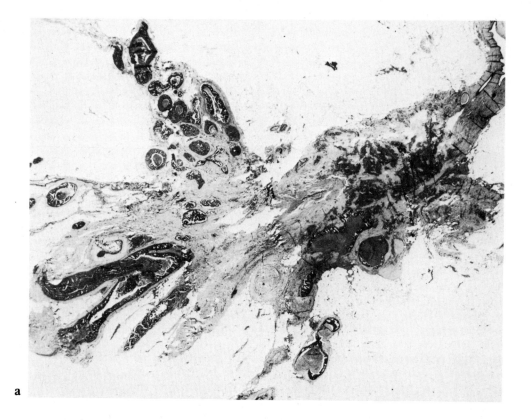

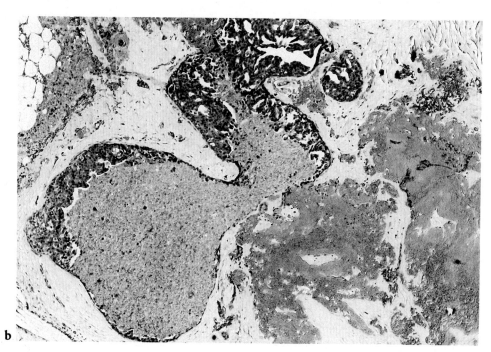

Fig. 9.17 (a) Elastotic radial scar with associated carcinoma in situ (CIS). (b) Deeper level of lower midfield of (a) shows comedo CIS separate from confluent elastosis (a × 10; b × 80).

for breast cancer (Andersen et al 1986; Nielsen et al 1987).

REFERENCES

Andersen J A, Gram J B 1984 Radial scar in the female breast: a long term follow-up study of 32 cases. Cancer 53: 2557–2560

Andersen J A, Carter D, Linell F 1986 A symposium on sclerosing duct lesions of the breast. Pathol Annu 21 (2): 145–179

Anderson T J, Battersby S 1985 Radial scars of benign and malignant breast: comparative features and significance. J Pathol 147: 23–32

Azzopardi J G 1979 Problems in breast pathology. Saunders, Philadelphia, p 174–187

Battersby S, Anderson T J 1985 Myofibroblast activity of radial scars. J Pathol 147: 33–40

D'Amore E, Montes E, Le M G et al 1985 Le centre de proliferation d'Aschoff. Ann Pathol 5: 173–182

Eusebi V, Grassigli A, Grosso F 1976 Lesioni focali scleroelastotiche mammarie simulant, il carcinoma infiltrante. Pathologica 68: 507–518

Fenoglio C, Lattes R 1974 Sclerosing papillary proliferations in the female breast. A benign lesion often mistaken for carcinoma. Cancer 33: 691–700

Fisher E R, Palekar A S, Kotwal N, Lipana N 1979 A nonencapsulated sclerosing lesion of the breast. Am J Clin Pathol 71: 239–246

Hamperl H 1975 Strahlige Narben und obliterierende mastopathie. Beitrage zur pathologischen histologie der mamma. XI. Virchows Arch (A) 369: 55–68

Linell F, Ljungberg O, Andersson I 1980 Breast carcinoma. Aspects of early stages, progression and related problems. Acta Pathol Microbiol Scand (A) (suppl) 272: 1–233

Lagace R, Grimand J A, Schurch W, Seemayer T A 1985 Myofibroblastic stromal reaction in carcinoma of the breast: variations of collagenous matrix and structural glycoproteins. Virchows Arch (A) 408: 49–59

Nielsen M, Christensen L, Andersen J 1987 Radial scars in women with breast cancer. Cancer 59: 1019–1025

Rickert R R, Kalisher L, Hutter R V P 1981 Indurative mastopathy: a benign sclerosing lesion of breast with elastosis which may simulate carcinoma. Cancer 47: 561–571

Semb C 1928 Fibroadenomatosis cystica mammae. Acta Chir Scand (suppl) 10: 1–484

Seemayer T A, Schurch W, Lagace R, Tremblay G 1979 Myofibroblasts in the stroma of invasive and metastatic carcinoma. A host response to neoplasia. Am J Surg Pathol 3: 525–533

Tremblay G, Buell R H, Seemayer T A 1977 Elastosis in benign sclerosing ductal proliferations of the female breast. Am J Sury Pathol 1: 1155–1158

Wellings S R, Jensen H M, Marcum R G 1975 An atlas of subgross pathology of the human breast with special reference to possible precancerous lesions. J Natl Cancer Inst 55: 231–273

Papilloma and related lesions

Anatomical pathology

Papillomas are often lesions of true ducts presenting within the large ducts of the subareolar area. They are also found in the periphery distant from the nipple, in smaller ducts, where they are more often multiple and associated with common patterns of hyperplasia. Papillomas of the lactiferous sinus and adjacent large ducts are well-delimited lesions within grossly identifiable ductal spaces. As these may present with nipple discharge when they are only 2–3 mm in dimension, careful surgical techniques including identification of the draining duct are often necessary (Azzopardi 1979). Lesions may extend along ducts for quite a distance, giving them an elongated shape. Haemorrhagic debris may be present in the duct adjacent to the lesions. When papillomas become large (they may attain the size of several centimetres) they appear to be encysted and are sometimes multilobulated. Focal sclerotic areas and haemorrhagic foci are common, but many specimens are uniform and soft.

Histologically, the lesions are true papillomas with stalk attachment to wall and epithelium covering usually arborescent fronds of fibrovascular stroma (Figs 10.1 and 10.2). The body of a papilloma may, however, have few branches and appear almost solid (Figs 10.3 and 10.4). The covering epithelium is usually of the normal two-cell population with cuboidal or columnar cells at the outer aspect which may occasionally demonstrate apocrine features. The inconstant basal or myoepithelial cells are more rounded, have a clearer cytoplasm, and are placed between the luminal cells and the basement membrane. The associated epithelium may present many faces (Figs 10.5–10.7). Haemorrhagic infarction is often focally present (Fig. 10.8), and is the commonly accepted reason for haemorrhagic nipple discharge. Areas of hyaline sclerosis may be seen within the stroma, and apparently result from remote ischaemic injury (Fig. 10.9).

Differential diagnosis

One of the most difficult areas of differential diagnosis in breast pathology is the evaluation of epithelial hyperplasia associated with true papillary lesions. When the epithelium is more than two cells thick and includes features of atypical hyperplasia or carcinoma in situ, the lesions must be extensively evaluated microscopically and these changes diagnosed when present (Fig. 10.7). The same criteria involved in the differential diagnosis of carcinoma in situ from atypical hyperplastic

Table 10.1 Differential diagnosis of papilloma vs non-invasive papillary carcinoma

Papilloma	Non-invasive 'encysted' papillary carcinoma
Regular two cell layer or pattern of epithelial hyperplasia of usual type covering fibrovascular fronds	Pattern of cribriform, micropapillary or (rarely) solid carcinoma in situ OR tall hyperchromatic cells
Varied cellular pattern	Homogeneous cellular pattern and uniform cytological feature
Low nuclear/cytoplasmic ratio	Hyperchromatic nuclei
May demonstrate apocrine change	Lacks apocrine features (May have eosinophilic cytoplasm)
'Pseudoinfiltration' of similar epithelium confined to the scar-like connective tissue enclosing the lesion	Surrounding tissue has carcinoma in-situ

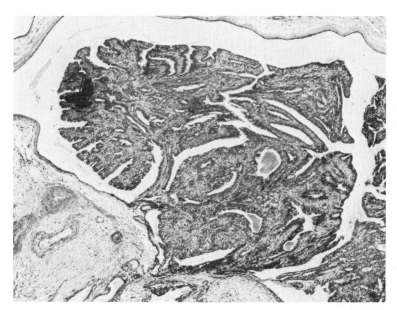

Fig. 10.1 A broad network of supporting stroma is presented in this papilloma. Note tethering stalk at lower left ($\times$ 50).

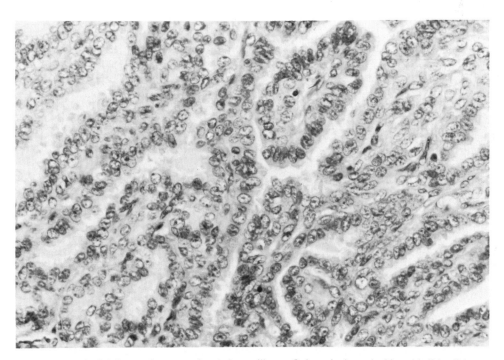

Fig. 10.2 Classical pattern of delicate arborescent fronds in papilloma. Only a single or double epithelial cell layer covers the fibrous fronds ($\times$ 300).

lesions are utilized, and the classic paper of Kraus & Neubecker (1962) remains a useful cornerstone in differential diagnosis (see Table 10.1 and also 'Non-invasive papillary carcinoma'). Areas of fibrosis and hyaline sclerosis surrounding the large lesions often have entrapped epithelium within the scar (see also 'Nipple adenoma', below), more appropriately interpreted as a pseudoinfiltration

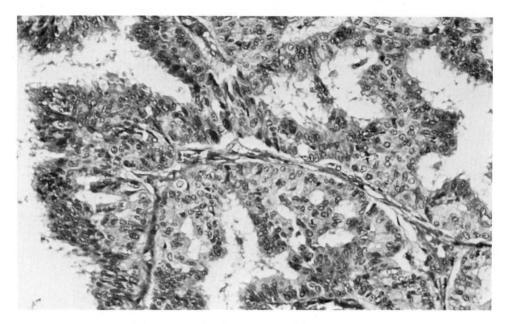

Fig. 10.3 These delicate, arborescent, fibrovascular fronds support a proliferated, benign epithelium (× 225).

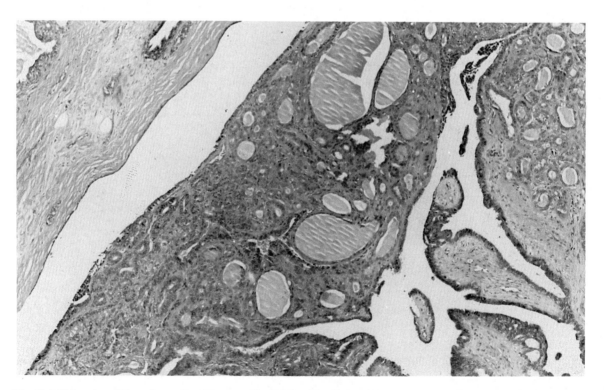

Fig. 10.4 This quite solid specimen of papilloma could not be so identified except at low power. The body of the lesion resembles adenosis (× 75).

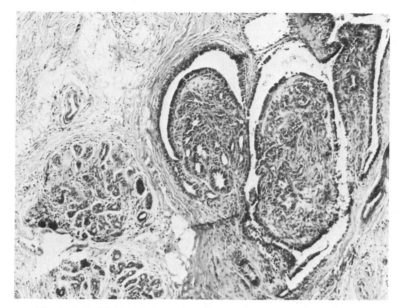

Fig. 10.5 Multilobulated form of papilloma is evident at right (× 75).

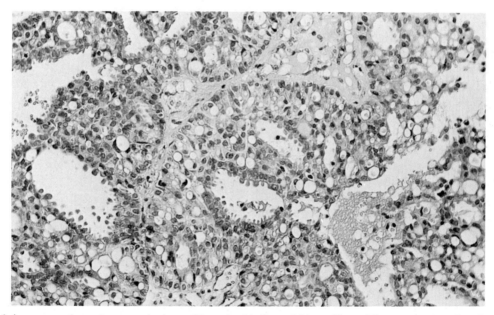

Fig. 10.6 A secretory change is present in the proliferated epithelium of this papilloma. The secretory vacuoles often contain central eosinophilic material (× 200).

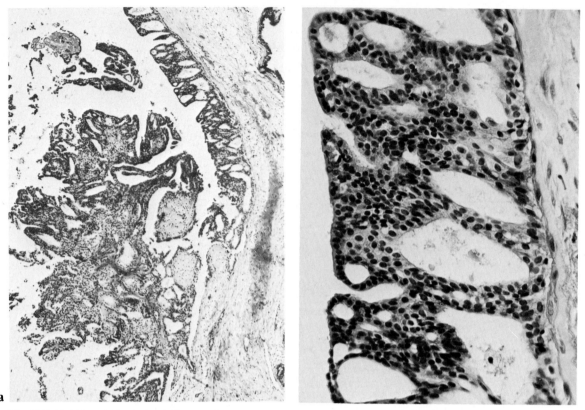

a   b

Fig. 10.7 (a) Although the large papillary configuration has equivocal malignant features, the elongated arcades at the top mark this as non-invasive carcinoma. (b) These delicate, yet rigid-appearing arcades have features of micropapillary and cribriform carcinoma in situ (high power of **a**) (**a** × 50; **b** × 320).

than true infiltration (Fenoglio & Lattes 1974). This interpretation may be difficult. Similarity of the potentially invasive epithelium to adjacent benign cell populations is strong assurance of benignity. In addition, if suspicious clusters of cells have the same stromal relationships as nearby deformed, benign glands, they are probably benign also. In general, if worrisome epithelial elements are contained within the fibrous tissue which surrounds and encloses the major papillary lesions, invasive malignancy is only mimicked. Patterns of ductal carcinoma in situ are diagnosed as such even when contained in these fibrous areas.

The late changes of infarction in papillomas (Flint & Obermann 1984) may produce appearances worrisome of carcinoma with compressed and distorted epithelium separated into isolated clumps. Squamous metaplasia may also be seen in this setting, and in the absence of established criteria for malignancy, is not cause for concern. Foci of squamous metaplasia may be extensive, particularly in larger, seemingly encysted lesions with quite solid epithelial masses (Reddick et al 1985).

Adenoma or florid papillomastosis of the nipple is probably not a specific lesion as it presents diverse histological patterns. It overlaps the histological appearances of papilloma, usual hyperplasia and adenosis (Rosen & Caicco 1986), and may be associated with an adjacent papilloma. This term, however, has been used for any lesion presenting under the nipple which produces a mass effect and is benign. Thus, a localized area of hyperplasia of usual type intermixed with fibrous and cystic changes may be termed an adenoma of the nipple or subareolar papillomatosis among other similar synonyms. Any of these lesions, by definition, is well defined and presents immediately beneath the nipple, often producing a smoothly or finely

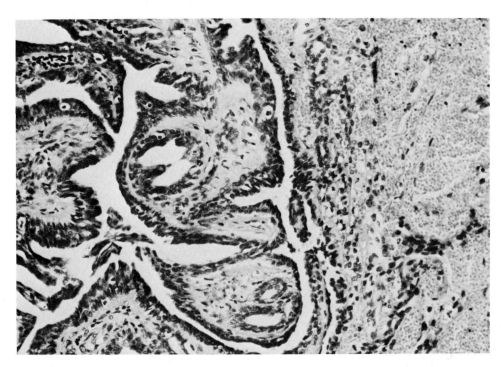

Fig. 10.8 Infarcted papilloma has atrophic epithelial elements at right, with marked stromal haemorrhage. Fronds at left are not infarcted (× 150).

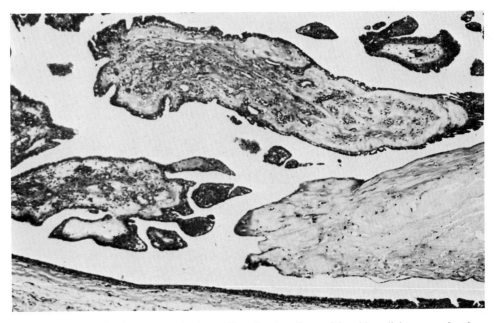

Fig. 10.9 The late effects of infarction are seen in the papillary fronds at lower right with acellular connective tissue at far right (× 75).

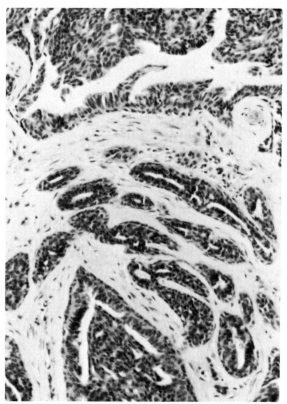

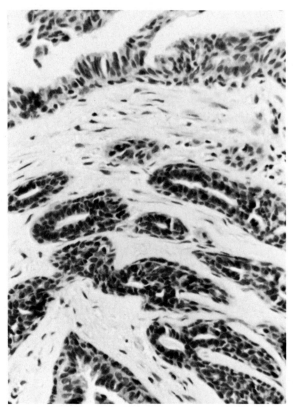

Fig. 10.10 Adenoma of the nipple with deformed ductular elements centrally between two larger spaces with benign hyperplasia (× 150).

Fig. 10.11 Higher power of Figure 10.10. Note evenness of two-cell population in ductular elements and tendency to parallel array in these elements. These features are indicative of benignancy (× 275)

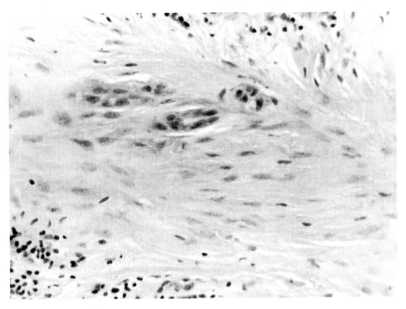

Fig. 10.12 Pseudoinfiltration of glandular constituents in a nipple adenoma. Identical cytology to more evidently benign adjacent epithelium avoids misinterpretation of malignancy (× 275).

pebbled and protuberant lesion at the nipple surface. Paget's disease may be suspected clinically, but eczematous features are absent. These lesions are usually less than 1 cm in size at the time of presentation. Histologically, they have mixtures of papilloma formation, usual hyperplasia and, frequently, normal-appearing glandular spaces and lobular units within a varied fibrous stroma (Figs 10.10–10.12). Frequently these lesions of the subareolar area have a distinctive pattern of epithelial hyperplasia with thin fronds of cells projecting a short distance into spaces (Figs 10.13 and 10.14). This pattern of epithelial hyperplasia is similar to that displayed in gynaecomastia. Because of a tendency toward nuclear hyperchromasia and relatively high nuclear-cytoplasmic ratio as well as considerable fibrosis, these lesions are often found worrisome

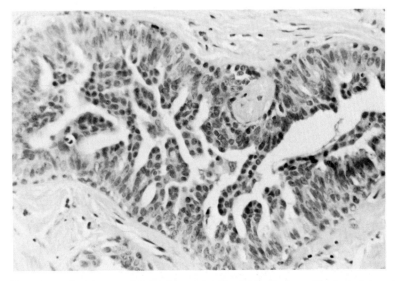

Fig. 10.13 Lining cells appear to bud into an elongated space in this nipple adenoma. The buds have a similar appearance to each other, and differ from patterns of usual hyperplasia with or without atypia (× 275).

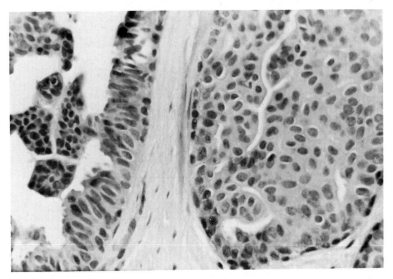

Fig. 10.14 Hyperplasia in a nipple adenoma. Note that bulbous cellular aggregates at left perch on lining cells which have a different appearance. Also benign is the more solid proliferation at right (× 275).

(Perzin & Lattes 1972). The regularity of pattern throughout much of the lesion, and lack of presentation of the fully developed examples of ductal carcinoma in situ, will avoid a mistaken diagnosis of malignancy. However, these lesions have occasionally been associated with carcinoma within the lesion (Gudjonsdottir et al 1971; Rosen & Caicco 1986), attesting to the necessity for complete histological sampling.

It is the concurrence of many small spaces containing complex patterns of epithelial hyperplasia enveloped by fibrosis which may lead to a mistaken diagnosis of malignancy, in situ or invasive. Careful attention to evaluation of hyperplastic patterns not qualifying for CIS as well as entrapped glands in sclerosis mimicking invasive tumour will avoid overdiagnosis of malignancy (Oberman 1984).

Ductal adenoma was christened by Azzopardi & Salm (1984) and is presented here because the lesion has probably most often been diagnosed as a sclerotic papilloma in the past. These lesions as reported demonstrate a variety of histological patterns in well-confined lesions with a dominant pattern of glandular proliferation or adenosis (Figs 10.15–10.17). Many of the lesions were

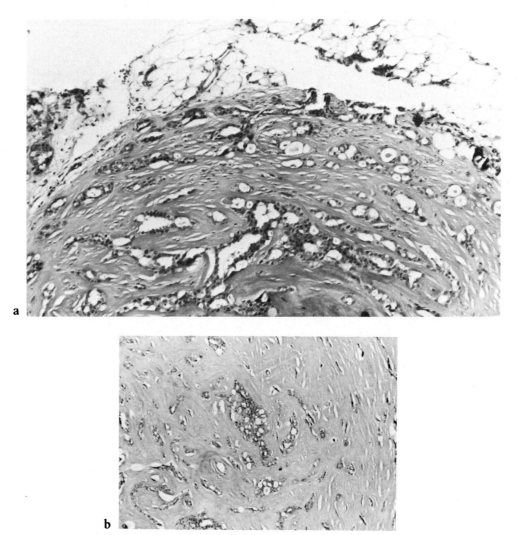

Fig. 10.15 (a) This is from the edge of a well-defined, mass lesion and demonstrates sharp demarcation from surrounding fat. The central portion of the same lesion is presented in (b). Such benign lesions may be recognized by several terms. Glandular elements are enclosed in dense fibrous tissue (a × 150; b × 40).

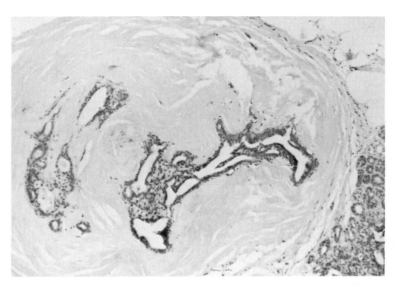

Fig. 10.16 This paucicellular lesion, manifestly benign, is difficult to classify, and consists of dense fibrous tissue primarily (× 40).

multifocal in two dimensions, yet closely clustered, and the overall size was up to 3 cm. Cases were characterized by an increase in closely clustered glandular units with ordered association of epithelial and myoepithelial cells. Most were delimited by an outer fibrous wall not so sharply demarcated as that of a fibroadenoma. Despite the fact that this outer fibrous sheath of parallel lamellae of collagen is impelling evidence of benignancy, focal eccentric peripheral fibrous border with included glandular elements may be misinterpreted as carcinoma (Fig. 10.18). Often, the central, glandular epithelium is unusually arrayed and may have irregular sclerosis (Figs 10.19 and 10.20). The presence of an apocrine-like cytology is common. When variation in nuclear size, as seen in papillary apocrine change, is present the histology may be worrisome (Fig. 10.21). With mixed features of sclerosing adenosis, tubular fibroadenoma, and papilloma, as well as dense scars similar to complex sclerosing lesions, it is clear that they are muddling lesions of which the nature and confines of definition are not clear. We believe that calling attention to them is valuable in avoiding overdiagnosis of malignancy. Our current approach to reporting is to regard them as sclerosing and adenotic variants of papilloma, nodular sclerosing adenosis or complex

sclerosing lesions depending on which they most resemble. This admittedly loose approach may be supported by appeal to the adage, 'Call them anything you like as long as you don't call them cancer'.

Solitary or central papilloma versus multiple or peripheral papillomas. The separation of these two patterns of papillary lesions has been popularized by Haagensen (1986), who has supported an increased risk for subsequent carcinoma development in the latter lesions, but not the former. The multiple papillomas by Haagensen et al's descriptions (1981) are more than simple papillomas, and are associated with epithelial proliferation beyond the fibrous tissue fronds. They illustrate that this proliferation often has atypical features approaching and reaching that of carcinoma in situ. We feel it important to stress that any risk of malignancy to be associated with these lesions can be assessed from the degree of atypical pattern or cytology present within or associated with it. This helps to explain the increased risk of later carcinoma suggested by Haagensen et al (1981) in a group of patients with multiple papillomas followed for 19 years. The illustrations depict associated proliferative changes that are categorized as malignant (usually duct CIS), many of which are absent from a more recent publication (Haagensen 1986).

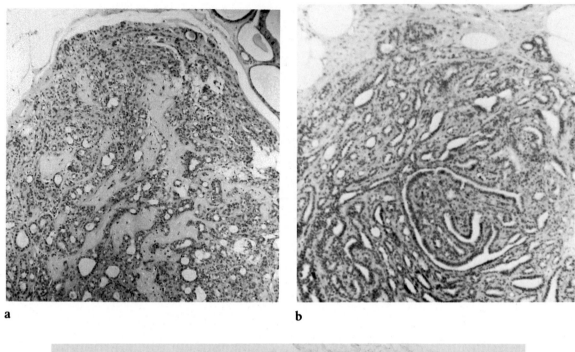

a   b

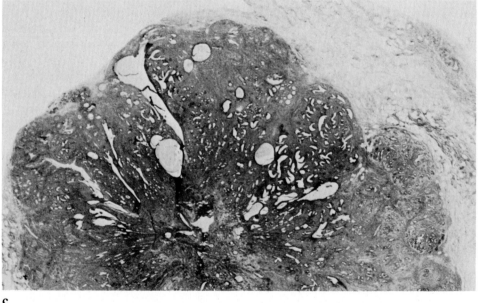

c

Fig. 10.17a–c Seemingly proliferated glandular, or adenotic, epithelium constitutes most of these 'ductal adenomas' (**a, b** × 40; **c** × 12).

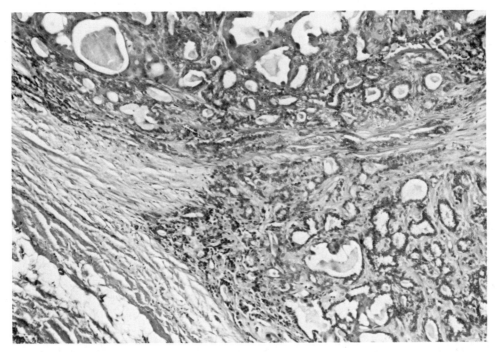

Fig. 10.18 Outer edge and fibrous capsule of this well-demarcated lesion is seen at lower left. Irregularities in interface between inner adenotic elements and fibrous capsule, seen in mild form here, may simulate invasion. Such a benign lesion could be termed nodular adenosis ($\times$ 100).

An interesting and useful approach to this problem has been proposed by Ohuchi et al (1984a) consequent to three-dimensional reconstruction of histological study of papillomas. They propose the terms *central* and *peripheral* for two varieties of papilloma. The central lesions are single and are confined to large ducts, while the peripheral lesions are usually multifocal and continuous with hyperplastic lesions of usual and frequently atypical type. The latter originate within lobular units, extend along small ducts, and merge with the epithelium covering fibrous supporting cores of peripheral papillomas. Ohuchi et al (1984b) found that these peripheral, multifocal papillomas were frequently associated with foci of borderline malignancy and carcinoma in situ of ductal type (DCIS). Only a single example of solitary papilloma contained DCIS. Some of the most difficult problems in the diagnosis of borderline lesions are seen in such cases. Careful attention to extensive sampling is mandatory as frequent foci of atypicality may be seen and the defining features of carcinoma in situ of ductal type may be approached or reached (see 'Carcinoma in situ'). Because of the association of the peripheral papilloma with epithelial proliferative disease, its association with subsequent breast cancer risk is definite and should be predicted on the basis of patterns of proliferation present (see 'Hyperplasia', Ch. 11). It must be emphasized that minute, solitary papillomas may be found peripherally, and their association with subsequent cancer risk after identification at biopsy is not demonstrated.

Clinical significance and prognostic implications

The solitary papilloma is not thought to have premalignant significance by most pathologists. However, a study from the Johns Hopkins Hospital (Carter 1977) found in careful follow-up of such women that carcinoma developed subsequently in a significant proportion. It was suggested that epithelial proliferative disease throughout the breast accompanying papilloma

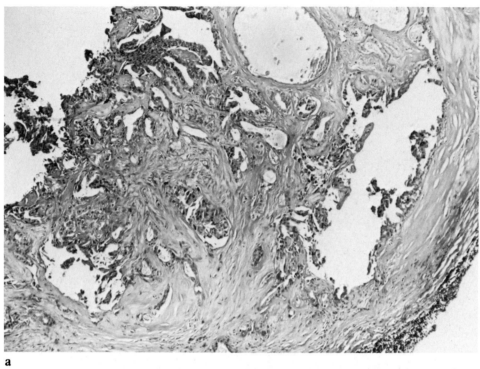

Fig. 10.19a, b Outer demarcation of this complex lesion is at lower right of (a). Deformity of central glandular elements as seen in (b) could suggest carcinoma. Such a benign local abnormality could be termed a complex sclerosing lesion (a × 100; b × 350).

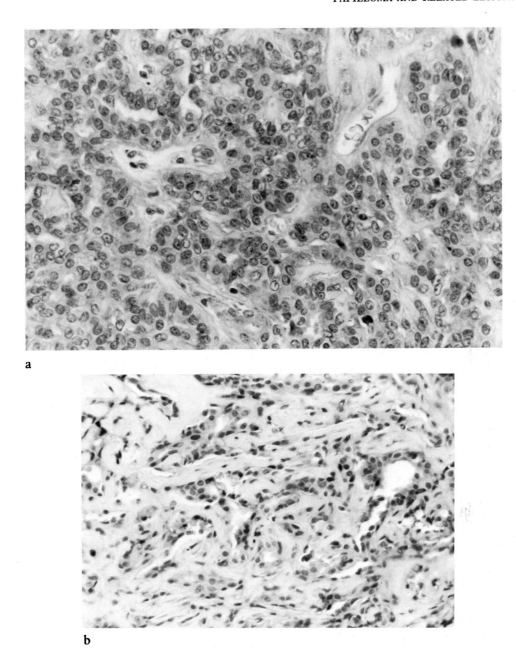

a

b

Fig. 10.20a, b Areas within nodular sclerosis or 'ductal adenomas' may show unusual organization of glandular elements and somewhat irregular sclerosis. Disorganization is not as manifest as in carcinoma (**a** × 350; **b** × 250).

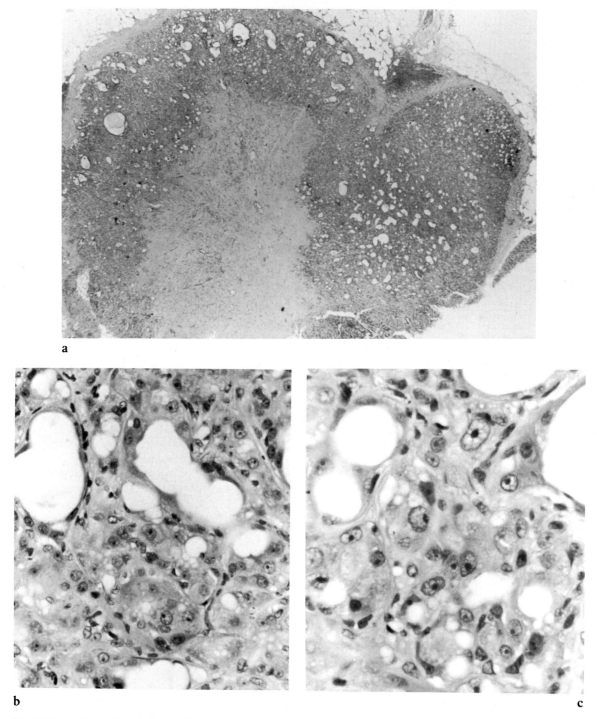

Fig. 10.21a–c These photographs are from a well-delimited breast mass. Note central scar in (a), and evident adenotic pattern extending to outer limits. Higher power views demonstrate an irregular, glandular array of cells with apocrine features including occasional enlarged nuclei. This cytological pattern is that of benign apocrine change. The lesion could be termed 'nodular adenosis' or a complex nodular sclerosing lesion (**a** × 15; **b** × 350; **c** × 450).

elevated the subsequent risk of carcinoma. Others (Haagensen 1986) have long felt that women with multiple papillomas have an increased risk for subsequent carcinoma development and, as pointed out above, many of these cases appear to be associated with epithelial proliferative changes of atypical type. It would seem, then, that the women with central, single or lactiferous sinus papillomas have a lesser risk of subsequent carcinoma than those with more extensive lesions. This prediction is consistent with studies of subsequent carcinoma risk after other hyperplastic lesions of breast. We feel that it makes intuitive sense that a woman who has demonstrated the ability to develop a true neoplasm within the breast, albeit benign, presenting as a papilloma, should be regarded as meriting careful subsequent follow-up. However, the risk undoubtedly is less for women with solitary or central papillomas than for women with combined patterns of hyperplasia.

Papillomas occur primarily in middle age, but may present, rarely, even in the second decade. Many of these lesions occurring in children and young adults will be associated with adjacent hyperplasia (Rosen 1985) and/or will have a complex sclerosis (Fenoglio & Lattes 1974). Haemorrhagic nipple discharge is the hallmark of clinical presentation for most central papillomas, necessitating careful surgical approach and histopathological evaluation for the possibility of atypical changes or changes qualifying for diagnosis of carcinoma in situ.

At the time of intraoperative frozen section diagnosis, identification of a large papillary lesion with epithelial hyperplasia should make the pathologist acutely aware of the difficulty of interpreting these changes. It is our frequent practice, when faced with such a situation, to defer a definitive diagnosis because of the necessity for multiple sampling, and suggest wider local excision of the area so that this extensive histological evaluation of margins and adjacent tissue can be done (see 'Non-invasive papillary carcinoma'). Encysted papillary lesions, even associated with histological changes of non-invasive malignancy, are usually seen in older women and

are low grade lesions seldom, if ever, associated with metastasis (see 'Non-invasive papillary carcinoma'). In most patients, wide local excision is probably adequate therapy for such lesions, and most often in this situation a subsequent operative procedure for mastectomy may be avoided because of the proof of the restricted nature of the lesion by the wider excision. This will mean, in the great majority of cases, the avoidance of a second operative procedure.

REFERENCES

Azzopardi J G 1979 Problems in breast pathology. Saunders, Philadelphia, p 150–166
Azzopardi J G, Salm R 1984 Ductal adenoma of the breast: a lesion which can mimic carcinoma. J Pathol 144: 11–23
Carter D 1977 Intraductal papillary tumors of the breast: a study of 78 cases. Cancer 39: 1689–1692
Haagensen C D 1986 Diseases of the breast, 3rd edn. Saunders, Philadelphia, p 136–191
Haagensen C D, Bodian C, Haagensen D E Jr 1981 Breast carcinoma risk and detection. Saunders, Philadelphia, p 146–237
Fenoglio C, Lattes R 1974 Sclerosing papillary proliferations in the female breast. Cancer 33: 691–700
Flint A, Oberman H A 1984 Infarction and squamous metaplasia of intraductal papilloma: a benign breast lesion that may simulate carcinoma. Hum Pathol 15: 764–767
Gudjonsdottir A, Hagerstrand I, Ostberg G 1971 Adenoma of the nipple with carcinomatous development. Acta Pathol Microbiol Scand (A) 79: 676–680
Kraus F T, Neubecker R D 1962 The differential diagnosis of papillary tumors of the breast. Cancer 15: 444–455
Oberman H A 1984 Benign breast lesions confused with carcinoma. In: McDivitt R W, Oberman H A, Ozzello L, Kaufman N (eds) The breast. Williams and Wilkins, Baltimore, p 1–33
Ohuchi N, Abe R, Takahashi T, Tezuka F 1984a Origin and extension of intraductal papillomas of the breast: a three-dimensional reconstruction study. Breast Cancer Res Treat 4: 117–128
Ohuchi N, Rikiya A, Kasai M 1984b Possible cancerous change of intraductal papillomas of the breast: a 3D reconstruction study of 25 cases. Cancer 54: 605–611
Perzin K H, Lattes R 1972 Papillary adenoma of the nipple (florid papillomastosis, adenoma, adenomatosis): a clinicopathology study. Cancer 29: 996–1009
Reddick R L, Jennette J C, Askin F B 1985 Squamous metaplasia of the breast. Am J Clin Pathol 84: 530–533
Rosen P P 1985 Papillary duct hyperplasia of the breast in children and young adults. Cancer 56: 1611–1617
Rosen P P, Caicco J A 1986 Florid papillomatosis of the nipple. A study of 51 patients, including nine with mammary carcinoma. Am J Surg Pathol 10: 87–101

Epithelial hyperplasia

Background and terminology

The fundamental feature of epithelial hyperplasia is an increased number of cells relative to that normally found above the basement membrane. The normal number in the breast is two and, therefore, three or more cells above the basement membrane define hyperplasia in the breast. These collections of hyperplastic cells tend to fill up or protrude into epithelial-lined spaces. The term does not, however, include conditions in which glandular elements are increased in number whilst the cells maintain a normal relation to the basement membrane. This latter condition has been termed, appropriately, *adenosis.*

Each type of epithelial hyperplasia (see Table 11.1) has a spectrum of change from mild to severe, presenting an escalating scale of complexity beginning with focal increases of typical cells of three or four in thickness and ending with patterns diagnostic of carcinoma in situ. The mild end of the spectrum begins when one is confident on histological grounds that there are increased numbers of epithelial cells. Severe changes are those which show great increase in cell number

Table 11.1 Epithelial hyperplasia of the breast.

1. Lobular type
        Atypical lobular hyperplasia (ALH)
        Ductal involvement by cells of ALH

2. Usual type ('ductal')
        Mild
        Moderate and florid (proliferative breast disease without atypia, (PDWA)
        Atypical hyperplasia of usual or 'ductal' type (ADH)

3. Apocrine type
        Papillary apocrine change

and a pronounced tendency to expand the space within which they reside. Qualitative changes of cells and histological pattern are separately assessed from quantitative. When epithelial hyperplasia has bizarre or unusual features, either in pattern of cell relationships or of nuclear appearance which approach that seen in carcinoma in situ (CIS), they may be termed 'atypical'. Atypical hyperplasia, as used in this book, is a term with specific histopathological meaning. The clinical significance of these changes must be determined separately from any histological mimicry of carcinoma in situ, most convincingly by follow-up studies after biopsy.

Problems of definition in these conditions are intrinsically obvious as changes in numbers of cells, size of spaces, nuclear pattern and cellular relationship do not vary in parallel. Despite this difficulty, various students of this problem have proposed classification schemes which are largely compatible although they use different terminology (Black & Chabon 1969; Wellings et al 1975). All of these systems recognize an escalating scale of quantitative and qualitative changes beginning with the most mild (that is, close to the usual or normal appearance of breast epithelia), and ending with severe changes which demonstrate some but not all of the features which define carcinoma in situ. The most completely detailed report which utilized stereomicroscopic tissue analysis (Wellings et al 1975; Jensen et al 1976) classified such parenchymal alterations as atypical lobules. The usual type of hyperplasia was termed atypical lobules type A, or ALA. They presented lesions of usual hyperplasia in an escalating scale of combined quantitative and qualitative changes from ALA-1 (columnar alteration of lobules, Ch. 5) to ALA-5 (carcinoma in situ of ductal type, DCIS, Ch. 12). The ALA-3 and 4 categories include lesions presented here as moderate and florid hyperplasia of usual type. Atypical 'ductal' hyperplasia, discussed below, would also be largely included in the ALA-4 category (Page et al 1986; Alpers & Wellings 1985). The system presented in this chapter separates quantitative changes of increased cell numbers from qualitative changes of pattern and cytology that have some features of CIS (atypical hyperplasia). We have found that this separation of qualitative from quantitative features enhances precision and reproducibility of diagnosis.

Terms such as 'epitheliosis' and 'papillomatosis' have been used for the most common or usual changes to be discussed in this chapter. Epithelial hyperplasia of usual type, often termed 'papillomatosis', has long been regarded as one of the component parts of the 'fibrocystic disease complex'. It is thought to be the change most likely to produce the elevated cancer risk considered to attend fibrocystic disease (Foote & Stewart 1945). The term 'papillomatosis' is potentially confusing and certainly inexact because of the evident derivation from the term 'papilloma', inasmuch as many examples of common type epithelial hyperplasia bear no resemblance to papillary patterns. We expect that three generations of pathologists familiar with this term will continue to perpetrate its use. It is commonly applied to examples of moderate and florid epithelial hyperplasia. The use of the term *epitheliosis* is similarly confusing because some use it for more severe forms of epithelial hyperplasia that have some resemblance to carcinoma in situ. Others advocate its usage to distinguish a confluent hypercellularity that is not cancer (Azzopardi 1979). It appears, then, to have lost its utility to call attention to proliferations associated with concern (Dawson 1933). In the situation where there is a medically meaningful increase in risk of cancer development, we prefer to apply the term *atypical hyperplasia* with the implicit assumption that there are forms of hyperplasia which are not atypical, i.e. that are typical or usual. Because the specificity of the terms 'epitheliosis' and 'papillomatosis' has been blurred, having included too many different changes within the broad confines of their definitions, we propose they be aban-

doned. The simpler and more widely applied term *hyperplasia* may be used without carrying the historical impediments of the other words whilst allowing qualification as 'mild, moderate, florid or atypical' to place individual examples in a spectrum of escalating change.

These hyperplastic lesions have unfortunately been lumped together under terms such as 'preneoplastic' or 'premalignant breast disease'. The application of such terms to an individual case without careful definition, particularly without understanding of the level of cancer risk implied, is to be deplored. The diagnostic phrase 'epithelial proliferative disease of the breast (EPDB)' (Rogers & Page 1979) or proliferative breast disease has been proposed in order to avoid this problem — 'proliferative' being used as an alternative to the analogous word *hyperplastic*, and combined with *disease* in order to specify that some abnormality such as increased risk of cancer is present (see 'Prognostic implications'). Thus, histologically proliferative conditions without linkage to increased cancer risk or other 'disease' would not be recognized as EPDB.

Three types of epithelial hyperplasia are recognized (Table 11.1). One of these, involving cells with apocrine features, is discussed in Chapter 4. The other special type of epithelial hyperplasia occurring in the breast is termed *lobular* because of its pronounced tendency to occur within lobular units and because it is associated with a type of infiltrating carcinoma termed *lobular*. The third and most common form of mammary epithelial hyperplasia is often termed 'ductal'. There is no evidence that these last lesions arise from ductal cells, there is rather only the solid evidence that they differ histologically and biologically from the atypical lobular hyperplastic lesions. For this reason and in keeping with the approach used for the common invasive carcinomas, we prefer the terms 'of usual type' or 'of no special type' for all hyperplastic epithelial lesions of non-lobular and non-apocrine type other than papilloma. The term *ductal hyperplasia* will probably be retained by many pathologists for these lesions because of the force of historical habit, and it is for this reason that we have retained the term 'ductal' for the analogous atypical and CIS lesions. However, it should be recognized that the term 'ductal' in these contexts denotes patterns of hyperplasia and not proven site of origin or cell type. The term 'ductal' for these hyperplastic lesions of no special type was chosen about 50 years ago to denote lesions other than those of lobular pattern. The important subgross analyses of Wellings and Jensen (Wellings et al 1975) have demonstrated that these 'ductal' pattern lesions usually occur within lobular units, and less often in terminal ducts. Proliferative lesions in true ducts are unusual and are most often truly papillary (see 'Papilloma').

The acceptance of the diagnostic category of atypical hyperplasia is strongly supported by long-term follow-up studies after biopsy (Page et al 1985) in which risk of subsequent invasive carcinoma development was one-half that of carcinoma in situ (CIS). In a diagnostic approach which would distinguish only CIS and benign, without an intervening borderline category, the atypical lesions would be distributed in both groups with more cases diagnosed as benign than as CIS (see Fig. 12.18). Thus, cases placed in the atypical hyperplasia categories are recruited from both the benign and CIS categories of a dichotomous (cancer yes–cancer no) system (Page 1986). Recognition of an 'atypical' category with consistent criteria was supported in papers by Fisher (1982), Ashikari et al (1974) and Ackerman & Katzenstein (1977). Azzopardi (1979) discussed atypical hyperplasia and was reticent to accept it because of uncertainty as to clinical implications. These are presented in the section on prognostic implications.

EPITHELIAL HYPERPLASIA OF USUAL TYPE ('DUCTAL')

Anatomical pathology

This series of lesions is recognized by an increased number of epithelial cells within spaces surrounded by a basement membrane. These changes may occur in solitary spaces which are usually terminal ducts, but more often occur diffusely throughout individual lobular units. For practical purposes of diagnosis, there is no impelling reason to separate the lesions on the basis of the presumed site in which they occur, whether large duct, terminal

duct, or lobule. The work of Wellings et al (1975) has demonstrated that most of these lesions are found in lobular units and the terminal ducts which connect units to the larger true duct system. The component cells of this form of hyperplasia do not have the cytological appearance of lobular or apocrine lesions, and are termed *of usual type* because they represent the most common form of hyperplasia seen in the breast. The cytoplasm tends to be less granular and eosinophilic than in apocrine change and, in contrast with both atypical lobular hyperplasia and apocrine change, the nuclear contours may vary considerably from cell to cell. The component cells of a given hyperplastic lesion may form a variety of histological patterns. There are small, barely definable papillary projections of cells at the mild end of the spectrum while at the other there may be masses of cells virtually filling the involved space. A multiplicity of intermediate forms exist, exhibiting solid, fenestrated and irregularly intertwined papillary structures which may variably and imperfectly mimic the cribriform patterns seen in ductal carcinoma in situ.

The common or usual pattern of hyperplasia found in the human breast is, other than cyst formation, the most frequent alteration recognized as abnormal. Usual patterns of hyperplasia are found in almost 50% of biopsies from perimenopausal women. Despite its frequency, this conformation is defined by exclusion, representing any hyperplastic focus which lacks lobular, apocrine and atypical features.

Mild hyperplasia

Mild hyperplasia of usual type is recognized primarily to distinguish it from the more marked changes which have been demonstrated to have relevance with regard to increased risk of breast cancer (Dupont & Page 1985). Thus, mild foci of hyperplasia, having no implication which is medically meaningful, may be ignored in most clinical reporting of individual biopsies, i.e. proliferative disease as defined above is absent.

Mild hyperplasia of usual type is defined at its minimal end by the recognition of at least three cells above the basement membrane. This presence of an extra cell layer (normal thickness is only two cells) may be focal or present evenly throughout a space. If focal, there is a corrugated (wrinkled or furrowed) appearance. Lobular units are usually regularly and uniformly involved, while adjacent units may appear quite different.

These mildest lesions do not present cell masses which cross over the involved space unless the spaces are little distended (Figs 11.1 and 11.2). One approach to the separation of mild and moderate hyperplasia is to accept three to four cells above the basement membrane as mild, and five or more as defining moderate or florid hyperplasia (Hutter et al 1986). The diagnostic histopathologist must be confident that the increased numbers of epithelial cells are not an illusion produced by sectioning artefact. This problem most frequently presents itself in evaluation of elongated, duct-like spaces (Fig. 11.3) in contrast to more spherical spaces within the lobular unit.

An epithelial alteration which masquerades as a mild hyperplasia is a seeming increase in epithelial cell number produced by the intermixing of foam cells and/or chronic inflammatory cells with ductal or terminal ductal epithelium (Fig. 11.4). Such an appearance may not be viewed as a hyperplastic lesion with confidence. Partial desquamation of epithelial strips into the lumen may be conceptualized as 'inflammatory pseudohyperplasia'.

Mild hyperplasia may be also mimicked in atrophic breast tissue where the ducts or ductules may assume a somewhat corrugated appearance (Fig. 11.5) and lend themselves more frequently to interpretational problems produced by sectioning artefact. This problem of apparent hyperplasia is usually resolved by recognizing that the component cells are not individually different from the adjacent non-hyperplastic epithelium, the cells having the same scant pale cytoplasm and small round to slightly ovoid densely staining nuclei found elsewhere in the atrophic ductal system.

Moderate and florid hyperplasia

Moderate and florid hyperplasia of usual type will be found in over 20% of biopsies. This moderate end of the usual hyperplasia spectrum begins with cellular alterations similar to mild hyperplasia, but with a tendency to distension of involved spaces

and crossing of the space by hyperplastic cells (Figs 11.6–11.12). The lesions are often comprised of cells resembling those seen in columnar alteration of lobules or mild, usual hyperplasia. This moderate hyperplastic lesion may coexist in a lobular unit with some ductules which, although not hyperplastic, have columnar alteration. Florid hyperplasia of usual type is recognized when distension and filling of spaces is of marked degree and the combined cytological and pattern features of atypical hyperplasia and CIS are absent (Figs 11.13–11.25). We recommend no special attention to separation of the moderate and florid categories as their relevance to cancer risk prediction is the same (see 'Prognostic implications', below).

The histological and cytological features of usual hyperplasia are most succinctly stated as variable; a variability which exists both within lesions and between them. Most importantly with regard to the possibility of misdiagnosis with atypical ductal hyperplasia (ADH) or DCIS, the nuclei in the benign lesions tend to vary one from another in degrees of roundness. Nuclear patterns are varied, tending often to be bland with delicate nuclear membrane, light staining chromatin, and often have small nucleoli. Mitoses are occasionally found and are of no diagnostic significance. Cytoplasm is usually lightly eosinophilic, but, again, varies greatly from deeply eosinophilic to clear. Occasionally, the cytoplasm is somewhat granular, approaching that of apocrine-like cells. Only when a lesion is purely apocrine (see Ch. 4) should it be so identified. Foci of usual hyperplasia may merge with apocrine change with either abrupt or gradual transition. Cell borders are often inapparent. Luminal aspect of cells frequently has a protrusion into the lumen, commonly termed a 'snout'.

Of defining significance with regard to this diagnosis are the patterns created by cellular groups, specifically: (1) the manner in which neighbouring cells relate to each other — varying and often locally parallel orientation; and (2) the intercellular spaces are irregular, differently shaped, often slit-like, and tend to appear in greatest number at the periphery of an involved space. The first phenomenon has been termed 'streaming' (Azzopardi 1979) or 'swirling'. This

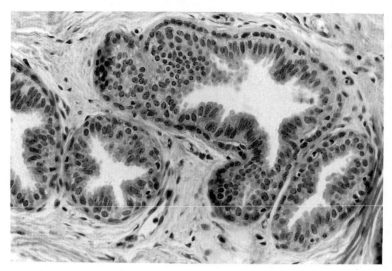

Fig. 11.1 Mild hyperplasia of usual type with heaped-up cells which have no tendency to cross over the spaces in this lobular unit. Note at lower centre an artefact of histological sectioning which produced apparent filling of a portion of the space (× 225).

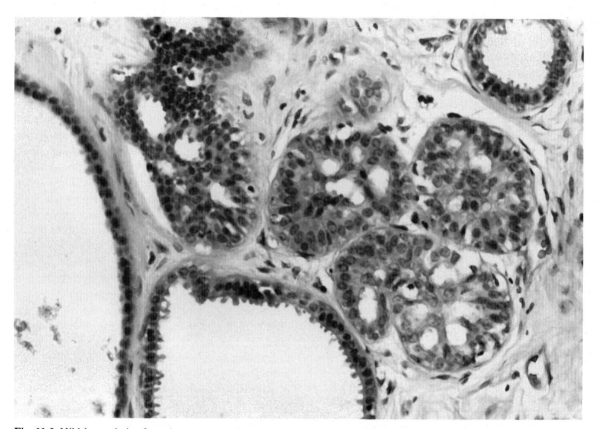

Fig. 11.2 Mild hyperplasia of usual type demonstrates tendency to cross slightly dilated spaces. Note that one cannot with confidence say that there are more than four cells above the basement membrane. Note also that the adjacent acinar space at lower left is a mild example of columnar alteration with apical snouting (× 400).

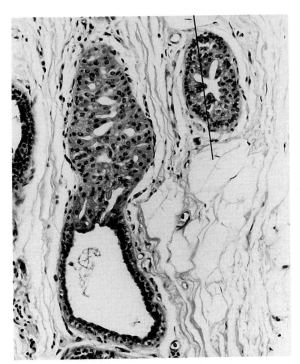

Fig. 11.3 Most of the bridging across the elongated and larger ductule appears to be a sectioning artefact produced by the undulation of the ductule through the plane of section. The cross-section shown in the upper right is probably closer to the actual appearance of this mild hyperplasia, and the line through this upper space demonstrates how the appearance of filling may be produced (× 175).

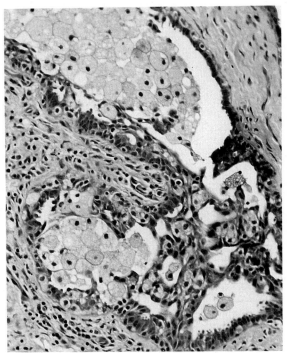

Fig. 11.4 This focus of apparent increase in ductal or ductular cells has attenuated and partially desquamated thin strands of cells intermixed with foam cells. It is not recognized as an example of hyperplasia (× 200).

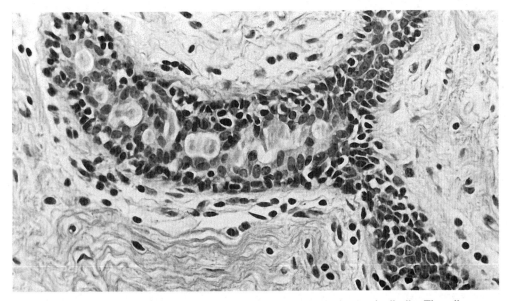

Fig. 11.5 This mild increase in cell number is primarily-due to artefact of sectioning longitudinally. The cells appear small and inactive. This pattern, most common in older women, is not recognized as hyperplastic (× 200).

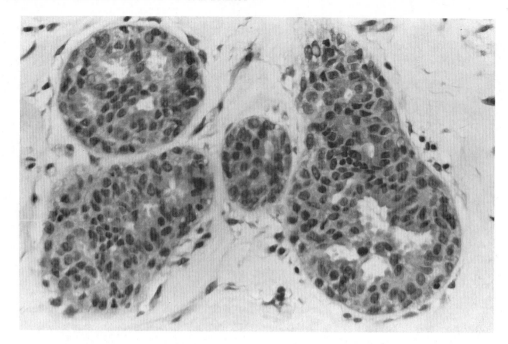

Fig. 11.6 These ductules or acini have a tendency towards filling without marked distension by a somewhat heterogeneous cell population characteristic of usual hyperplasia. This is, then, moderate hyperplasia and a common pattern of proliferative disease without atypia (× 350).

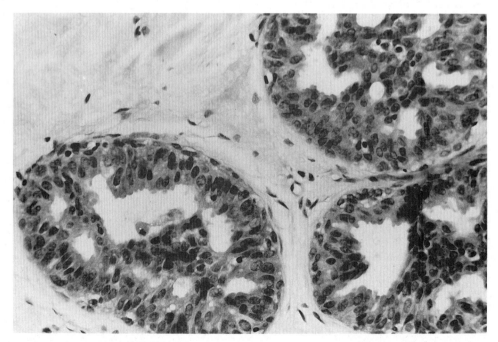

Fig. 11.7 Ductules are partially filled with irregular arcades of cells. In this example of moderate hyperplasia of usual type, the central cell groups are irregularly clumped together and are not recognized as atypical despite evident hyperchromasia (× 350).

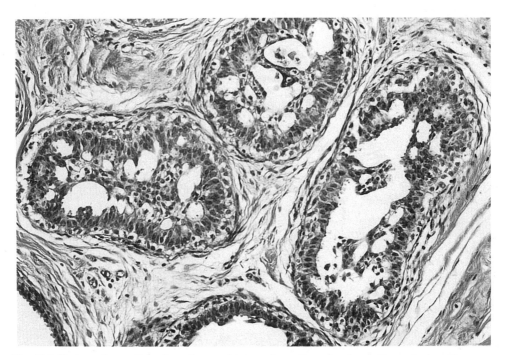

Fig. 11.8 Moderate hyperplasia of usual type with irregular and tapering bars of hyperplastic cells (× 225).

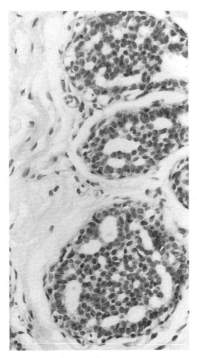

Fig. 11.9 As the duct-like spaces or acini begin to fill with cells the secondary lumina tend to be peripheral to the central cell mass and exhibit irregular contours, features of usual (non-atypical) hyperplasia (× 200).

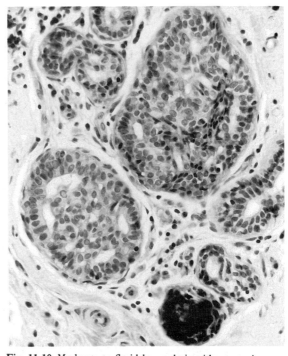

Fig. 11.10 Moderate to florid hyperplasia without atypia. The spaces are almost filled but there is a heterogeneous population of cells with some swirling and peripheral slit-like secondary lumina. Note calcification in acinus at bottom right (× 200).

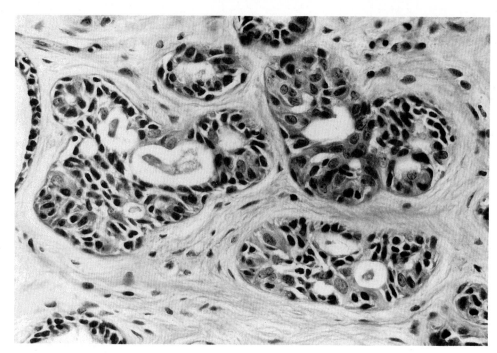

Fig. 11.11 Polymorphism of cytological features is quite extreme in this example of usual hyperplasia (× 400).

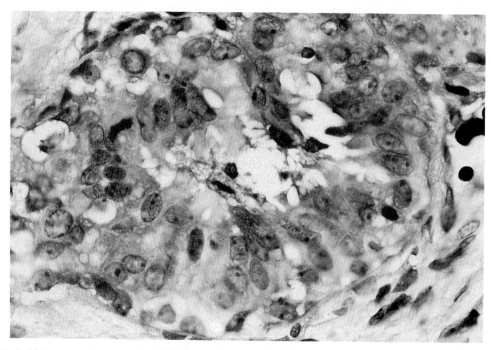

Fig. 11.12 At high power, the nuclear variability in usual hyperplasia is manifest. Nuclei vary from vacuolated to hyperchromatic and some have enlarged nucleoli. Note the absence of advanced or definitive features of cytological atypia (× 900).

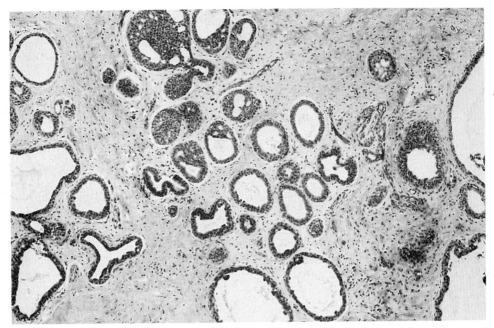

Fig. 11.13 Low power view of the variability so frequent in benign breast biopsies. Mild hyperplasia, early cystic dilatation and apocrine change are present to left, right, and lower centre. Upper centre has proliferative disease, demonstrated at high power in Figure 11.14 (× 75).

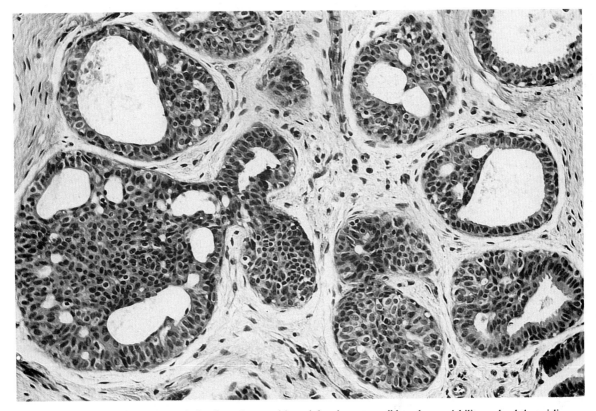

Fig. 11.14 Moderate to florid hyperplasia of usual type with peripheral spaces, mild nuclear variability and subtle swirling. Irregularity and peripheral placement of secondary lumina also support lack of atypical features (× 225).

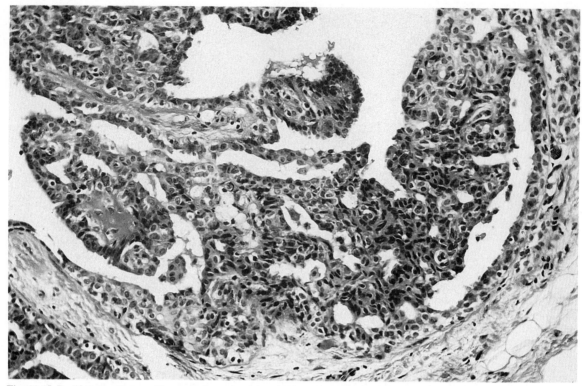

Fig. 11.15 Proliferative disease without atypia at the right of this greatly dilated space is in continuity with the formation of a papilloma with slightly hyaline fibrovascular stroma at left (× 25).

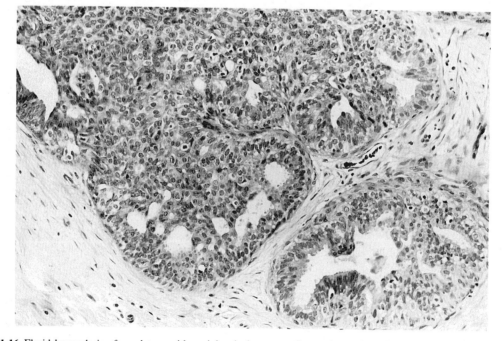

Fig. 11.16 Florid hyperplasia of usual type with peripheral placement of secondary spaces. Nuclei and cytoplasmic contour are predominantly heterogeneous. A few clusters of rounded cells with pale cytoplasm and the central placement of seemingly solid clusters of cells are insufficient to consider a diagnosis of atypia (× 175).

Fig. 11.17 Florid hyperplasia of usual type with small peripheral spaces remaining and very small intercellular spaces in the large central cellular mass. Note heterogeneity of nuclear chromasia and contour (× 225).

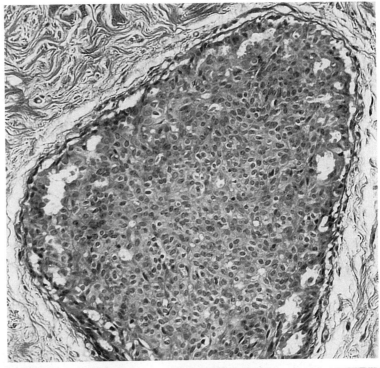

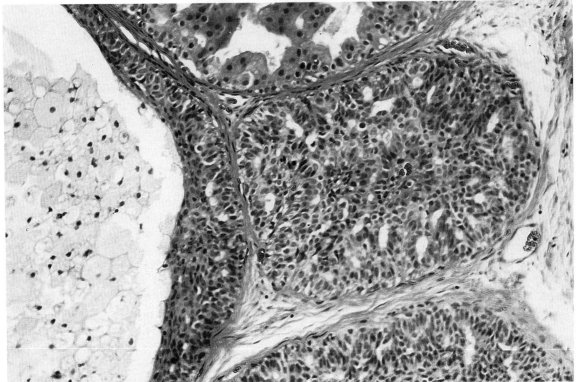

Fig. 11.18 Florid hyperplasia of usual type. Note focal streaming and parallelism of hyperchromatic nuclei. Papillary apocrine change is present above (× 225).

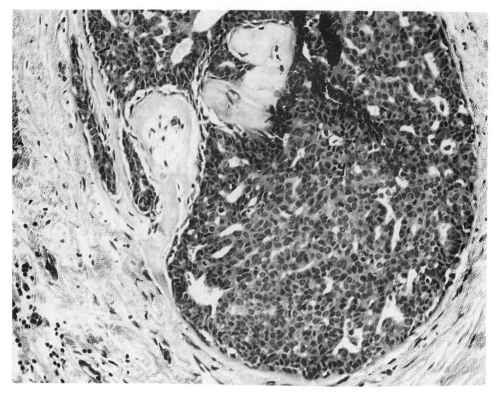

Fig. 11.19 Florid hyperplasia with well-developed, narrow slit-like lumina. Note pseudofiltration adjacent to main cellular mass at upper left (× 225).

tendency of the elongated cells of usual hyperplasia to swirl may be regarded as analogous to the 'squamous eddies' of benign epidermal neoplasms. The presence of swirling or streaming is strong and impelling evidence for benignancy. Slit-like and irregular intercellular spaces are also positive evidence for benignancy. Note that the spaces may be quite small, i.e. 10 microns or less in width when cells are closely packed. In this last situation, ALH or LCIS may be mimicked, but should not be diagnosed. When intercellular spaces are large, arches or bridges of cells appear to cross spaces. These will lack the uniformity of width and cell placement which characterize cribriform DCIS. The narrower cellular extensions of usual hyperplasia will taper, becoming thinner as they extend away from the major cell mass. Cell placement in these arches is irregular or spindled with long axis of cells parallel to the long axis of the bridge (Azzopardi 1979).

Solid patterns of usual hyperplasia without intercellular spaces are occasionally seen, but almost without exception partially fill involved spaces. In those rare situations when solid cell masses fill spaces, swirling of cells and lack of features of CIS will produce an appropriate recognition of benign hyperplasia. Most of the time, however, solid masses are only apparently so, and careful perusal of thin histological sections will reveal slit-like intercellular spaces.

Foam cells may be seen in association with these lesions, most often centrally in the involved space. The recognition of these foam cells as of no significance will avoid mistaken impressions of lobular neoplasia or necrosis. Necrosis of cells, usually in the middle of these proliferative lesions, may be found and should not be interpreted as indicating comedo carcinoma in the absence of other features of CIS. Usually, when necrosis of central cells in usual hyperplasia is mimicked, the apparently necrotic cells are pyknotic and appear to be similar one to another.

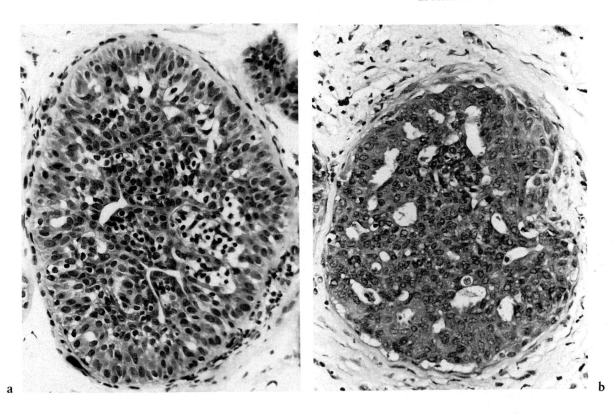

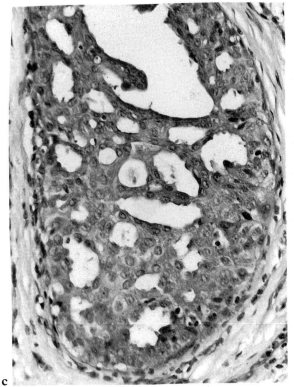

Fig. 11.20a–c Each of these spaces demonstrates florid hyperplasia with some elements suggestive of atypia. In general, the presence of many irregularly contoured spaces between the cells is the most consistent feature denying an assignment of atypia to an individual lesion (**a, b** × 225; **c** × 300).

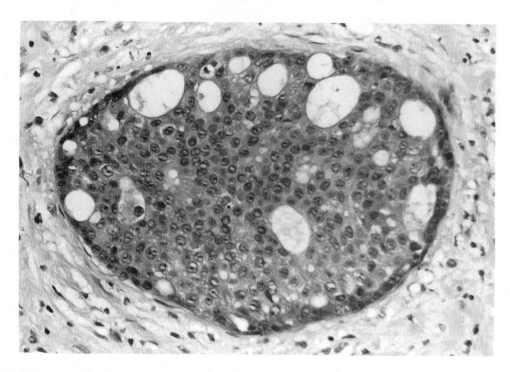

Fig. 11.21 Although a solid cellular area is present centrally, this is not atypical because the cytology is similar to that of non-atypical cells present peripherally. Also, irregularly sized secondary spaces are present peripherally in this example of florid hyperplasia (× 250).

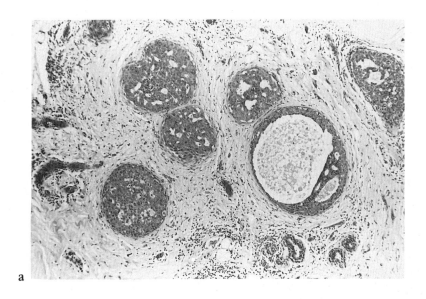

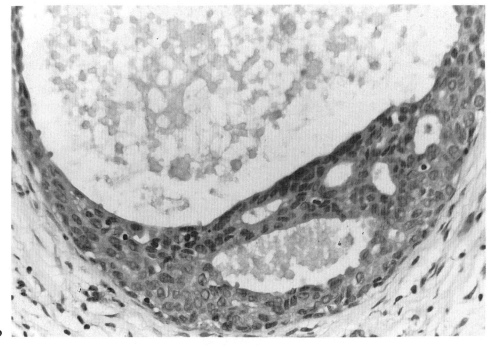

Fig. 11.22 (a) Usual patterns of hyperplasia are seen with characteristic, sinuous, interconnecting strands of cells separated by irregular and often slit-like spaces. The largest space at right of centre is suspicious and may be seen more closely in (b).
(b) This oval contains secondary spaces which are insufficiently crisp and the cell population too heterogeneous for atypia despite the suspicious presentation of the somewhat rigid and narrow bar of cells. Note the cells appear somewhat compressed and although hyperchromatic, do not have the even placement characteristic of atypia and carcinoma in situ. The apparent cellular debris present between the cellular groups does not change this conclusion (a × 75; b × 300).

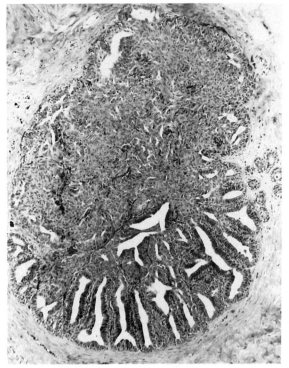

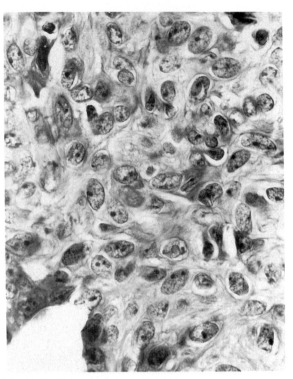

Fig. 11.23 This large focus of florid hyperplasia appears solid at the right and has fibrovascular stalks like a papilloma at the left. However, even at this low power, the many slit-like spaces are apparent (× 75).

Fig. 11.24 High power view of Figure 11.23 demonstrates mild nuclear variability and swirling characteristic of benign hyperplasia of usual type (× 800).

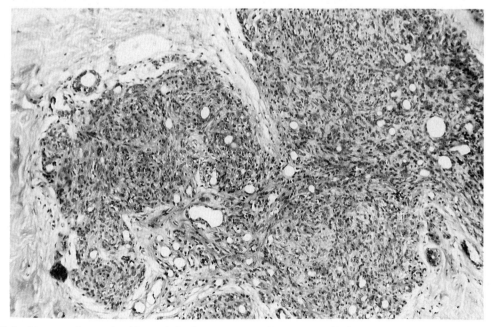

Fig. 11.25 In this unusual example of hyperplasia the component cells are very spindled. It is probable that myoepithelial features predominate in these cells, but their prognostic implications are included within proliferative disease without atypia (× 75).

Atypical ductal hyperplasia (ADH)

Atypical hyperplasia of 'ductal' or no special type is diagnosed when either cytological or pattern criteria of ductal carcinoma in situ (DCIS) are met, but both are not present in full flower (see CIS, Ch. 12). Atypical hyperplasia is also diagnosed if criteria of DCIS are present, but not uniformly so throughout at least two spaces.

ADH is recognized within the series of usual hyperplasias when there are some of the qualitative histological features which characterize DCIS (Figs 11.26–11.36). However, not all of the major features of DCIS are present (see Table 12.1). Many features, diagnostic and otherwise, of DCIS have been and may be cited in this context. However, some are more specific and sensitive than others. It is those which are present most often and most indicative of DCIS which should be emphasized (Page et al 1985): (1) a uniform population of cells, (2) smooth geometric spaces between cells or micropapillary formations with even cellular placement, and (3) hyperchromatic nuclei. ADH has some of these features, but lacks the full measure of these criteria for DCIS. Any case having one or the other of the first two (major) criteria with the second present in only suggestive form will be diagnostic of ADH. The third criterion may be viewed as contributory, but neither specific nor sufficient for a diagnosis of ADH. A swirling cellular pattern or irregular and slit-like intercellular spaces as seen in usual hyperplasia will deny the diagnosis of ADH. Thus, all examples of ADH must have a population of relatively uniform cells.

A frequent pattern recognized as ADH has a central population of evenly spaced cells with hyperchromatic nuclei. This pattern simulates CIS in the presentation of a uniform group of cells, resembling a neoplastic population of cells. This feature is noted as cellular monotony in grade IV lesions by Jensen (1981). Other examples of ADH will have a slightly varied cytology, but with patterns of intercellular spaces identical to those seen in DCIS. Occasionally, both pattern and cell population appear diagnostic, but portions of the space will be lined by cells maintaining a normal columnar layer of luminal cells. Even less frequently, DCIS is strongly suggested but is denied because the central cell population has a high nuclear cytoplasmic ratio that is gradually lost towards the outer layer of proliferated cells. Also, in order to foster interobserver agreement, the study of Page et al (1985) adopted an arbitrary rule for DCIS that two spaces had to be completely involved by a uniform population of cells demonstrating a diagnostic pattern. Therefore, presence of a single space with diagnostic features of DCIS is diagnosed as ADH. However, very few cases of ADH will be resolved in this fashion. Note that the basalar or myoepithelial cell layer is not decisive, and may be apparent or absent as a separate cell population in ADH or DCIS. Note also that cytological atypia per se as ordinarily assessed has little relevance to the diagnosis of ADH, rather it is a population of uniform cells which is most often indicative of ADH.

Both the experienced histopathologist and the tyro alike may be frustrated by the complex permutations of lesions which are found. This frustration is produced because the cytological changes and the architectural (histological) patterns do not vary in parallel. Thus, there are many 'shades of grey' discomfort zones between usual hyperplasia and DCIS which the histopathologist may encounter all too frequently. For example, a lesion viewed at low power may be strongly suggestive of the cribriform pattern typical of duct carcinoma in situ, while higher power examination exhibits some of the cytological variability of usual hyperplasia rendering a diagnosis of carcinoma unacceptable. On the other hand, in a hyperplastic lesion with papillary features which exhibits few if any of the architectural features of duct carcinoma in situ, there may be a remarkable resemblance of the component cells to those seen in ductal carcinoma in situ. Each example is properly diagnosed as atypical hyperplasia because the cytology or the architecture of a hyperplastic lesion exhibits some, but not all, features of ductal carcinoma in situ. Atypicality, then, may be found in any quantitatively assessed example of mild, moderate, or florid hyperplasia, and recognizes qualitative cytological and/or histological pattern features of CIS.

Differential diagnosis

Hyperplasia with atypia is one of the most

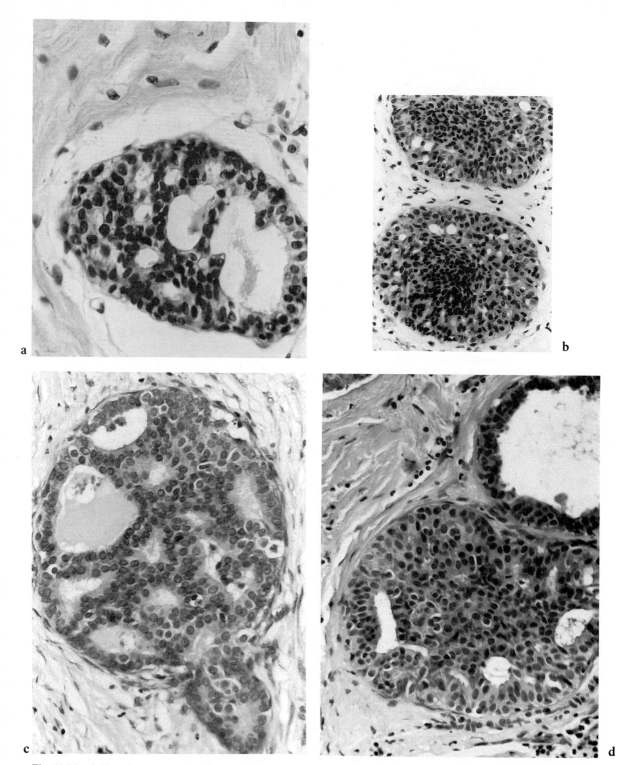

Fig. 11.26a–d These lesser examples of atypical ductal hyperplasia demonstrate an advanced degree of regularity of spaces or cellular arcades, and/or areas of relatively uniform cytological pattern without intercellular lumina. (**a** × 300; **b** × 175; **c** × 225; **d** × 225).

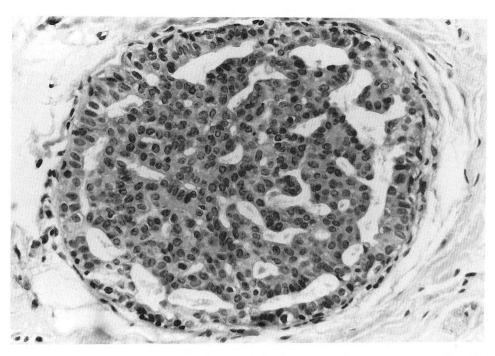

Fig. 11.27 This finely reticulated or filigree pattern of spaces is of sufficient regularity to suggest atypia. The cells are quite homogeneous with somewhat clear cytoplasm, identifiable cytoplasmic borders, and regularly oval nuclei. Thus, both pattern and cytology are suggestive of carcinoma in situ. As they are insufficient for a CIS diagnosis, this is ADH (× 225).

significant problems for the diagnostic histopathologist. It is clear from the definition (some, but not all, defining features of CIS) that various appearances will qualify for this designation. This is because various histological and cytological changes combine to imperfectly resemble ductal carcinoma in situ. Despite the seeming lack of clarity or firmness of the definition, we believe that experienced surgical pathologists and histopathologists frequently recognize such a category in terms of 'worrisome' or 'when I first saw this lesion I felt that duct carcinoma in situ should be ruled out'. If, then, after careful analysis, the lesion does not qualify as carcinoma in situ on either cytological or histological grounds, then it is usually and appropriately considered to represent an example of atypical hyperplasia. Atypicality is most commonly seen with florid hyperplasia. However, the degree of filling of the duct-like space is almost irrelevant in the differential diagnosis of atypical hyperplasia and duct carcinoma in situ. The features which best distinguish hyperplasia from atypical lesions or

non-comedo CIS are irregular nuclear conformation, and irregular slit-like luminal spaces with ragged borders. This nuclear irregularity is a mild degree of pleomorphism, and does not include advanced cytological features of malignancy as seen in comedo CIS.

Juvenile papillomatosis is a term proposed by Rosen et al (1980) for localized, multinodular masses with many cystic spaces and histological features characterized as: 'Although the individual microscopic features were not unique to this entity, the constellation did prove remarkable.' Hyperplasia of usual type, often florid, occurs with papillary apocrine change and adenosis. Thus a complex and 'busy' histological picture is produced. The hyperplasia may have narrow bars and many fairly regular spaces, approaching and reaching patterns of ADH. With an average age of about 20 years, patterns of atypia in this setting should be interpreted with caution. However, there may be an association between juvenile papillomatosis, family history of breast cancer and breast cancer risk elevation (Rosen et al 1985).

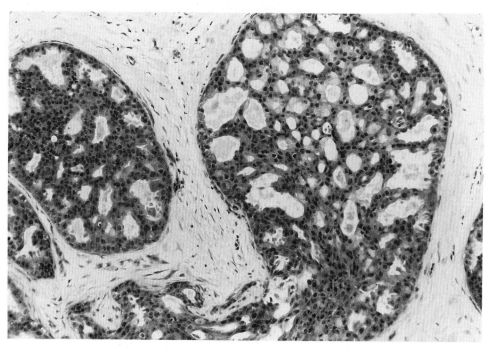

Fig. 11.28 Atypical ductal hyperplasia with diagnostic pattern at left. The more dishevelled pattern at the right would not be diagnostic of atypia (× 175).

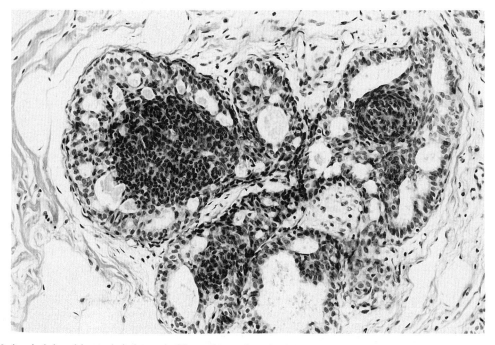

Fig. 11.29 Atypical ductal hyperplasia because of hyperchromasia and relative homogeneity of cytological pattern in space at uppermost left. Note the similar cell groupings in the picture with swirling which would not be so diagnostic (× 175).

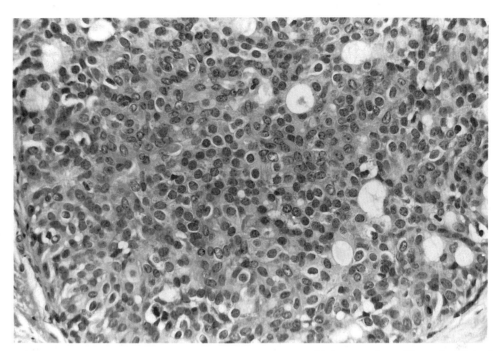

Fig. 11.30 Atypical ductal hyperplasia recognized solely on the basis of relative homogeneity and hyperchromasia of central cellular mass (× 400).

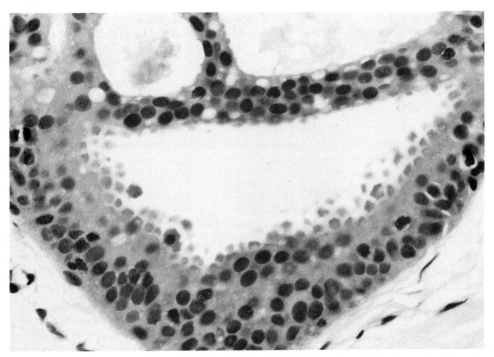

Fig. 11.31 Rigid bar crossing the space in upper central portion of the photograph would be diagnostic of ductal carcinoma in situ if the cell pattern were maintained throughout the remainder of the space. Note evident polarity with increased apical cytoplasmic compartment in most of the cells of the lower portion of the space, a finding which indicates ADH rather than DCIS (× 400).

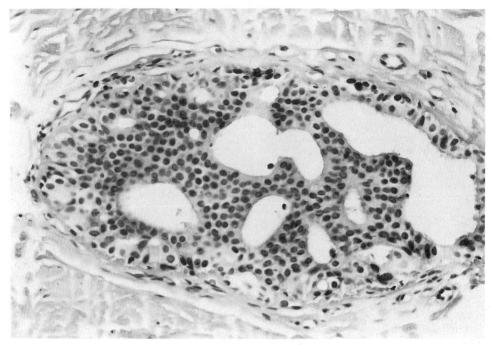

Fig. 11.32 This well-developed example of atypia is arguably diagnostic of DCIS in its central portion. However, the remaining cells of the space are clearly different and are polarized (in the manner of normal cells) at the right (× 300).

Clinical relevance and prognostic implications

Moderate and florid hyperplasia (PDWA)

Moderate and florid hyperplasia of usual type may be included in the term 'proliferative disease without atypia' (PDWA) for convenience. The major utility of the cumbersome diagnostic phrase 'PDWA' is that it states that a condition is present and that atypia has been sought, but not found. In the frequent clinical setting in which the absence of atypical hyperplasia is as much sought for as its presence, the assurance that atypical hyperplasia is absent is definitely appropriate.

The clinical significance of PDWA or usual hyperplasia of moderate and florid degree rests in the positive demonstration of a risk of subsequent invasive carcinoma of 1.5–2 times that of the general population (Dupont & Page 1985). Such a small elevation of risk is usually interpreted as indicating only a greater degree of enthusiasm for screening by mammography. This finding is consistent with the few similar prospective studies which have been done (Kodlin et al 1977), and consistent with concurrent studies relating a greater incidence of such changes in breasts containing cancer as compared to cancer-free breasts (Jensen et al 1976).

Clinical significance of ADH

Atypical ductal hyperplasia (ADH) stands in an intermediate position both histologically and as a cancer risk indicator between PDWA and DCIS. Without this designation, some of these lesions would be recognized as DCIS and others would be regarded as benign. They have long been regarded as examples of 'worrisome' histological patterns, worrisome because they rest at the balance point of the scale between benign and malignant diagnostically and prognostically. Long-term follow-up after biopsy alone (Page et al 1985) has demonstrated an intermediate risk of invasive cancer development between benign lesions and DCIS (Table 11.2).

The clinical significance of identifying and diagnosing ADH in a breast biopsy specimen rests in the prognostic significance of breast cancer risk. Women followed after biopsy alone for 15 years

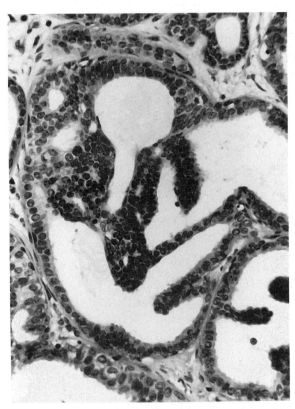

Fig. 11.33 Markedly atypical hyperplasia of ductal type with bulbous, micropapillary structures and trabecular bars, without involvement of the complete space by the population of hyperchromatic cells (× 225).

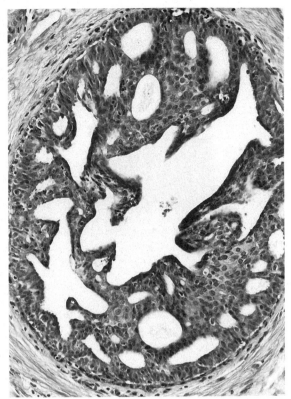

Fig. 11.34 While there is evident uniformity of some clear intercellular spaces, the cellular prolongations tend to taper and there is a definite tendency for peripheral placement of secondary spaces. Besides the suggestion of pattern criteria for DCIS, there also are areas of relatively homogeneous, evenly placed cells. However, the pattern and cytological criteria for DCIS are clearly not uniform and this is an excellent example of ADH (× 200).

Table 11.2 Risk of subsequent invasive carcinoma development after identification at biopsy.

Moderate and florid hyperplasia (of usual type)	1.5–2 ×
ADH	4 ×
ALH	4 ×
Ductal involvement by cells of ALH (with diagnostic ALH)	7 ×
LCIS	10–11 ×
DCIS (Note, this relates to small examples, see Ch. 12)	10–11 ×

develop invasive breast cancer about four times as often as women in the general population, controlling for age (Page et al 1985). This relative risk translates into an absolute risk which indicates about 10% of women with ADH will develop invasive carcinoma of either breast within 10 years of that biopsy. Note that this magnitude of risk is the same as that found for the contralateral breast after mastectomy for invasive carcinoma (see 'Bilaterality', Ch. 16). This latter clinical situation is a more familiar one and for which surgical intervention is seldom undertaken. Risk of subsequent carcinoma is further elevated, approximately doubled to eight to 10 times, if there is a family history of breast carcinoma in a first degree relative, i.e. mother, sister, or daughter (Page et al 1985).

The incidence of ADH in a biopsied population (prior to the introduction of mammography) is about 2% with rare examples identified prior to the age of 35–40. Incidence is about 4% in the perimenopausal age group, rising to 6% in the late 60s. This age distribution is similar to that of the analogous disease, DCIS.

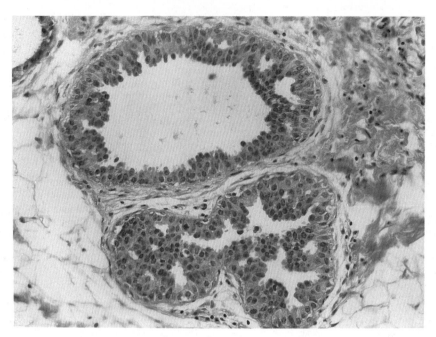

Fig. 11.35 This example of ADH suggests the micropapillary type of ductal carcinoma in situ. Note that the rigidity and uniformity of micropapillary DCIS is not maintained throughout, and that a polarized second population of cells is present focally at the interpapillary areas ($\times$ 200).

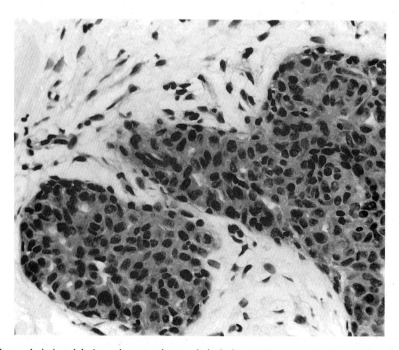

Fig. 11.36 Atypical hyperplasia in a lobular unit presenting a relatively homogeneous population of hyperchromatic cells. While atypical lesions of lobular type are suggested, the slight irregularity of cell placement and presence of intercellular spaces favours a diagnosis of atypical ductal hyperplasia ($\times$ 350).

McCarty et al (1978) evaluated epithelial hyperplasia in breasts contralateral to those containing carcinoma. They recognized cribriform and papillary-cribriform patterns of epithelial hyperplasia which were highly statistically associated with patients having had carcinoma. These patterns of epithelial hyperplasia are closely analogous to ADH, and McCarty et al's findings (1978) must be taken as evidence of concurrent association of ADH with carcinoma.

Note that ADH defines a histologic, spectrum of resemblance to DCIS from minimal to almost identical, i.e. slightly worrisome to very worrisome. No further prognostic significance may be drawn from recognition that a patient may be assigned to either end of the ADH spectrum. However, the follow-up study noted above (Dupont & Page 1985) did recognize a histological pattern reminiscent of ADH felt to be insufficiently developed to occasion a diagnosis of ADH. Most of these cases demonstrated slightly bulbous groups of cells tethered to the luminal surface of normally polarized, luminal cells (Figs 11.37 and 11.38). These cases of 'minimally atypical ductal hyperplasia' did not demonstrate an incidence of breast cancer greater than that of proliferative disease without atypia (Ch. 11). It is not our practice to diagnose these minimal changes in biopsy reports.

ATYPICAL LOBULAR HYPERPLASIA (ALH)

Anatomical pathology

Atypical lobular hyperplasia (ALH) is presented as a single entity rather than a series of lobular changes. This is because definition of such a series has been difficult. Wellings et al (1975) attempted to define such a series as atypical lobules type B (ALB), but few such examples hampered the clear demonstration of a series from mild hyperplasia to LCIS as was possible for mild usual hyperplasia to DCIS. For many years, mammary histological patterns reminiscent of LCIS, but falling short of the well-developed pattern have been termed ALH. However, specific criteria to differentiate ALH from LCIS have seldom been offered.

Histological criteria for the diagnosis of LCIS are presented in Chapter 12. When identical cytological appearances are found in lobular units, but less than one-half of the acini in a unit are filled, distorted and distended with a uniform population of characteristic cells, then ALH is diagnosed (Figs 11.39–11.44). Most often the criterion for LCIS which is not met, thus leading to a diagnosis of ALH, is filling of acini, i.e. intercellular spaces are present. Care must be taken not to misinterpret intracellular lumina (see 'LCIS', Ch. 12) as intercellular spaces. Well-fixed and stained histological preparations are mandatory for the reliable identification of these changes.

The cytology of ALH is usually quite bland, with round, frequently somewhat lightly stained nuclei and cytoplasm evenly spaced one from another without evident pattern or polarity. Small nucleoli may be present. It is the uniformity and roundness of the cell population which is the major guide-post to a diagnosis of ALH. Within lobular units, the presence of a cell population cytologically different from ALH cells is strong evidence against a diagnosis of LCIS, and should prompt reserve in the diagnosis of ALH (see 'ductal involvement by cells of ALH', below). Occasionally, most cells in usual hyperplasia will be rounded, mimicking the cells of lobular neoplasia. If the pattern is otherwise characteristic of usual hyperplasia, it should be regarded as such. *If any lobular unit meets the criteria for LCIS, then that diagnosis overrides any presence of ALH.*

Reliable criteria of diagnosis demand that each end of a spectrum be set. The upper end of ALH borders on LCIS, and the lower end borders on quite non-specific lobular appearance for which no diagnostic term is proposed. Thus, we do not recognize lobular hyperplasia as a diagnostic term because of imprecision of histological definition and current lack of clinical relevance. The least developed but diagnostic examples of ALH must have a group of almost identical, characteristic cells, evenly spaced relative to each other which are definitely increased in number over that normally present in an acinus. This approach assists the diagnosis of ALH when fixation artefact or mammary involution produces a loss in polarity of acinar cells which may mimic ALH (Figs 11.45 and 11.46). Also avoided, is the possibility of mistaking similarly altered foci of mild hyperplasia

Fig. 11.37 Bulbous collections of somewhat pyknotic cells appear to perch upon an otherwise unremarkable, columnar luminal cell population. This appearance does not appear to carry implications of increased cancer risk (× 300).

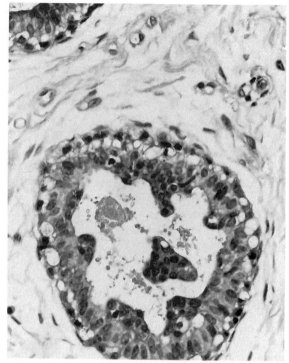

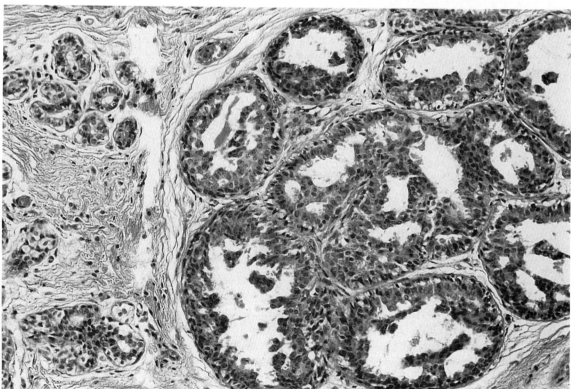

Fig. 11.38 'Minimally atypical ductal hyperplasia' similar to that in Figure 11.37 resembles patterns of hyperplasia found in gynaecomastia (× 225).

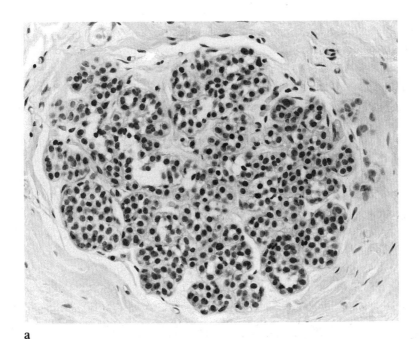

a

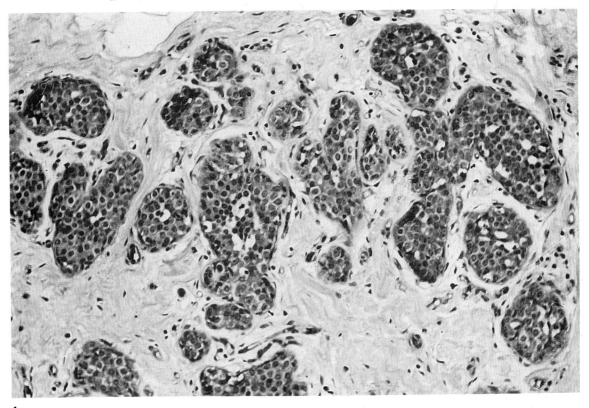

b

Fig. 11.39a,b These examples of atypical lobular hyperplasia may be considered 'gold standard'. The resemblance to lobular carcinoma in situ is great, but it is evident that uniform filling and distension of individual acini are not present in more than 50% of the lobular units demonstrated (**a** × 225; **b** × 225).

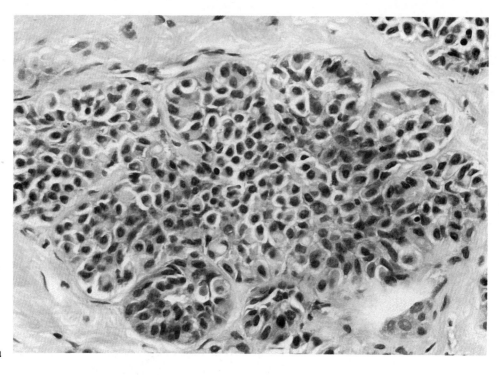

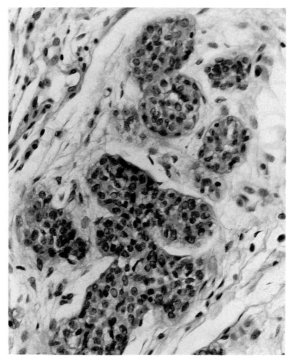

Fig. 11.40 (a) Atypical lobular hyperplasia demonstrates a greater degree of cellular pleomorphism than usually seen in that diagnosis. Intracytoplasmic lumina are evident. (b) Here is a more common example of the cytology of atypical lobular hyperplasia than (a). Note some suggestion of cytological variability, but with a dominance of similar population of rounded cells (**a, b** × 300).

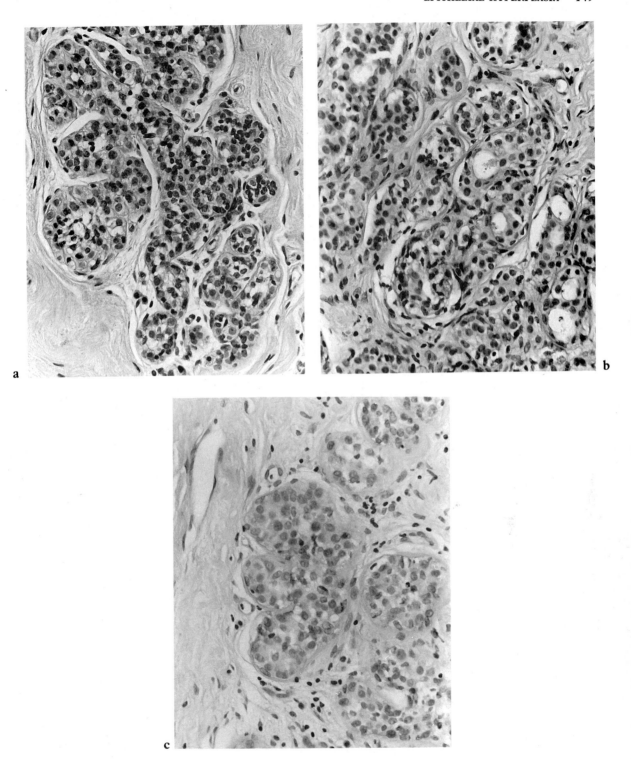

Fig. 11.41a–c Cells with characteristic cytology are somewhat intermixed with a second cell population in these examples of atypical lobular hyperplasia. Note in (**b**) that the lobular unit is somewhat deformed, occasionally presenting difficulties in diagnosis. In (**b**), distortion and distension of some acini are readily apparent, however, they are not filled because remnants of lumina are frequently apparent (**a–c** × 250).

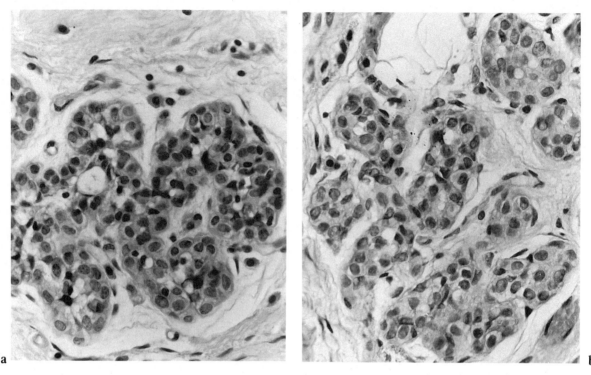

a   b

Fig. 11.42a,b These high power views of advanced examples of atypical lobular hyperplasia reveal occasional clear spaces immediately adjacent to nuclei which by special stains are revealed to be intracytoplasmic lumina (**a, b** × 350).

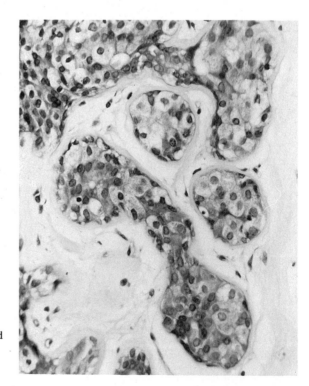

Fig. 11.43 Although unusual, occasionally the collections of cells with characteristic cytological features of ALH form cellular groups or clumps interspersed between an attenuated second cell population. Nuclear alterations will aid in differentiation from the rare cell clear change of no known significance (× 300).

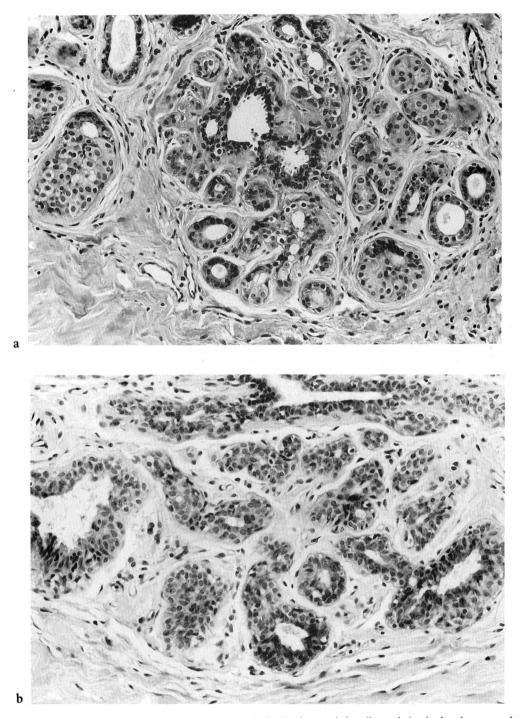

Fig. 11.44a,b In these examples of atypical lobular hyperplasia the characteristic cell population is sharply separated from a presumably remnant normal cell population as seen in several acini. In (**b**), the pattern is more subtle and is seen most readily in the involved acinar spaces at far left and far right (**a, b** × 225).

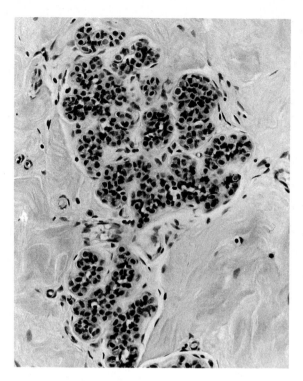

Fig. 11.45 This is a truly borderline example of minimal atypical lobular hyperplasia or no atypia at all. There is a suggestion that more than two of the rounded cells are present adjacent to one another, but in the absence of certainty, atypical lobular hyperplasia is better left undiagnosed (× 225).

of usual type for ALH. Occasionally a clear separation of ALH from atypical ductal hyperplasia is difficult (Figs 11.47–11.49). Fortunately, the currently recognized prognostic implications are so similar that it matters little which type of atypia is diagnosed in this situation.

Cells of ALH may involve ducts in much the same way as LCIS (Fig. 11.50). The histological, patterns produced are usually more subtle than the pagetoid or mural pattern of LCIS (Fechner 1972) and the solid pattern of LCIS involvement of ducts is not seen with ALH. Such a finding may be termed ductal involvement by ALH.

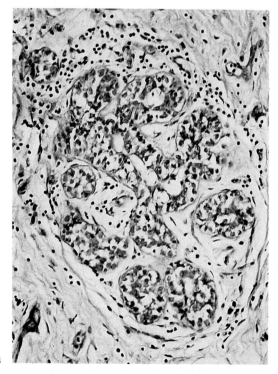

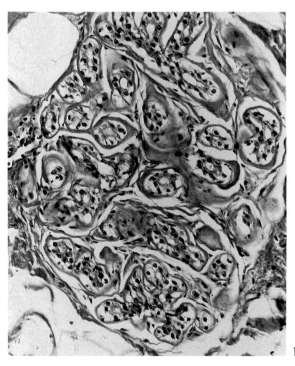

a   b

Fig. 11.46a,b These lobular units present patterns which mimic atypical lobular hyperplasia because of loss of polarity of cells within acini. Whether this is because of a natural phenomenon, or a fixation artefact is often not apparent (**a, b** × 225).

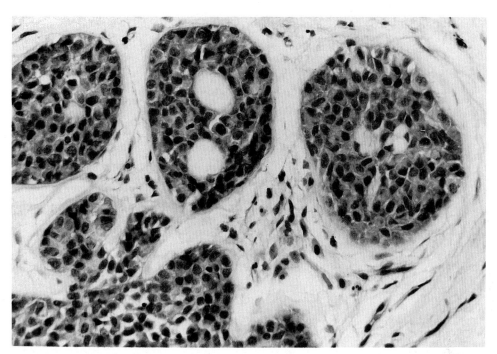

Fig. 11.47 Atypical hyperplasia is recognized because of extreme hyperchromasia and resemblance to some intermediate appearance between atypical ductal and atypical lobular hyperplasia. Thus this is not clearly an example of either. The irregular cell placement and seeming formation of intercellular lumina favour a diagnosis of atypical ductal hyperplasia (× 350).

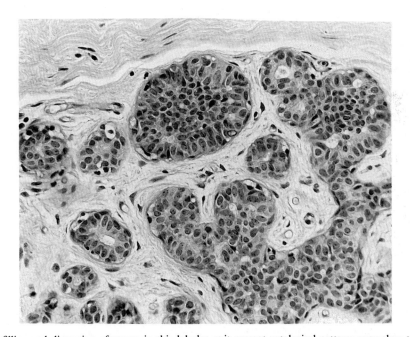

Fig. 11.48 Partial filling and distension of spaces in this lobular unit present cytological patterns very close to atypical lobular hyperplasia at lower right whereas the pattern closely resembling atypical ductal hyperplasia is seen in the upper centre. As the resemblance to atypical lobular hyperplasia with clusters of round cells with clear cytoplasm is a 'better fit' at the lower right, ALH is the favoured diagnosis (× 225).

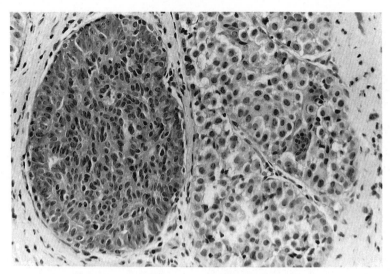

Fig. 11.49 Varied patterns of atypical hyperplasia (AH) rarely occur adjacent to each other. A 'ductal' pattern AH is at left with a focus unresolvable between ALH and ADH at right. The cytology is so characteristic of lobular hyperplasia to the right that ALH must be noted in the diagnosis. Combined ADH and ALH should probably be diagnosed (× 225).

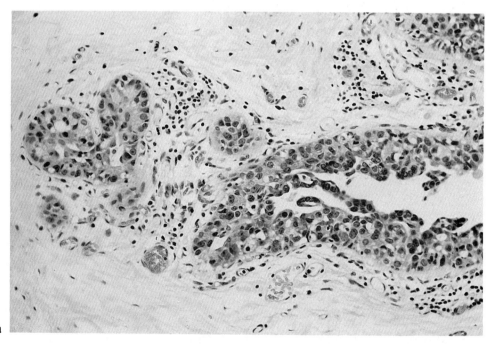

Fig. 11.50a–d These are all examples of cells of atypical lobular hyperplasia undermining a different luminal 'ductal', cellular population. In some examples the second cell population is very attenuated. In (d) a 'clover-leaf' pattern is apparent. Identical appearances may be seen in lobular carcinoma in situ, with the defining diagnostic features separating LCIS from ALH being present in the lobular units (a × 200; b × 225; c × 400; d × 200).

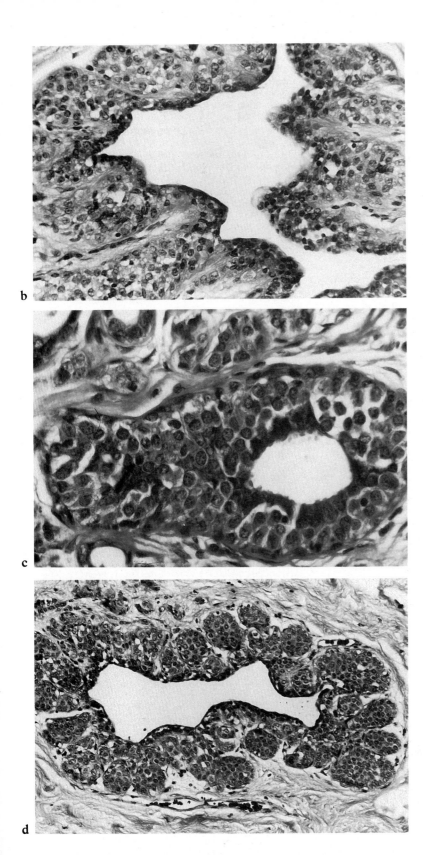

Clinical and prognostic correlates

The spectrum from lesser examples of ALH up to and including LCIS may be fruitfully termed 'lobular neoplasia', an approach fostered by Haagensen et al (1978). Adoption of the degree of filling, distortion and distension of lobular acini as determinant criteria for the separation of ALH from LCIS in biopsies has revealed a relative risk of subsequent invasive carcinoma development for ALH to be four times that of the general population in two separate studies (Page et al 1978, 1985). This magnitude of risk elevation contrasts with that of about 10 times found when LCIS is not further treated after biopsy.

Other than the magnitude of subsequent carcinoma risk (see above) ALH does not differ from the analogous CIS lesions (LCIS) in clinical correlates and implications (Page et al 1985). The incidence of ALH in benign biopsies is somewhat over 1% and the great majority of cases are found in women in the perimenopausal ages, with a decreasing incidence with advancing age after menopause. The subsequently developing invasive carcinomas may appear in either breast and are more likely to be of tubular or invasive lobular type (Haagensen et al 1978; Page et al 1985). As with ADH, there appears to be a remarkable risk interaction with a strong family history of breast cancer. Women with a family history of breast cancer in a first-degree relative (mother, sister, or daughter) as well as ALH at biopsy, double their risk of subsequent invasive carcinoma over that of ALH alone.

Ductal involvement by cells of ALH was found by Page et al (1987) to elevate slightly the subsequent risk of carcinoma when found together with ALH over that of ALH alone (see Table 11.2).

REFERENCES

Ackerman L V, Katzenstein A L 1977 The concept of minimal breast cancer and the pathologist's role in the diagnosis of 'early carcinoma'. Cancer 39: 2755–2763

Alpers C E, Wellings S R 1985 The prevalence of carcinoma in situ in normal and cancer-associated breasts. Hum Pathol 16: 796–807

Ashikari R, Huvos A G, Snyder R E 1974 A clinicopathologic study of atypical lesions of the breast. Cancer 33: 310–317

Azzopardi J G 1979 Problems in breast pathology. Saunders, Philadelphia, p 113–123, 213–233

Black E M, Chabon A B 1969 In-situ carcinoma of the breast. Pathol Annu 4: 185–210

Dawson E K 1933 Carcinoma in the mammary lobule and its origin. Edinb Med J 40: 57–82

Dupont W D, Page D L 1985 Risk factors for breast cancer in women with proliferative breast disease. N Engl J Med 312: 146–151

Fechner R E 1972 Epithelial alterations in the extralobular ducts of breast with lobular carcinoma. Arch Pathol 93: 164–171

Fisher E R 1982 The pathology of breast cancer as it relates to its evolution, prognosis and treatment. Clin Oncol 1: 703–734

Foote F W, Stewart F W 1945 Comparative studies of cancerous versus noncancerous breasts. Ann Surg 121: 6–53, 197–222

Haagensen C D, Lane N, Lattes R, Bodian C 1978 Lobular neoplasia (so-called lobular carcinoma in situ) of the breast. Cancer 42: 737–769

Hutter R V P and others 1986 Consensus meeting. Is 'fibrocystic disease' of the breast precancerous? Arch Pathol Lab Med 110: 171–173

Jensen H M 1981 Breast pathology, emphasizing precancerous and cancer-associated lesions. In: Bulbrook R D, Taylor D J (eds) Commentaries on research in breast disease, vol 2. Liss, New York, p 41–86

Jensen H M, Rice J R, Wellings S R 1976 Preneoplastic lesions in the human breast. Science 191: 295–297

Kodlin D, Winger E E, Morgenstern N L, Chen U 1977 Chronic mastopathy and breast cancer: a follow-up study. Cancer 39: 2603–2607

McCarty K S Jr, Kesterson G H D, Wilkinson W E, Georgiade N 1978 Histologic study of subcutaneous mastectomy specimens from patients with carcinoma of the contralateral breast. Surg Gynecol Obstet 147: 682–688

Page D L 1986 Cancer risk assessment in benign biopsies. Hum Pathol 17: 871–874

Page D L, Vander Zwaag R, Rogers L W, Williams L T, Walker W E, Hartmann W H 1978 Relation between component parts of fibrocystic disease complex and breast cancer. J Natl Cancer Inst 61: 1055–1063

Page D L, Dupont W D, Rogers L W, Rados M S 1985 Atypical hyperplastic lesions of the female breast. A long-term follow-up study. Cancer 55: 2698–2708

Page D L, Dupont W D, Rogers L W 1986 Breast cancer risk of lobular-based hyperplasia after biopsy: "ductal" pattern lesions. Cancer Detect Prevent 9: 441–448

Page D L, Dupont W D, Rogers L W 1987 Ductal involvement by cells of atypical lobular hyperplasia in the breast Hum Pathol (in press)

Rogers L W, Page D L 1979 Epithelial proliferative disease of the breast. A marker of increased cancer risk in certain age groups. Breast Dis Breast 5: 2–7

Rosen P P, Cantrell B, Mullen D L, DePalo A 1980 Juvenile papillomatosis (Swiss cheese disease) of the breast. Am J Surg Pathol 4: 3–12

Rosen P P, Holmes G, Lesser M L, Kinne D W, Beattie E J 1985 Juvenile papillomatosis and breast carcinoma. Cancer 55: 1345–1352

Wellings S R, Jensen H M, Marcum R G 1975 An atlas of subgross pathology of the human breast with special reference to possible precancerous lesions. J Natl Cancer Inst 55: 231–271

Carcinoma in situ (CIS)

The establishment of in situ mammary carcinoma as an entity distinct from hyperplasias and invasive disease was gradual through the first half of this century, but it is now firmly accepted and includes several subtypes with differing natural histories. In general, carcinoma in situ (CIS) is characterized histologically by disturbed cellular orientation, hyperchromasia and pleomorphism which mimic the cellular appearance of infiltrating carcinoma, but without evidence of invasion. The abnormal cells are contained within the sites where epithelial cells are normally found although lobular units and ducts may be greatly deformed. The prognostic importance of this diagnosis rests largely on the supposition that similar areas remaining within the breast, following identification of these changes in a biopsy, will often progress to invasive carcinoma in a significant percentage of patients so characterized. Some types of carcinoma in situ may be thought of as markers of increased subsequent risk of cancer development. There is no conclusive evidence that CIS is an obligate precursor of invasive disease.

Three types of mammary carcinoma in situ are recognized. Each is associated with a specific histological appearance as well as different prognostic implications with regard to both the ipsilateral and contralateral breast. Generally, carcinoma in situ of comedo type must be considered most closely related to infiltrating carcinoma both histologically and prognostically. The remaining two types of CIS, non-comedo ductal CIS and lobular CIS have lesser degrees of cytological atypia and less direct association with invasive carcinoma. Although most cases of carcinoma in situ fall into one or another of the three diagnostic categories, coexistence of two and, rarely, three histological types may be seen. Paget's disease of the nipple is discussed here because it usually represents carcinoma in situ of the subareolar ducts which has gained access to the adjacent nipple surface. Because this does not involve stromal invasion, the process must be regarded as in situ. Non-invasive papillary carcinoma, a lesion closely related to CIS, is also discussed in this chapter.

Atypical patterns of epithelial hyperplasia, histologically defined as having some of the features of CIS, are discussed in this chapter to aid in the presentation of differential diagnosis. The clinical relevance of these changes with regard to breast cancer risk is presented in Table 11.1.

COMEDO CARCINOMA IN SITU

Classification and terminology

Many recent studies include the comedo type of carcinoma in situ with the other two patterns (micropapillary and cribriform) of CIS considered ductal (DCIS) (Ashikari et al 1971; Contesso & Petit 1979). We feel that comedo CIS should be separately categorized from micropapillary and cribriform types because of its probably greater malignant potential, larger size and increased ease of clinical and mammographic detection. Cell kinetic studies have supported this separation (Meyer 1986).

We reserve the term comedo CIS for lesions without stromal invasion and always make this clear by adding the phrase in situ. This has been a source of confusion in the past as cases reported as comedo carcinoma have had definite foci of invasion (Lewis & Geschickter 1938; Gillis et al 1960).

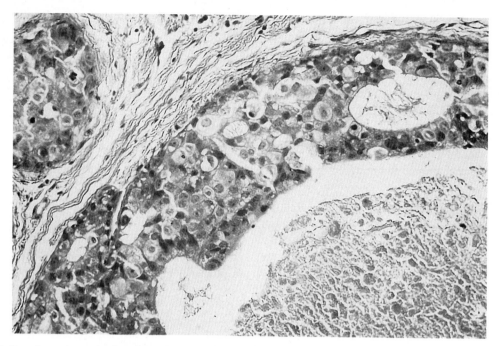

Fig. 12.1 Comedo carcinoma in situ with maintenance of intercellular spaces. Necrotic cells have lost their recognizable form in the 'comedo' material at upper left (× 225).

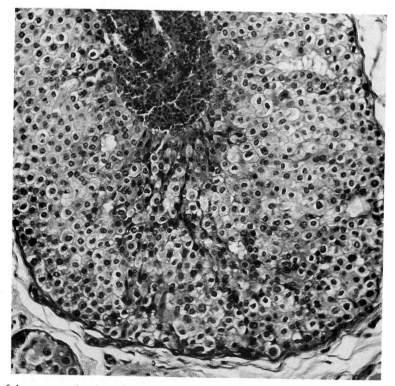

Fig. 12.2 Because of the near complete loss of space or gland forming capacity as well as because of the central necrosis this example of carcinoma in situ should be viewed as of comedo type. Cytological atypia and pleomorphism are not as advanced as is usually seen (× 225).

Anatomical pathology

The feature characterizing this type of in situ carcinoma is the presence of necrotic cellular debris in ductal and lobular spaces. As these spaces are commonly 2 and even 3 mm in diameter, the soft, cheese-like, necrotic material may be appreciated by the naked eye, and it is this feature that led to the naming of this tumour type by its resemblance to the common comedone. Histologically, the necrotic debris is usually centrally placed presenting varying degrees of cellular disruption or dissolution including the total loss of cellular detail (Figs 12.1–12.2). Viable cells are present in solid or perforated masses adjacent to the duct wall surrounding the necrotic debris. The cells are large with markedly atypical nuclear features and often have a large amount of cytoplasm. This advanced degree of cytological atypia is as characteristic a feature of the comedo CIS as is the necrosis.

Differential diagnosis

The cytological features of malignancy are well developed in these cases and histological diagnosis usually presents little difficulty. Note that this advanced nuclear atypia includes the classic criteria of malignancy, and not the mild nuclear variability which characterizes hyperplasia of usual type. Occasionally, when necrosis is particularly marked and few viable cells are present, the diagnosis may be missed. When such areas are present, extensive sampling must be pursued. As areas of micropapillary and cribriform in situ are often intermixed with comedo carcinoma in situ (Fig. 12.3), this can present problems in classification. In general, these are best resolved by rendering a diagnosis either of comedo carcinoma in situ or intraductal carcinoma of mixed type with comedo pattern predominating, etc. In other words the diagnosis of comedo CIS should be favoured when its histological features are present.

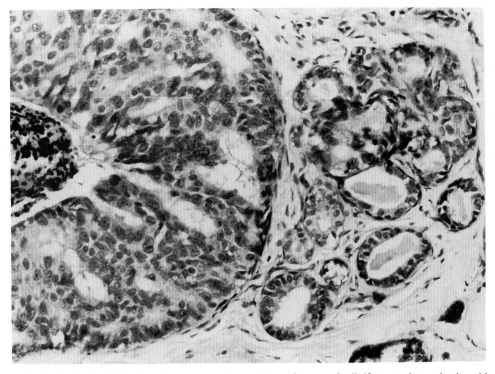

Fig. 12.3 This sample of comedo carcinoma in situ also has prominent features of cribriform carcinoma in situ with well-formed, rigid spaces. Note involvement of a portion of the lobular unit at right (× 300).

Highly pleomorphic cells may extend into readily definable lobular units (Fechner 1971), a phenomenon termed 'cancerization of lobules' by Azzopardi (1979). As in other circumstances, sclerosed and deformed lobules will present difficulties in diagnosis because infiltrating carcinoma may be mimicked. We demand demonstration of infiltrating cancer beyond definable lobular units before making such a diagnosis (see Ch. 16).

A solid pattern of in situ carcinoma with involved spaces completely filled with cells is recognized by some (Ozzello & Sanpitak 1970; Ashikari et al 1971), but as its histopathological definition is not well defined, and it is usually found mixed with other patterns, we feel that its separate distinction is not warranted. Thus, the diagnostician should attempt to place such cases in recognized categories by their closest resemblance. This solid pattern of CIS has expanded ducts or ductules filled with cells which often appear cytologically intermediate between lobular CIS and comedo CIS without central necrosis (Figs 12.4–12.5); which is to say, these solid variants are more pleomorphic than lobular CIS, and less than comedo CIS. Happily, these patterns

are very rare; however, for that reason their clinical implications are not known. This solid pattern would include at least some of the organoid and carcinoid-like cases of CIS reported by Cross et al (1985). We consider it prudent to diagnose both lobular and ductal CIS in this setting if the cytology of lobular lesions is present (Figs 12.33–12.36). Thus, clinical implications of each diagnosis will be applied in the absence of certainty as to which is most appropriate. With occasional foci of necrosis we feel such cases should be reported as comedo carcinoma in situ, particularly when the nuclear atypia is well developed. The presence of well-formed gland-like spaces removes a case from consideration as an example of solid or comedo type except in situations in which necrosis and cytological atypia are well developed. (Figs 12.1 and 12.2). It must also be noted that foam cells (Fig. 12.6) and focal necrosis may be seen without justifying a diagnosis of comedo CIS. Specifically, small foci of pyknotic, necrotic cells present in otherwise characteristic patterns of usual hyperplasia, LCIS or non-comedo DCIS will not change the diagnosis established by the characteristic patterns.

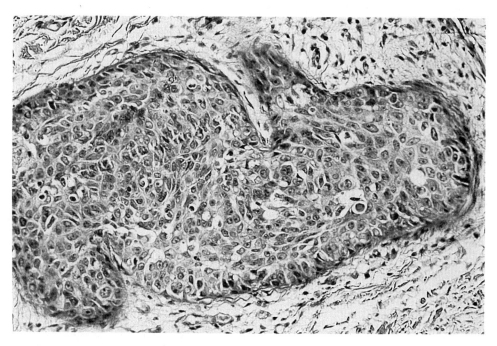

Fig. 12.4 This undeniable example of carcinoma in situ lacks distinctive features as to type and is often termed 'solid' for evident reasons (× 225).

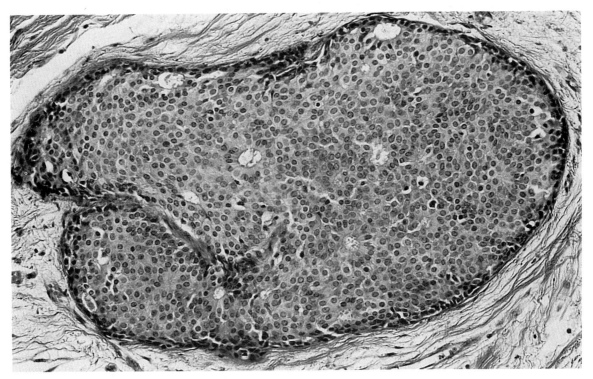

Fig. 12.5 This example of carcinoma in situ has few of the usual clean-cut architectural or cytological features of that diagnosis. The uniformity of cell population and crispness of definition of small gland-like formations qualify this as a non-comedo type of ductal carcinoma in situ (× 225).

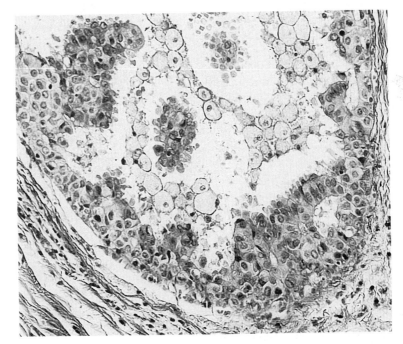

Fig. 12.6 Ductal carcinoma in situ. The central foam cells do not qualify for a diagnosis of comedo type carcinoma in situ (× 225).

Clinical features and prognostic correlates

A large percentage of these cases present clinically with masses up to 5 cm in diameter (Millis & Thynne 1975). Even though invasion may not be detected by careful and extensive histological examination, 1–2% of these cases (primarily larger ones) may be associated with metastases in axillary lymph nodes. This does not include those biopsied cases in which separate foci of invasive carcinoma are revealed elsewhere in the breast in subsequent mastectomy — a finding in a significant number (perhaps as many as 5%) of cases (Carter & Smith 1977; Rosen et al 1980).

Microinvasion, as described in Chapter 16, is particularly common with comedo in situ carcinoma. It is certainly more common than with other types of CIS. However, we and others (Millis & Thynne 1975) have seen cases of comedo carcinoma in situ treated by wide local excision with five to 15 years follow-up with no evidence of further breast disease. How often this might happen is not known with certainty because the few studies which have reported women treated by local excision of CIS have not regulary separated comedo from the other patterns of DCIS. The natural history of these lesions is also imperfectly known, because they have been traditionally treated by mastectomy with the high expectation of cure. Experience from the middle of this century (Lewis & Geschickter 1938; Geschickter 1943) indicates that comedo CIS presenting as a large palpable mass is highly likely to recur after local excision.

Detection and diagnosis of this type of in situ carcinoma by mammographic study, particularly in screening programme, are often possible as the central necrotic debris frequently calcifies and is detected in linear arrays (Millis 1979). This is less often true of the other types of in situ carcinoma.

CRIBRIFORM AND MICROPAPILLARY CARCINOMA IN SITU (non-comedo DCIS)

Terminology

The terms 'cribriform' and 'micropapillary' denote patterns of epithelial proliferation which have been recognized as malignant for almost as many decades as has comedo CIS, and are currently more frequently diagnosed than comedo CIS. We feel that the use of the term 'ductal' and hence DCIS for all of these lesions is justified only in order to point out that they differ from the lobular lesions. This terminology will probably continue to be both used and useful; however, we feel there are compelling reasons to separately report comedo and non-comedo DCIS.

It is not a common practice to evaluate separately the different types of ductal carcinoma in situ (DCIS). The reason for this is, undoubtedly, that they are rare conditions and lumping them together under the rubric of DCIS has been a common practice. Thus, a Mayo Clinic study (Gillis et al 1960) as well as the series from M.D. Anderson Hospital (Westbrook & Gallager 1975) have grouped together comedo, micropapillary and cribriform, and intracystic carcinomas. We believe there are reasons to keep these types of breast disease separate, as their malignant potential is probably different. We would therefore encourage future reports of in situ mammary carcinoma to document, as Millis & Thynne (1975) have done, the type of ductal carcinoma in situ present and whether a dominant mass was present or not.

We believe that those minute examples of non-comedo DCIS reported recently by Betsill et al (1978) and Page et al (1982) need to be identified separately from more extensive disease. Both of these recent reports document the review of a large number of biopsies initially reported as benign. About 1 in each 400 biopsies contained small foci of non-comedo DCIS. The follow-up of these women, detailed below, indicates a very different prognosis from that generally associated with large examples of comedo CIS (see 'Clinical and prognostic implications'). As emphasized by Azzopardi (1979), it is important to separate different types of ductal carcinoma in situ. The current problem, however, is that many reported series have not done this, and although the papers noted above reporting patients treated by mastectomy may include primarily women with more extensive disease, there is no guarantee of this.

Anatomical pathology

Occasionally these lesions produce a palpable

lump. More commonly, however, they are incidentally associated with a palpable or mammographic abnormality within the breast occasioning biopsy. Histologically, cribriform and micropapillary patterns are so often intermixed that they need to be discussed and considered together. A micropapillary pattern (less common than cribriform) presents papillary projections from the surface of lobular, ductal or cystic spaces, which tend to have regular size and shape. There is no fibrovascular stalk. Their papillae are smooth and bulbous, so that the rounded tip distant from the wall is broader than its base (Figs 12.7–12.9). It is the regularity, and crispness of definition of these papillations which make them distinctive on low power examination. The cribriform pattern is recognized by neat, punched-out spaces of similar size within a characteristic population of cells (Figs 12.10–12.13). It is the crispness of definition and the uniformity of cell population in both cytology and cell placement which are the essential elements. As the spaces become larger, and the strands of cells narrower, the cribriform

and micropapillary patterns merge to produce similar appearances. Small foci of necrotic cells may be seen in these lesions without occasioning a diagnosis of comedo CIS in the absence of the cytological features of that diagnosis.

Three-dimensional studies have shown that the crisp spaces of cribriform CIS are dispersed and do not interconnect, while those regular and slit-like spaces characterizing common hyperplasia are interconnected (Ohuchi et al 1985).

Differential diagnosis

In order to provide consistency and reliability in diagnosis, it is our practice to follow the simple rules presented in Table 12.1. While we recognize that they may seem arbitrary, they do provide objective guidelines conducive to intra- and inter-observer agreements. Biopsies presenting extensive areas of cribriform and micropapillary change are both more easily identified and more readily diagnosed as carcinoma. Cases with less extensive disease, as noted in the terminology section of this

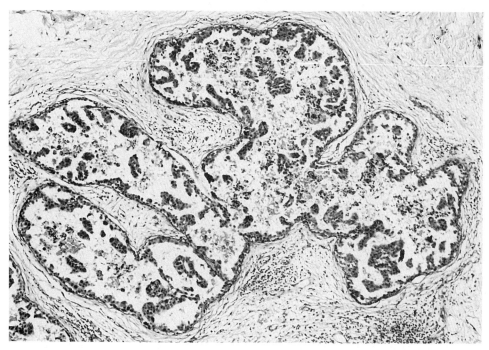

Fig. 12.7 This well-developed example of micropapillary carcinoma in situ is evidently present in an expanded lobular unit (× 75).

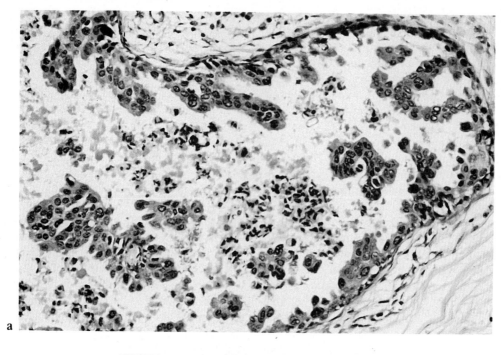

a

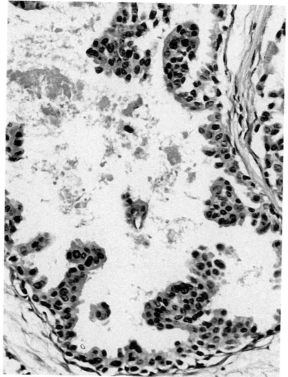

b

Fig. 12.8a, b Bulbous and non-attenuating fronds of hyperchromatic cells in micropapillary carcinoma in situ (**a, b** × 225).

Fig. 12.9 Clear cells similar to those of lobular carcinoma in situ do not detract from a diagnosis of micropapillary ductal carcinoma in situ because of the characteristic fronds of the latter diagnosis (× 225).

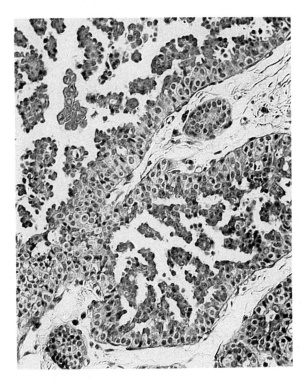

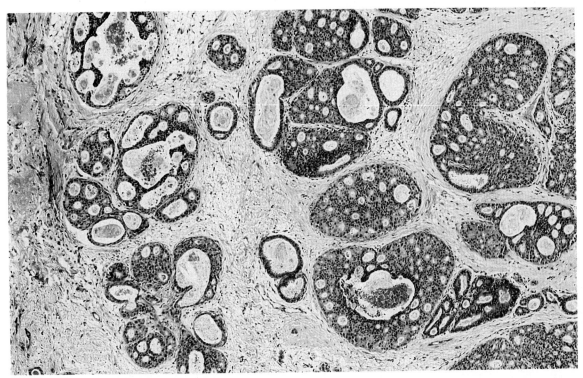

Fig. 12.10 Characteristic cribriform ductal carcinoma in situ fills many spaces. Occasional foci of central cell necrosis do not occasion a diagnosis of comedo carcinoma in situ (× 75).

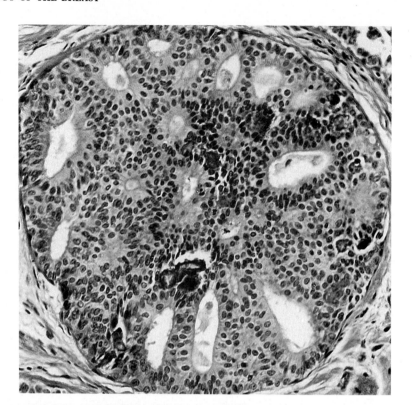

Fig. 12.11 Cribriform ductal carcinoma in situ with focal calcifications seen as dark intercellular concretions (× 225).

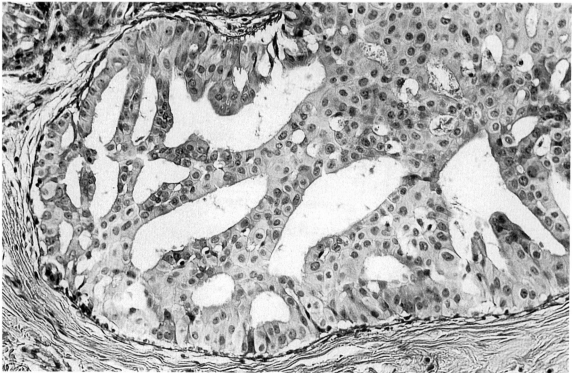

Fig. 12.12 The rigid arches of similar cells support a diagnosis of cribriform ductal carcinoma in situ. Note the apocrine appearance of the cells (× 225).

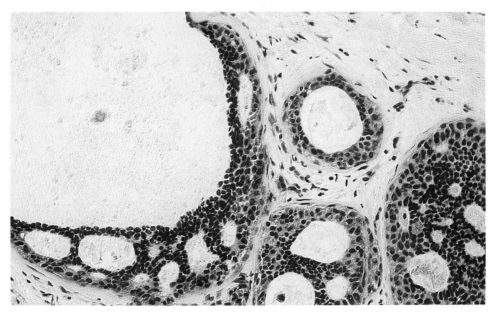

Fig. 12.13 These hyperchromatic cells may be recognized as part of a cribriform ductal carcinoma in situ because of non-tapering, rigid arches. Note some basalar cells differ slightly from more hyperchromatic and central cells. This feature suggests atypical ductal hyperplasia, but is insufficient to deny DCIS diagnosis (× 225).

Table 12.1 Histological criteria for cribriform and micropapillary carcinoma in situ (DCIS).

Uniform population of cells throughout entire area★

'Punched out', neatly rounded, geometric spaces or bulbous, well-defined, papillary fronds

Round, hyperchromatic, monotonous, randomly placed nuclei

Helpful: presence in many spaces (at least two)

Exception: nuclear atypia as seen in comedo throughout areas, while rare, establishes carcinoma in situ diagnosis without classic patterns or necrosis; cytoplasm often granular and eosinophilic

★Bounded by basement membrane.

chapter, often remain undiagnosed. This is a prime reason for our arbitrary, but helpful rule requiring that two spaces demonstrate all the diagnostic elements (Table 12.1). Confines of histologic definition are provided for rare, border-line lesions. Thus a consequence of requiring uniformity of both cell population and pattern is that extensive lesions will more often qualify as CIS than will those similar patterns found in fewer spaces. Examples of similar histological patterns

falling short of having each and every diagnostic feature of CIS and, therefore, diagnosable as atypical hyperplasia of ductal pattern (ADH) are exemplified in Figures 12.14–12.16. The debate in an individual borderline case between diagnoses of carcinoma in situ and atypical hyperplasia may be aided by reference to patterns presented in Figure 12.18. Following these rules, we, like Betsill et al (1978), find an incidence of micro-papillary and cribriform carcinoma in situ of about 0.25% in biopsies originally diagnosed as benign. The atypical ductal hyperplasia cases come largely from lesions which would otherwise (without recognizing an atypical category) be termed benign, but a few ADH cases are recruited from cases which would be recognized as DCIS without rigorous application of diagnostic criteria (Fig. 12.17).

Small clusters of necrotic cells may be seen in spaces involved by these types of carcinoma. However, if more than two or three spaces with necrosis are seen, and there is nuclear atypia of any degree, the diagnosis of comedo carcinoma should be considered. We designate some of these cases as ductal carcinoma in situ with comedo features;

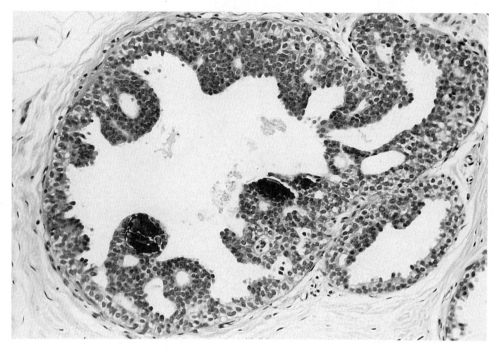

Fig. 12.14 This extremely atypical proliferative lesion lacks the uniformity of features diagnostic of ductal carcinoma in situ, and therefore is an example of atypical ductal hyperplasia. Note epithelium along wall of primary space with normal polarity focally. Compare to Figures 12.9 and 12.13 (× 200).

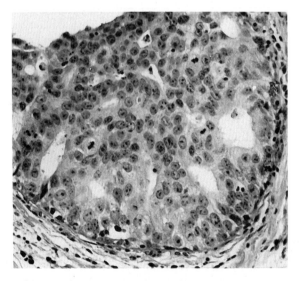

Fig. 12.15 Atypical ductal hyperplasia is diagnosed rather than ductal carcinoma in situ because of irregular placement of component cells, irregularity of spaces and lack of uniform cell population (× 330).

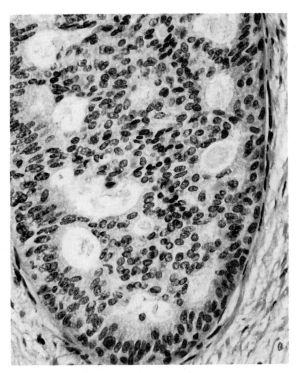

Fig. 12.16 Criteria for ductal carcinoma in situ are not attained in this example of atypical ductal hyperplasia because the bands of cells are often thinned or attenuated. Slight irregularities in cell placement and appearance are also seen (× 320).

defining extent and other pattern of disease in a commentary. Thus, reporting of these cases should include some indication of the extent of disease and, in the microscopically detected lesions, the extent of sampling utilized within the laboratory.

A histological variant of DCIS has been described in which a signet ring cytology (see Ch. 16) is found (Fisher & Brown 1985). These are often found in association with other forms of CIS, and any separate or distinct clinical implication is unknown.

Rosen & Scott (1984) have described an apparent histological variant of DCIS termed 'cystic hypersecretory duct carcinoma of the breast'. Two patients had concomitant invasive carcinoma and six patients had non-invasive lesions only. The lesions present multicystic foci containing secretory material and lined by an epithelium resembling micropapillary CIS with vacuolated cytoplasm (Fig. 12.19). Longer follow-up (longest was two years) and study of additional cases will be necessary to determine if this lesion has distinctive clinical characteristics.

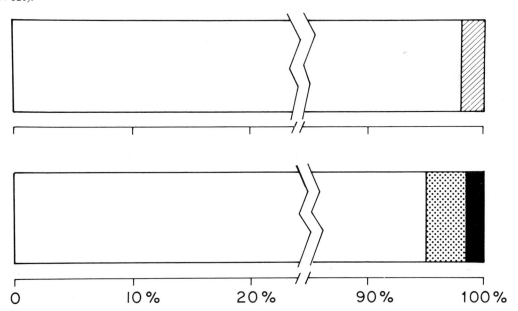

Fig. 12.17 Above, a dichotomous model applied to breast biopsies, either benign or in which a dominant mass is not produced by carcinoma in situ (CIS), shows a 2% incidence of CIS (dark band). In the lower graph, a diagnostic model accepting atypical hyperplasia (AH, ductal and lobular) shows a 3.5% incidence of AH (dotted band) and a 1.5% incidence of CIS (black band). Note, most cases of carcinoma in situ are lobular carcinoma in situ and that the remainder of the biopsies (clear bands) indicate subsequent risk of cancer of less than two times the general population. Thus the atypical cases are recruited from both the benign and CIS categories (from Page et al 1986 with permission of Saunders, Philadelphia).

Fig. 12.18 Architecture or pattern of the full series of hyperplastic lesions of usual, common or 'ductal' type: these secondary patterns of cell groupings are presented independently of cues of cytology and cell placement. Most of these patterns might be recognized as atypical if the cell population supported that diagnosis. However, in general those pattern cues presented here will be diagnosed as hyperplasia without atypia in examples 1 and 2 with escalating likelihood of atypia up to examples 15 and 16 which would be almost without exception diagnostic of ductal carcinoma in situ. Note also that cues of ductal or acinar size are removed in this distribution. In general, the mild hyperplasias are present in small spaces, and the remainder occur in expanded spaces.

Mild hyperplasia of usual type in patterns 1 and 2 have small mounds and tufts of cells. The projections of cells do not usually completely traverse the lumen. As with all other lesions of usual hyperplasia the nuclei will tend to be heterogeneously ovoid, and luminal borders irregularly ragged or ruffled, often by apocrine-like 'snouts'.

Moderate hyperplasia of usual type in patterns 3–6 have aggregates of cells occupying somewhat over 50% of the lumen. The bands of cells irregularly traverse the lumen. If thin cellular strands are present, the cells not only maintain the irregularity of shape and placement characteristic of benign hyperplasia, but the nuclei frequently are elongated, curved or fusiform. Pattern 6 overly dramatizes the attenuation of trabeculae which are a cue to benignancy. The trabeculae appear to have been stretched beyond their limits of elasticity leaving beaded, wisp-like tendrils, irregularly moth-eaten rather than regularly lace-like as in cribriform ductal carcinoma in situ.

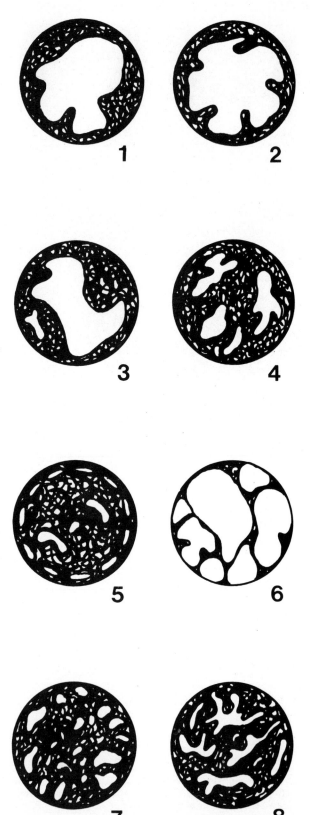

In florid hyperplasia of usual type (patterns 5–9 and 10) the component cells may virtually obliterate the primary lumen with secondary luminal structures frequently present as irregularly collapsed circles, slit-like structures at the edge of the primary lumen, or as unpredictably serpentine, maze-like passages. Increasing degrees of smoothness, regularity, and roundness progressively support the likelihood that these cellular patterns will support a diagnosis of atypia as seen in patterns 11–14. The extreme regularity and crispness of pattern definition of 15 and 16 will almost without exception be found diagnostic of ductal carcinoma in situ.

Atypical hyperplasia in this series takes many forms, usually with a few, smooth, crisp trabecular arcades or a solid focus of uniform cells in an otherwise typical hyperplastic lesion. If cytological features are reminiscent of ductal carcinoma in situ but histological pattern is intermediate between that of usual hyperplasia and ductal carcinoma in situ, the lesion is atypical.

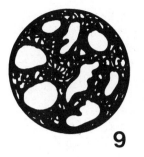

9

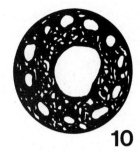

10

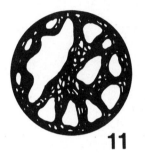

11

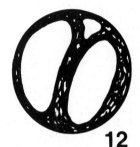

12

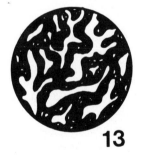

13

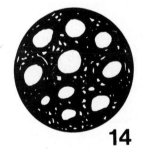

14

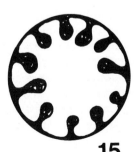

15

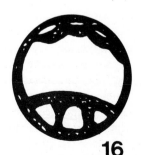

16

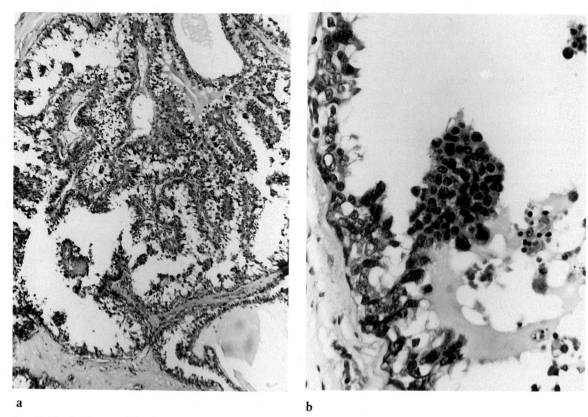

a   b

Fig. 12.19a, b These proliferative changes are atypical because of relatively uniform cytology and hyperchromasia as well as focal tendency to bulbous formations as in micropapillary carcinoma in situ. This pattern is similar to those which have been recognized as secretory ductal carcinoma, non-invasive. Note secretory features are mimicked (**a** × 75; **b** × 275).

The variety of hyperplastic patterns found in breasts is so diverse, that generally applicable rules of diagnosis will fail in the face of occasional unusual patterns. Page et al (1982) accepted two examples of non-comedo DCIS (28 total cases) which lacked papillary and cribriform features as well as the necrosis of comedo. These cases had advanced nuclear atypia as seen in comedo CIS. Note well: nuclear patterns seen in apocrine change with large nucleoli are not reason to establish a diagnosis of CIS (Fig. 12.20).

Any lesion of non-comedo DCIS must be considered as potentially having an invasive focus. The diagnosis of invasion is occasionally difficult, but is usually recognized only when the in situ disease is extensive. Rare examples of probable or possible microinvasion are confined to cases in which it is not clear whether uneven and irregularly spaced cell groups are within pre-existing units or outside the confines of parenchymal units.

Truly invasive foci most often have a slightly different cytology and pattern from the in situ disease, and are definitely within the supporting stroma and fat and outside the specialized connective tissue of lobular units.

Clinical and prognostic implications

As noted above, it is probable that more extensive examples of DCIS have greater invasive potential than more focal examples. We do know, however, that 25–30% of women with only microscopic foci will, if left untreated by other than biopsy, develop an invasive carcinoma within 15 years. These subsequent tumours will appear in the same place within the breast as the original lesions (Betsill et al 1978; Page et al 1982). This represents a magnitude of risk elevation of 10–11 times the general population matched for age. The risk is undoubtedly higher for larger and palpable

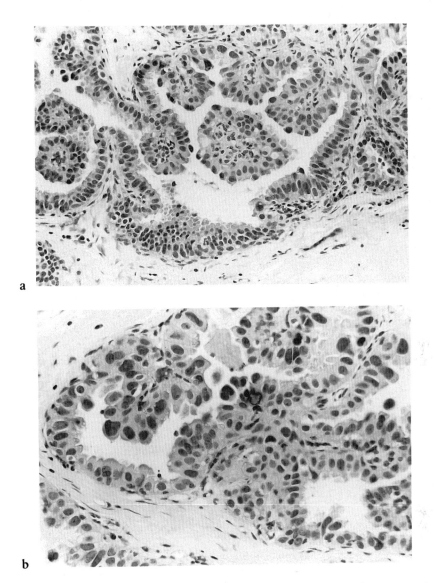

a

b

Fig. 12.20a, b Very rarely, lobular units with cytology suggestive of apocrine type will have foci with greatly enlarged and hyperchromatic nuclei without much internal detail. Although unusual, the foci cannot be recognized as atypical in the sense of indicating heightened risk of subsequent carcinoma development at this time (**a** × 200; **b** × 250).

examples of DCIS treated by excisional biopsy alone. The risk of contralateral breast cancer after DCIS may not be different from that of the general population (Webber et al 1981).

Death from carcinoma in situ of any type treated by mastectomy without invasive carcinoma identified in the mastectomy specimen or lymph nodes is not recorded (Brown et al 1976). Note is made of two unique cases in the literature, each palpable and of comedo DCIS type, in which radiation therapy for DCIS was followed by metastases and death of the patient (Wulsin & Schreiber 1962; Millis & Thynne 1975). This provides further evidence for separately recording the different types of CIS. Likelihood of recurrence (usually non-invasive disease) following planned local excision of these lesions is more common if they exceed 2 cm in diameter (Lagios et al 1982, 1986). These follow-up studies provide strong evidence that the extent of DCIS is a prime determinant of local recurrence after excision, and that smaller lesions are amenable to conservative therapy. The regular monofocality of DCIS is also supported by the observations of this group (Lagios et al 1986) because recurrences have all been in the same quadrant as the original lesion. This reinforces the need for recording type and extent of disease. A randomized clinical trial assessing local excision of DCIS with and without radiotherapy is in progress (Fisher et al 1986).

An understanding of CIS is fostered by recognizing histological patterns similar to, but falling short of, diagnostic CIS. The category of atypical ductal hyperplasia (ADH) provides confines of definition to DCIS as well as a useful diagnostic category for cases otherwise recognized as borderline. ADH carries clinical implications of increased cancer risk after biopsy of about four to five times that of the general population matched for age (see Ch. 11). The category is also useful in that the term 'cancer' is avoided for a finding which elevates risk of invasive cancer to less than one-half that of DCIS. This is a histologically and clinically satisfactory resting place for cases difficult to call 'benign' or 'malignant'; they are clearly neither, but are truly borderline (Page 1986). The diagnosis of ADH should be reserved for a small number of cases, just over 1% of biopsies in our experience.

LOBULAR CARCINOMA IN SITU

Historical development

Lobular carcinoma in situ (LCIS) was first described and named by Foote & Stewart (1941). This designation for the change is still preferred by most histopathologists. The term intra-acinous carcinoma suggested by Muir in the same year (1941) is no longer used, and probably included examples of other types of carcinoma in situ. Many studies have followed the initial description, and there is now general agreement that LCIS signifies a degree of multifocality and bilaterality greater than that identified by any other diagnosis of malignancy in the breast.

The year 1978 was important in the development of knowledge concerning LCIS. Two institutions recorded their experience with extended follow-up information on patients after treatment by biopsy only (Haagensen et al 1978; Rosen et al 1978). Despite the use of slightly different terminology and a disagreement regarding therapy, it is quite clear that these two groups are in substantial agreement about when to record a diagnosis of lobular carcinoma in situ (which Haagensen et al 1978 preferred to call lobular neoplasia) and in complete agreement as to what this means for a woman with such a change identified at biopsy.

Although there continues to be controversy over terminology and diagnostic criteria (Andersen et al 1980) there is general agreement about implications of increased cancer risk associated with LCIS. The term 'lobular neoplasia' may be used synonymously, primarily to avoid the term 'carcinoma' but we prefer the term LCIS largely because it has been used in most publications. We do diagnose 'atypical lobular hyperplasia' (ALH) in related lesions of lesser severity (see Ch. 11), and do use the term 'lobular neoplasia' to denote the full spectrum of LCIS and ALH. However, we do not use 'lobular neoplasia' as a diagnostic term in clinical reports.

Anatomical pathology

LCIS is not palpable in tissue and is invisible to the naked eye.

Histologically, a group or cluster of ductules (lobular unit) is filled by cells demonstrating a lack of regular cohesion or orientation (Figs 12.21–12.25). The nuclei are rounded for the most part, or at least oval, usually without hyperchromatism. The cytoplasm tends to be somewhat clear. A remarkable similarity in cellular appearance and placement with regard to each other is important in recognition of LCIS. Distension and distortion of the involved spaces completes the histological definition of LCIS.

The presence of clear vacuoles in the cytoplasm is a helpful marker for LCIS as they are frequently present (Andersen & Vendelboe 1981). These crisp spaces are clear with haematoxylin and eosin, but stain with Alcian blue and/or PAS (see 'Invasive lobular carcinoma', Ch. 13). These 'intracytoplasmic' lumina are often subtle, but may be prominent (Fig. 12.26).

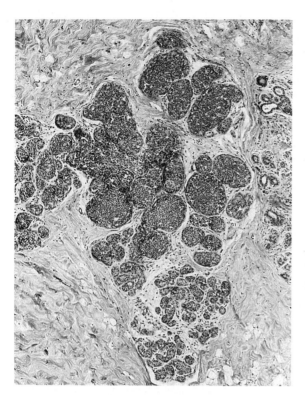

Fig. 12.21 Lobular carcinoma in situ with both extreme (central) and mild (at left and below) distension of acinar elements. Changes are not diagnostic in the lobular unit at left; however, the case is recorded as lobular carcinoma in situ because criteria for lobular carcinoma are met in centre of picture (× 50).

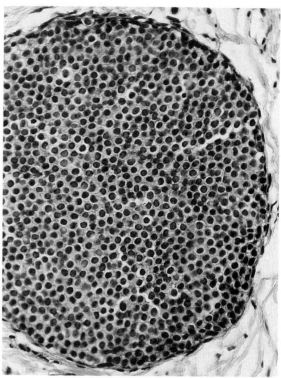

Fig. 12.22 Extreme distension of acinus in advanced and classical example of lobular carcinoma in situ. Note regularity of cytology and cell placement (× 320).

Multicentricity is a prime feature of LCIS with many cases having the disease demonstrable by biopsy in the contralateral breast at time of initial diagnosis (Rosen et al 1981). LCIS is not evenly distributed among the mammary quadrants, but appears to follow the distribution of parenchymal elements, favouring the central region beneath the nipple and the upper, outer quadrant (Lambird & Shelley 1969).

Differential diagnosis

A 'classic' case of LCIS would, then, contain similar cells throughout each involved and distorted space. As lesser examples of this 'full-blown' phenomenon are encountered, the designation atypical lobular hyperplasia (ALH) is appropriate (see Ch. 11). The presence of apparent spaces separating the cells, so that one may not say the units are 'full' will support a designation of atypical lobular hyperplasia rather than LCIS. Furthermore, the lack of apparent distension of the involved spaces as well as the intermixture of other cell types would support a diagnosis of ALH.

Consistency in diagnosis of LCIS is fostered by requiring that each of the following criteria be fulfilled:

1. The characteristic and uniform cells must comprise the entire population of cells in a lobular unit.

2. There must be filling (no interspersed, intercellular spaces between cells) of all the acini (terminal ductules).

3. There must be expansion and/or distortion of at least one-half the acini in the lobular unit.

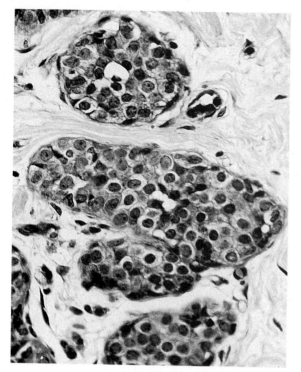

Fig. 12.23 Example of somewhat greater cytological pleomorphism in lobular carcinoma in situ than seen in Figure 12.22 (× 450).

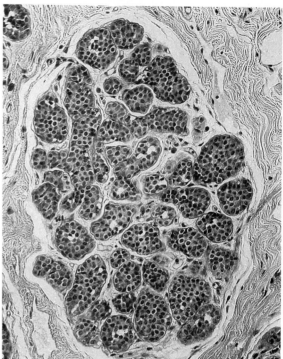

Fig. 12.24 Criteria for lobular carcinoma in situ of cell population and distortion of at least 50% of acini are met in this lobular unit (× 160).

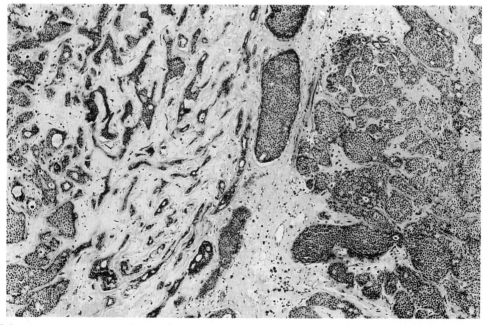

Fig. 12.25 Involvement of sclerosed lobular units by lobular carcinoma in situ may present difficulties and uncertainty in diagnosis. This example should be accepted as lobular carcinoma in situ because distension, etc., are well developed at periphery at left and at right (× 50) (Courtesy of R. Fechner.)

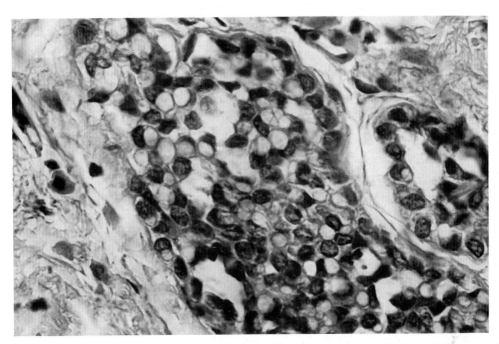

Fig. 12.26 Rarely, cases of lobular carcinoma in situ may have pronounced cytoplasm vacuolization, which are cytoplasmic lumina (× 600).

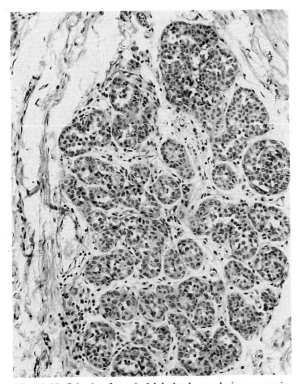

Fig. 12.27 Criteria of atypical lobular hyperplasia are met in this lobular unit, falling short of lobular carcinoma in situ (× 125).

We have found that observers in our laboratories will agree over 95% of the time on the diagnosis of LCIS when these rules are followed. Lesser degrees of involvement are diagnosed as atypical lobular hyperplasia (ALH, see Ch. 11), a diagnosis carrying a lesser risk of subsequent carcinoma. Illustrations of ALH are found in Figures 12.27–12.29.

We agree with McDivitt et al (1968) that focal involvement of ducts by cells of lobular neoplasia (see below) is an important warning sign for the presence of LCIS or ALH, but that establishment of the diagnosis must rest upon characteristic patterns within lobular units. This change in ducts related to ALH and LCIS has been called 'pagetoid' (Foote & Stewart 1941). Here, cells cytologically similar or identical to those seen in clusters of acini are found in single spaces which probably represent ducts (Figs 12.30–12.32). There is a marked tendency for these cells to present in groups immediately above the basement membrane, displacing or pushing toward the lumen another population of cells which are clearly different (Fechner 1972). This pagetoid pattern is often found in cases of LCIS and its

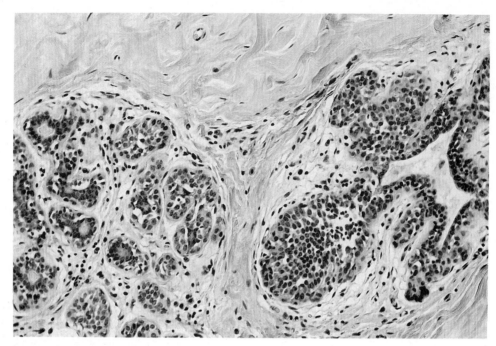

Fig. 12.28 Mild example of atypical lobular hyperplasia recognized by clusters of characteristic cells in acini at left centre. Compare to uninvolved acini at left periphery of photograph. Diagnostic certainty is fostered by presence of similar cells in duct at right ('pagetoid' spread) (× 200).

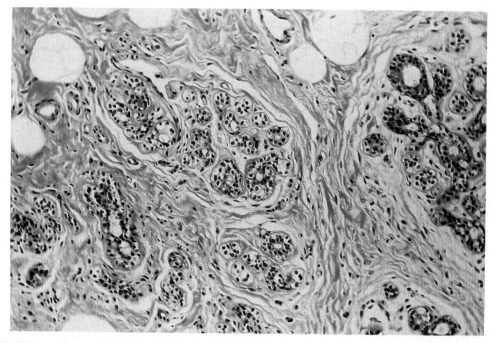

Fig. 12.29 Mimicry of atypical lobular hyperplasia is produced by loss of cellular polarity. This is not diagnosable as atypical lobular hyperplasia because increased cell numbers (more than two above basement membrane) are not reliably discerned (× 200).

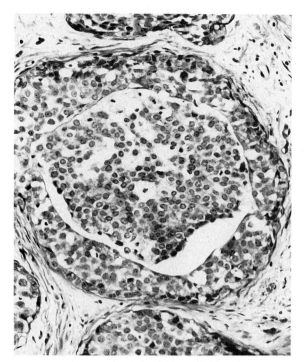

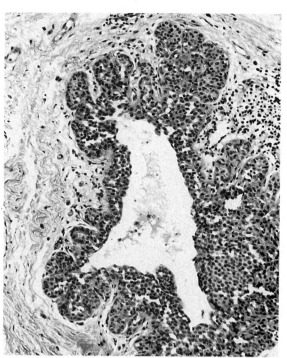

Fig. 12.30 Pagetoid spread of LCIS into duct at centre is an extreme 'mural' pattern approaching a solid pattern. Note thinned, strand-like remnants of ductal luminal epithelium (× 150).

Fig. 12.31 Duct with involvement by cells of atypical lobular hyperplasia showing the so-called 'cloverleaf' pattern (× 125).

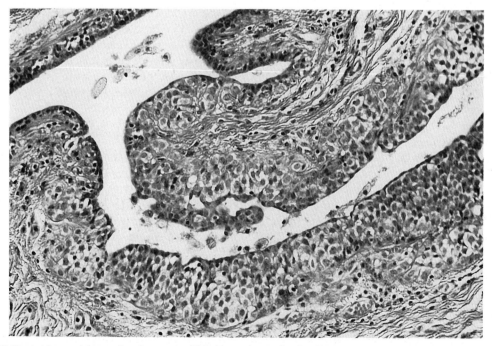

Fig. 12.32 Pagetoid spread into a duct in a case of lobular carcinoma in situ. Note flattened overlying luminal cells. Central cell mass is result of a fold in duct wall (× 225).

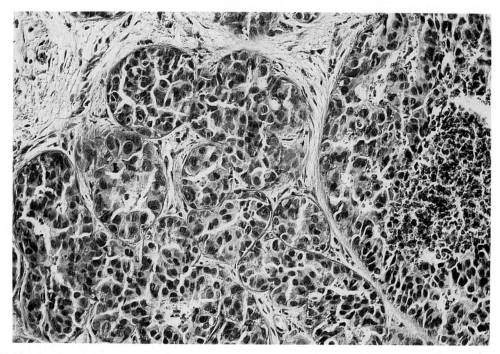

Fig. 12.33 Non-invasive carcinoma expands the acini of a lobular unit at left. The pleomorphism of cells and cytological similarity to comedo carcinoma in situ at right remove this lesion from the lobular carcinoma in situ group (× 225).

identification in a case without evident LCIS should indicate a careful search for diagnostic changes of LCIS or ALH elsewhere in the breast (Wheeler & Enterline 1976). Ductal involvement by cells of LCIS is both more frequent and usually more extensive than that of ductal involvement by cells of ALH. Note that the diagnosis of LCIS or ALH rests in the patterns found in lobular units. Occasionally cells with clear cytoplasm probably representing macrophages may mimic ductal involvement by cells of lobular neoplasia.

Another histological pattern which may be confused with lobular carcinoma in situ (see 'Comedo CIS, differential diagnosis') is one presenting involvement of lobular units by carcinoma in situ of 'ductal' type (Fig. 12.33–12.37). It is in such cases that the histopathologist may need to look to other areas to make a diagnosis by finding areas with more classic appearances. This does not deny the occasional necessity of diagnosing carcinoma in situ or atypical hyperplasia of both lobular and ductal type.

Lobular carcinoma in situ may present within fibroadenomas, and represents the most common

malignancy to be discovered in this manner. 65% of the 62 cases of cancer in fibroadenoma have been LCIS (Pick & Iossifides 1984). Although extent of disease as related to lobular unit involvement may not be available to the microscopist, extensiveness of involvement by characteristic cells usually facilitates diagnosis.

Clinical features and prognosis

The clinical implications of a diagnosis of lobular carcinoma in situ are derived from studies of the pathological content of breasts removed following the diagnosis as well as from studies of women followed after biopsy only. Careful examination of mastectomy specimens occasioned by the diagnosis of lobular carcinoma in situ at biopsy will usually reveal multifocal lobular carcinoma in situ, approximately 80% of which will appear in breast quadrants other than that in which lobular carcinoma was identified at time of biopsy. Approximately 6% of these breasts removed within several months following recognition of LCIS on biopsy will reveal invasive carcinoma (Carter & Smith

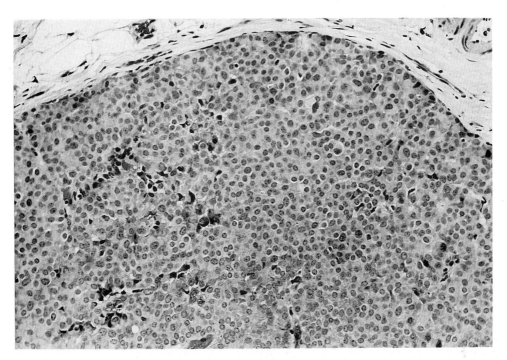

Fig. 12.34 This large space is involved by cells of the type seen in lobular neoplasia thus providing mixed cues for subcategorizing the type of CIS. The tendency to rounded, gland-like or rosette-like formation favours DCIS (× 200).

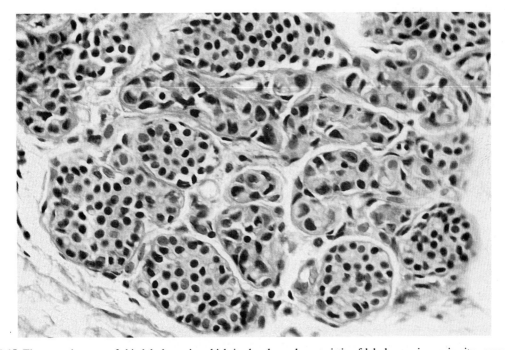

Fig. 12.35 The central spaces of this lobular unit, which is elsewhere characteristic of lobular carcinoma in situ, present a somewhat pleomorphic population of cells more reminiscent of ductal carcinoma in situ. A diagnosis of combined ductal carcinoma in situ and lobular carcinoma in situ should be considered (× 450).

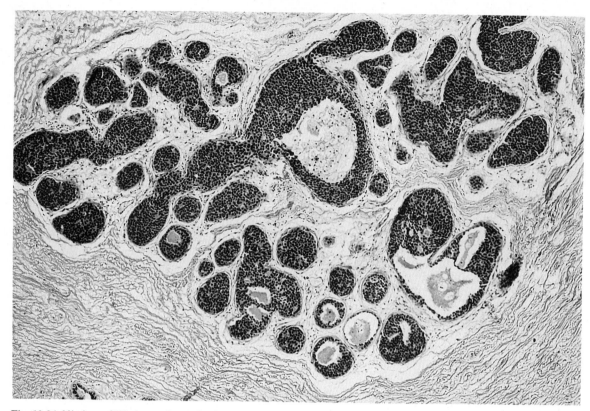

Fig. 12.36 Mimicry of lobular carcinoma in situ by the largely solid aggregates of cells in this cribriform ductal carcinoma in situ is evident in this lobular unit. Note tendency to formation of spaces and arches (× 75).

1977; Rosen et al 1979a, 1979b).

Follow-up of women not having mastectomy following biopsy recognition of lobular carcinoma in situ reveals that 20–30% of these women will develop invasive mammary carcinoma in the ensuing 15–20 years (Haagensen et al 1978; Rosen et al 1978) and that the incidence of carcinoma will be evenly distributed throughout the intervening years (Table 12.2). The most disturbing fact with regard to therapy is that almost 50% of these invasive carcinomas will occur in the breast opposite from that presenting with the lobular carcinoma in situ. Evidently LCIS is more of a marker for breast cancer risk than a direct precursor.

It is obvious that none of the several alternative choices for therapy is entirely satisfactory and that there is room for a considerable amount of clinical judgement and individual patient preference in decision-making. The therapeutic dilemma

Table 12.2 Features of lobular caricinoma in situ.

Anatomical (all recognized by Foote & Stewart 1941)
  Inconspicuous character on gross examination
  Characteristic occurrence in lobular units
  Multicentricity
  'Pagetoid' extension into larger ducts
  Association with a distinctive type of diffusely infiltrative
    carcinoma with similar cells
  Cytoplasmic mucoid globules/vacuole
  Coexistence with other forms of infiltrating cancer

Clinical
  Incidence varies — around 1% of breast biopsies
  No clinical or anatomical correlates aid in identifying
    women with LCIS
  Subsequent invasive carcinoma after biopsy only (follow-up
    period of 15 years): 15–20% in ipsilateral breast and
    10–15% in contralateral breast

associated with the diagnosis of LCIS can best be understood by considering the variety of therapeutic approaches currently recommended. The general practice at some institutions is to follow

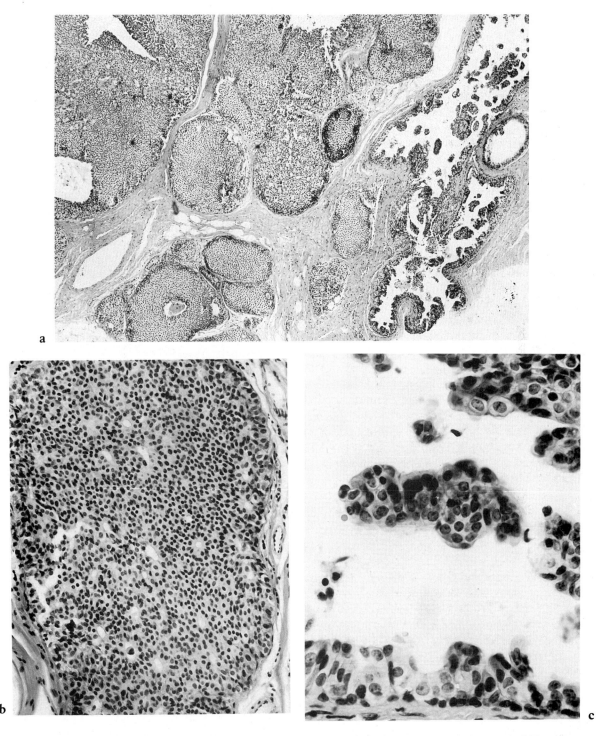

Fig. 12.37a–c These photographs from adjacent fields of a case of non-comedo ductal carcinoma in situ have variable patterns which may confound attempts at specific diagnosis. The micropapillary and cribriform patterns predominate. More solid aggregates mimic lobular carcinoma in situ at low power (**a**), but are found to contain small spaces at high power (**b**). The micropapillary pattern at high power includes a two-cell population of compact and clear cells (**c**), but each are characteristic of carcinoma in situ (**a** × 50; **b** × 150; **c** × 450).

women with this diagnosis carefully, in the belief that the great majority will be cured by treatment after clinical detection of invasive carcinoma (Haagensen et al 1978). At another institution it is felt that the recommendation for follow-up without further surgery should be considered an investigative procedure and the recommendation for the conservative approach should be made only if the patient and physician are prepared to accept the responsibility of lifetime surveillance (Rosen et al 1978). That institution considered it prudent in most cases to recommend ipsilateral mastectomy with low axillary dissection and concurrent biopsy of the opposite breast (Rosen et al 1981). This approach appears to have lowered the incidence of subsequent cancer as compared to follow-up without further surgery. We can only conclude that at this time several approaches are used in the clinical management of LCIS.

The special situation of LCIS presenting in a fibroadenoma is so rare, that prognostication is less certain than when LCIS occurs in breast parenchyma. However, there is evidence that LCIS in fibroadenoma should be regarded as having similar implications as the more common presentation (Fondo et al 1979). Note that the age incidence of LCIS in fibroadenoma approximates that of LCIS (Rosner et al 1980) (peaking in the fifth decade) and not the younger ages of fibroadenoma (Pick & Iossifides 1984).

PAGET'S DISEASE OF THE NIPPLE

Terminology

Paget's disease of the nipple is diagnosed when a patient presents with an eczematous lesion of the nipple which histologically demonstrates carcinoma cells in nipple epidermis. This term should not be viewed as a special type of breast cancer as it merely represents a phenomenon noted clinically when intraductal carcinoma reaches the nipple surface. This point is further strengthened by the fact that this pattern of disease in the nipple may or may not be attended by invasive cancer within the breast — a variability rendering prognostic implications almost invalid. The presence of Paget's disease of the nipple means that there is an in situ carcinoma present, at least of

the immediate nipple area. Mandatory assessment of the extent of disease may reveal extensive in situ carcinoma in the underlying breast and, quite possibly, invasive carcinoma as well.

Anatomical pathology

The histological diagnosis of Paget's disease of the breast is based upon the demonstration of carcinoma cells of adenocarcinoma type within the epidermis of the nipple. In its usual form, large cells with clear cytoplasm are intermixed both singly and in groups within the epidermis. This discrete placement of the so-called Paget's cells among epidermal cells of the nipple is the histological hallmark of this diagnosis (Fig. 12.38). Paget's disease of the nipple is also diagnosed when cells lacking clear and sharply defined cyto-

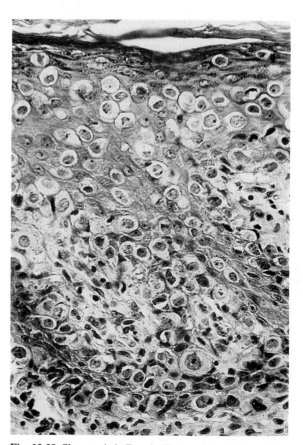

Fig. 12.38 Characteristic Paget's disease of the nipple. Note the crisp separation of enlarged, atypical cells from keratinocytes (× 320).

plasm tend to replace large areas of the epidermis (Fig. 12.39). In this latter situation the intra-epidermal collections of Paget's cells assume solid island-like or glandular configurations more closely mimicking patterns seen in the usual type of infiltrating mammary carcinoma.

Special stains for mucins are of use in this diagnosis as positive reactions are often, although not invariably, present in cytoplasm of Paget's cells. Alcian blue, PAS after diastase, muci-carmine and aldehyde fuchsin may all be of use. The Paget cells usually lack glycogen.

Differential diagnosis

Other conditions may mimic Paget's disease histo-logically with clear cells within the epidermis. Of little problem is the occasional presence of epidermal cells with clear cytoplasm (Fig. 12.40). Whether this picture represents a fixation artefact or some other phenomenon is not clear. However, these epidermal clear cells are easily differentiated from Paget's disease because the epidermal cells maintain their relationship to other epidermal cells and have similar nuclei to other epidermal cells. Occasional cells with clear cytoplasm in normal nipples did have altered local relationships (Toker 1970), but these cells were negative for mucin. Intraepidermal squamous dysplasia or carcinoma in situ and intraepidermal melanoma will present obvious problems in diagnosis. Fortunately, both conditions are very rare in the nipple. Paget's disease will present atypical cells interspersed between normal epidermal cells, while epidermal atypias will present no sharp demarcation from normal epidermal cells. Intraepidermal melanoma usually disturbs the epidermal cells less than Paget's cells. Note that melanin may be found in Paget's cells (Azzopardi & Eusebi 1977).

Recourse to mucin stains (see above) to mark Paget's cells will resolve most differential diag-nostic situations. Immunocytochemical stains for

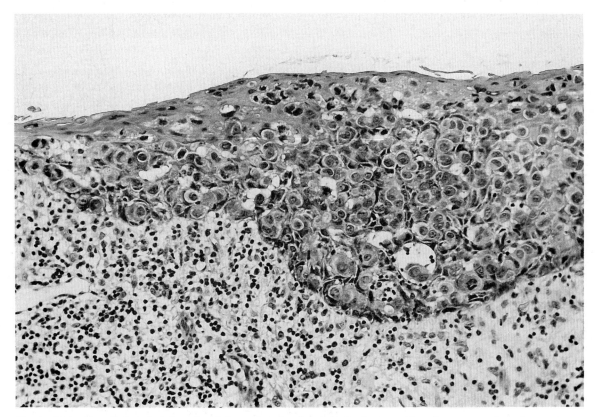

Fig. 12.39 Paget's cells have largely replaced the epidermal cells of nipple. Attenuated keratinocytes are almost inapparent between Paget's cells centrally, and are present as a pure population at far right (× 250).

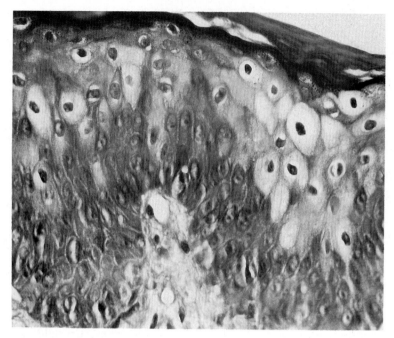

Fig. 12.40 Nipple epidermis with clear cytoplasm seen in occasional keratinocytes. Note that this appearance is easily distinguished from Paget's disease (× 400).

markers of melanoma and glandular cells may be necessary (Vanstapel et al 1984).

Clinical and prognostic implications

Clinically, Paget's disease presents as a reddened, eczematous area on the nipple. It is not merely keratotic or irregular, but presents as a moist area. The clinical suspicion of Paget's disease when followed by histological confirmation of the diagnosis necessitates a search for an underlying mammary carcinoma. This may be found confined to ducts or may have an invasive component (Ashikari et al 1970). Virtually all patients with palpable masses will have invasive disease, and somewhat less than one-half without masses will have invasive disease in the breast (Chaudary et al 1986). Prognosis depends upon the extent of tumour within the breast (Salvadori et al 1976). Thus, failure to find an invasive focus carries only the implications of carcinoma in situ. Rarely will an excisional biopsy of the nipple lesion be followed by an inability to demonstrate carcinoma within the underlying breast. Only 2/35 examples of Paget's disease in one series had only in situ

disease confined to the region of the nipple (Chaudary et al 1986). The association of Paget's disease with underlying mammary carcinoma is so complete, that in this situation one must assume that a small focus of intraductal carcinoma was confined to the area of ducts immediately under the nipple. Extensive and often multifocal intraductal carcinoma is found in the majority of cases including those with an infiltrating component.

NON-INVASIVE PAPILLARY CARCINOMA

Background

The understanding of malignant papillary lesions in the breast has long been confused because the term 'papillary' has been used for lesions of different pattern and prognosis. As a consequence, and because of recent studies clarifying this issue, we do not use the term unless further defined for clarification, i.e. invasive or non-invasive. The most frequent lesion indicated by the term *papillary carcinoma*, not further specified, had the underlying fibrovascular branching structure of a papilloma with epithelial atypia of several types. The classic paper of Kraus & Neubecker (1962), as well as other works, utilizes the term 'papillary carcinoma', not further specified, to include the micropapillary and cribriform patterns of ductal carcinoma in situ. While this is most comprehensible considering the frequent concurrent appearance of these lesions, their varied clinical presentation and prognostic implications merit separate distinction of the different patterns. Kraus & Neubecker (1962), furthermore, included foci of invasion and adjacent ductal carcinoma beyond the confines of the lesion in their list of diagnostic criteria, and did not separately identify patients with and without these features in their follow-up data.

Particularly because it gives specific confines of histopathological definition, and follow-up after local excision alone, the study of Carter et al (1983) has led the way in subclassifying non-invasive papillary carcinomas. They have demonstrated that the presence of carcinoma in situ in breast beyond the delimited papillary lesion has prognostic importance.

Anatomical pathology

Non-invasive papillary carcinomas have the fundamental structure of a papilloma, with sufficiently atypical epithelium surmounting the branched, fibrous tissue to qualify as carcinoma in situ. In one variety, elongated cells with spindle-shaped, hyperchromatic, usually monomorphic nuclei are closely packed, perpendicular to the fibrous papillary stalks (Figs 12.41 and 12.42). In other examples, patterns of cribriform ductal carcinoma in situ are seen in collections of cells between the fibrovascular fronds (Figs 12.43–12.45). Still further examples are as heterogeneous as the series of atypical ductal hyperplasia and ductal carcinoma in situ, but must have at least some areas diagnostic of CIS (see Table 12.1).

Grossly, these cases are usually well delimited from surrounding breast by an only slightly irregular fibrous covering (Figs 12.46–12.48). Thus, they may be said to be 'encysted', and that term may be added for diagnostic clarity. However, other patterns of carcinoma may be cystic (see Ch. 16). Despite the use of 'encysted',

internally there often is no fluid-containing space, and tightly packed epithelium and fronds of fibrous tissue fill the centre. Diameter at time of detection is most frequently 1–3 cm. Consistency is often soft, but will vary with the relative amount of firm connective tissue.

Careful sampling of the lesion and adjacent tissue is mandatory, because diagnostic areas of CIS as well as invasive carcinoma may be focal (see Ch. 10, 'Clinical implication'). A difficult diagnostic problem is presented when epithelium is within the outer, delimiting wall. It is most often enclosed epithelium of the in situ carcinoma within, and is not invasive carcinoma (Fig. 12.48).

Note that complex sclerosing lesions (CSL; Ch. 9) may have papillary foci (Fenoglio & Lattes 1974) and areas of pseudoinvasion into scar-like tissue. These latter lesions represent the most important differential diagnostic consideration for encysted, papillary carcinoma (Ch. 15) along with papilloma (Ch. 10). However, most CSLs do not have an outer fibrous sheath or cyst wall which probably represents a dilated duct (Carter et al 1983).

Clinical correlations and implications

The best information available concerning the clinical aspects of these papillary lesions comes from the work of Carter et al (1983). They reported 29 women who underwent mastectomy for these intracystic papillary lesions, and none developed metastases concurrently or in an average follow-up of five years. Eleven other women had local excision only, eight of whom had no ductal carcinoma in situ (DCIS) adjacent to the mass lesion and had no recurrence in follow-up averaging 10 years. The three patients experiencing recurrence of carcinoma (two invasive, one persistent DCIS) all had DCIS extending beyond the cyst into small and medium-sized ducts at initial treatment. Overall, 41% of their cases had extension of non-invasive carcinoma beyond the cyst. Therefore, careful evaluation of such lesions for associated foci of carcinoma in situ or invasive) adjacent to the dominant mass are mandatory. If such areas are lacking, local excision may be expected to be curative, but obviously must include sufficient surrounding tissue for evaluation of the presence of DCIS.

Fig. 12.41 Papillary fronds are covered by hyperchromatic, elongated cells in this non-invasive papillary carcinoma (× 150).

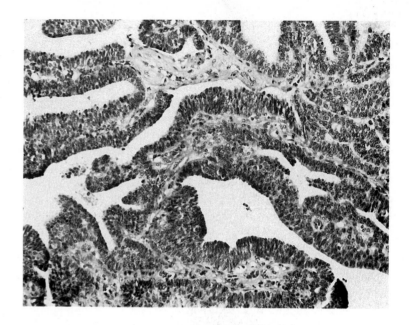

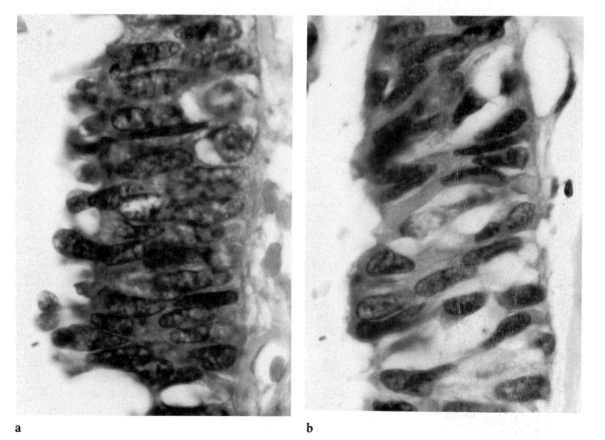

a

b

Fig. 12.42a, b Elongated, hyperchromatic nuclei, arrayed perpendicular to the stromal core of a papillary frond, characterize one pattern of non-invasive papillary carcinoma (**a,b** × 750).

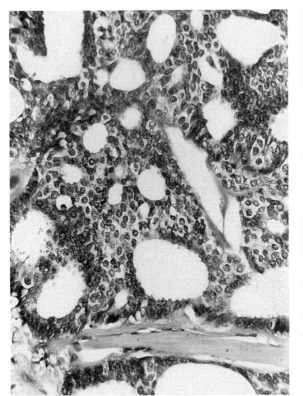

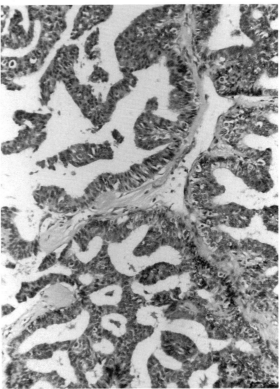

Fig. 12.43 Rigid, smooth patterns of cribriform carcinoma in situ are seen in a central area of a non-invasive papillary carcinoma (× 225).

Fig. 12.44 Central portion of a non-invasive papillary carcinoma. Note projecting, hyperchromatic cells forming cribriform and micropapillary patterns (× 150).

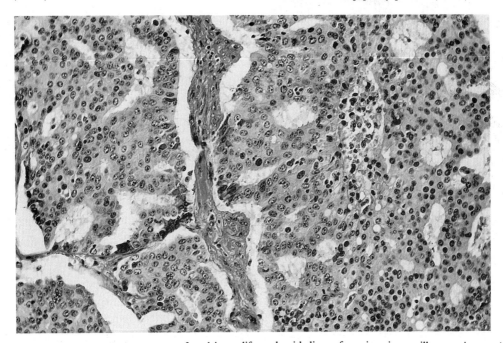

Fig. 12.45 Many varieties of cell placement are found in proliferated epithelium of non-invasive papillary carcinomas (× 200).

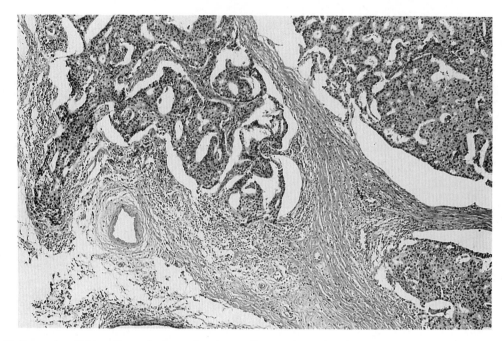

Fig. 12.46 Outer edge of this well-contained, non-invasive papillary carcinoma is at lower left, with evident irregularity (× 75).

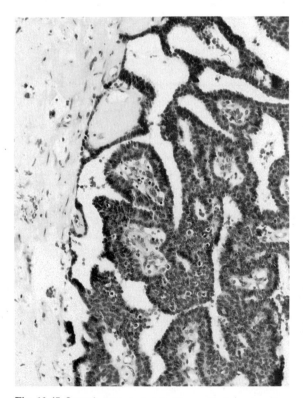

Fig. 12.47 Smooth outer and delimiting wall of non-invasive papillary cancer is at left (× 100).

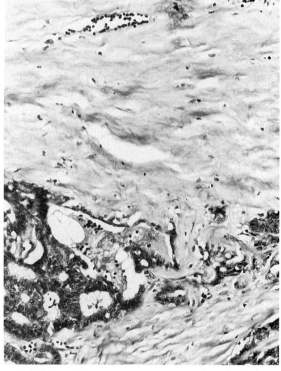

Fig. 12.48 Outer fibrous wall of a non-invasive papillary carcinoma has included epithelium. This does not represent invasive carcinoma (× 100).

REFERENCES

Andersen J A 1974 Lobular carcinoma in situ. A long-term follow-up in 52 cases. Acta Pathol Microbiol Scand (A) 82: 519–533

Andersen J A, Vendelboe M L 1981 Cytoplasmic mucous globules in lobular carcinoma in situ. Am J Surg Pathol 5: 251–255

Andersen J A, Fechner R E, Lattes R, Rosen P P, Toker C 1980 Lobular carcinoma in situ: (Lobular neoplasia) of the breast (a symposium). Pathol Annu 14(2): 193–223

Ashikari R, Park K, Huvos A G, Urban J A 1970 Paget's disease of the breast. Cancer 26: 680–685

Ashikari R, Hajdu S I, Robbins G F 1971 Intraductal carcinoma of the breast (1960–1969). Cancer 28: 1182–1187

Azzopardi J 1979 Problems in breast pathology. Saunders, Philadelphia p. 128–146, 192–233, 266–273

Azzopardi J G, Eusebi V 1977 Melanocyte colonisation and pigmentation of breast carcinoma. Histopathology 1: 21–30

Betsill W L Jr, Rosen P P, Lieberman P H, Robbins G F 1978 Intraductal carcinoma. Long-term follow-up after treatment by biopsy alone. J A M A 239: 1863–1867

Brown P W, Silverman J, Owens E, Tabor D C, Terz J J, Lawrence W J 1976 Intraductal 'non-infiltrating' carcinoma of the breast. Arch Surg 111: 1063–1067

Carter D, Smith R R L 1977 Carcinoma in situ of the breast. Cancer 40: 1189–1193

Carter D, Orr S L, Merino M J 1983 Intracystic papillary carcinoma of the breast. After mastectomy, radiotherapy or excisional biopsy alone. Cancer 52: 14–19

Chaudary M A, Millis R R, Lane E B, Miller N A 1986 Paget's disease of the nipple: a ten year review including clinical, pathological, and immuno-histochemical findings. Breast Cancer Res Treat 8: 139–146

Contesso G, Petit J Y 1979 Les adenocarcinomes intracanalaires non infiltrants du sein. Bull Cancer (Paris) 66: 1–8

Cross A S, Azzopardi J G, Krausz T, van Noorden S, Polak J M 1985 A morphological and immunocytochemical study of a distinctive variant of ductal carcinoma in situ of the breast. Histopathology 9: 21–37

Fechner R E 1971 Ductal carcinoma involving the lobule of the breast. Cancer 28: 274–281

Fechner R E 1972 Epithelial alterations in the extralobular ducts of breasts with lobular carcinoma. Arch Pathol 93: 164–171

Fenoglio C, Lattes R 1974 Sclerosing papillary proliferations in the female breast. A benign lesion often mistaken for carcinoma. Cancer 33: 691–700

Fisher E R, Brown R 1985 Intraductal signet ring carcinoma: a hitherto undescribed form of intraductal carcinoma of the breast. Cancer 55: 2533–2537

Fisher E R, Sass R, Fisher B et al 1986 Pathologic findings from the national surgical adjuvant breast project (protocol no 6). I. Intraductal carcinoma (DCIS). Cancer 57: 197–208

Fondo E Y, Rosen P P, Fracchia A A, Urban J A 1979 The problem of carcinoma developing in a fibroadenoma: recent experience at Memorial Hospital. Cancer 43: 563–567

Foote F W, Stewart F W 1941 Lobular carcinoma in situ. Am J Pathol 17: 491–495

Geschickter C F 1943 Diseases of the breast. Lippincott, Philadelphia, p. 502–507

Gillis D A, Dockerty M B, Clagett O T 1960 Pre-invasive intraductal carcinoma of the breast. Surg Gynecol Obstet 110: 555–562

Haagensen C D, Lane N, Lattes R, Bodian C 1978 Lobular neoplasia (so-called lobular carcinoma in situ) of the breast. Cancer 42: 737–769

Kraus F T, Neubecker R D 1962 The differential diagnosis of papillary tumours of the breast. Cancer 15: 444–455

Lagios M 1986 Biology of duct carcinoma in situ of limited extent. Prospective study of patients treated by tylectomy. Lab Invest 54:34A

Lagios M D, Westdahl P R, Margolin F R, Roses M R 1982 Duct carcinoma in situ. Relationship of extent of noninvasive disease to the frequency of occult invasion, multicentricity, lymph node metastases, and short-term treatment failures. Cancer 50: 1309–1314

Lambird P A, Shelley W M 1969 The spatial distribution of lobular in situ mammary carcinoma. Implications for size and site of breast biopsy. J A M A 210: 689–693

Lewis D, Geschickter C F 1938 Comedo carcinomas of the breast. Arch Surg 36: 225–244

McDivitt R W, Stewart F W, Berg J W 1968 Tumors of the breast. Atlas of tumor pathology, second series, fascicle 2. Armed Forces Institute of Pathology, Washington, D C, p 29–49

Meyer J S 1986 Cell kinetics of histologic variants of in situ breast carcinoma. Breast Cancer Res Treat 7: 171–180

Millis R R 1979 Mammography. In: Azzopardi J (ed) Problems in breast pathology. Saunders, Philadelphia p 437–459

Millis R R, Thynne G S J 1975 in situ intraduct carcinoma of the breast: a long term follow-up study. Br J Surg 62: 957–962

Muir R 1941 The evolution of carcinoma of the mamma. J Pathol Bacteriol 52: 155–172

Ohuchi N, Abe R, Takahashi T, Tezuka F, Kyogoku M 1985 Three-dimensional atypical structure in intraductal carcinoma differentiating from papilloma and papillomatosis of the breast. Breast Cancer Res Treat 5: 57–65

Ozzello L, Sanpitak P 1970 Epithelial stromal junction of intraductal carcinoma of the breast. Cancer 26: 1186–1198

Page D L 1986 Cancer risk assessment in benign breast biopsies. Hum Pathol 17: 871–874

Page D L, Dupont W D, Rogers L W, Landenberger M 1982 Intraductal carcinoma of the breast: follow-up after biopsy only. Cancer 49: 751–758

Pick P W, Iossifides I A 1984 Occurrence of breast carcinoma within a fibroadenoma. A review. Arch Pathol Lab Med 108: 590–594

Rosen P P, Scott M 1984 Cystic hypersecretory duct carcinoma of the breast. Am J Surg Pathol 8 31–41

Rosen P P, Lieberman P H, Braun D W Jr, Kosloff C, Adair F 1978 Lobular carcinoma in situ of the breast: detailed analysis of 99 patients with average follow-up of 24 years. Am J Surg Pathol 2: 225–251

Rosen P P, Senie R, Schottenfeld D, Ashikari R 1979a Non-invasive breast carcinoma. Frequency of unsuspected invasion and implications for treatment. Ann Surg 189: 377–382

Rosen P P, Seni R T, Farr G H, Schottenfeld D, Ashikari R 1979b Epidemiology of breast carcinoma: age, menstrual status, and exogenous hormone usage in patients with lobular carcinoma in situ. Surgery 85: 219–224

Rosen P P, Braun D W Jr, Kinne D E 1980 The clinical significance of pre-invasive breast carcinomas. Cancer 46: 919–925

Rosen P P, Braun D W Jr, Lyngholm B, Urban J A, Kinne D W 1981 Lobular carcinoma in situ of the breast: preliminary results of treatment by ipsilateral mastectomy and contralateral breast biopsy. Cancer 47: 813–819

Rosner D, Bedwani R N, Vana J, Baker H W, Murphy G P 1980 Non-invasive breast carcinoma. Results of a national survey by the American College of Surgeons. Ann Surg 192: 139–147

Salvadori B, Fariselli G, Saccozzi R 1976 Analysis of 100 cases of Paget's disease of the breast. Tumori 62: 529–536

Toker C 1970 Clear cells of the nipple epidermis. Cancer 25: 601–61

Vanstapel M-J, Gatter K C, DeWolf-Peeters C, Millard P R, Desmet V J, Mason D Y 1984 Immunohistochemical study of mammary and extra-mammary Paget's disease. Histopathology 8: 1013–1023

Webber B L, Heise H, Neifeld J P, Costa J 1981 Risk of subsequent contralateral breast carcinoma in a population of patients with in situ breast carcinoma. Cancer 47: 2928–2932

Westbrook K C, Gallager H S 1975 Intraductal carcinoma of the breast: a comparative study. Am J Surg 130: 667–670

Wheeler J E, Enterline H T 1976 Lobular carcinoma of the breast in situ and infiltrating. Pathol Annu 11 pt. 2: 161–188

Wulsin J H, Schreiber J T 1962 Improved prognosis in certain patterns of carcinoma of the breast. Arch Surg 85: 741–800

Infiltrating carcinoma: major histological types

Mammary carcinoma presents in a great variety of histological patterns, including specific types which have useful clinical correlates and prognostic implications. In general, these special types recognize neoplasms of lesser malignant potential (Dixon et al 1985). Currently, it is generally accepted that tubular and related neoplasms as well as mucinous carcinomas have an excellent prognosis (Gallager 1984). Medullary, pure lobular and those neoplasms with a predominant in situ component have an intermediate malignancy between the first noted group of neoplasms and the most frequent mammary carcinomas which are of no special type (often termed 'ductal'). In general, the first group with excellent prognosis has 90–95% five-year survival, the intermediate group has a 70–80% five-year survival, and the last group has a 60% or less five-year survival record. The special type cancers also have a relation to mode of detection, in that they are more common in mammographically discovered cancers as opposed to palpable lesions. In screening programmes using mammography the special type cancers are more frequent in prevalent cancers (those detected at first screen by mammography) than cases detected subsequently at yearly intervals (incident cases) (Anderson et al 1986). Conversely, cancers presenting in intervals between screening, presumably faster growing, are more likely to be poorly differentiated and not special type (von Rosen et al 1985).

Prognostication in breast carcinoma is becoming increasingly important as the therapeutic armamentarium broadens to include different chemotherapeutic, surgical and radiotherapeutic approaches. Stratification of groups of women on the basis of prognosis becomes extremely relevant.

This may be done by a combination of factors. We believe that special tumour types, extent of lymph node metastases, tumour size, necrosis within the tumour, and histological grading should all be considered. It is unfortunate that there continues to be a widespread tendency to regard any breast carcinoma as similar to the next, ignoring the well-established information that groups of excellent, poor and intermediate or indeterminant prognosis can be determined prospectively. It must be recalled that prognostication is an assessment of probability.

The accompanying Table 13.1 gives a general presentation of various classifications as applied to series of cancer cases. Note that the categories are quite similar. We have not included the rare types and patterns of carcinoma which are discussed in subsequent chapters. Succeeding chapters present cancer types which are rare, as well as patterns and features of carcinomas which should not be recognized as defining specific types of cancer. In large part, we recognize the WHO classification (Azzopardi et al 1981) and the work of McDivitt et al (1968).

Morphological classification of invasive breast cancer has been used for several decades. A variety of breast cancer classification schemes has been proposed utilizing either (1) a descriptive terminology for patterns of tumour growth (histological typing) or (2) a numerical grade based on degrees of glandular differentiation and nuclear characteristics (histological grading). This chapter includes discussions of the first approach. The second approach presumes a correlation between grade and survival, such that disordered growth pattern and bizarre nuclear features equate with poor prognosis. Histological grading that attempts

Table 13.1 Series of invasive mammary carcinomas.*

Rosen (1979) New York	Fisher et al (1975) USA	Fu et al (1981) Ohio	Wallgren et al (1976) Stockholm	Sakamoto et al (1981) Tokyo	Edinburgh Scotland §
75% Ductal	53% NOS†	48% NOS†	64% NST‡	47% Common (scirrhous)	70% NST‡
3% Minimally invasive ductal		13% Predominantly intraductal			3% Minimally invasive
10% Lobular	5% Lobular	11% Lobular	14% Lobular	2 % Lobular	10% Lobular (7% variants)
10% Medullary	6% Medullary	15% Medullary (10% variant)	6% Medullary	2% Medullary	5% Medullary (3% variants)
1% Tubular	1% Tubular	7% Tubular	7% Tubular		3% Tubular
2% Colloid	2% Mucinous	2% Colloid		4% Mucinous	2% Mucinous
0.5% Papillary	4% Mixed papillary and cribriform (adenocystic) and tubular	2% Papillary	9% Cribriform or papillary		1% Papillary
				22% Papillotubular	4% Cribriform
	28% Combined	5% Combined		20% Solid-tubular	2% Combined

* Revised to correct for in situ carcinomas.
† Not otherwise specified.
‡ No special type.
§ Authors' series.

to impose a single consistent and ordered classification system upon the full range of patterns seen in breast cancer is of limited reliability if applied generally; however, it may be particularly useful if applied only to those breast cancers which are of no special type, which is to say those not clearly identified by recognition of special histological types. Histopathological typing has separated a proportion of invasive carcinomas that have prognostic implications different from the remainder. Yet the largest percentage of breast cancers (between 70 and 80%) will fall within a group which, although varied in pattern, presents difficulties in further subclassification on the basis of histological type. It is within this group of breast cancers of no special type that a grading system of nuclear atypia and glandular differentiation will be most useful (see Ch. 17).

Mixtures of various tumour types present problems in classification. For example, how should a breast cancer be classified if 80% is of no special type (NST), 10% is of mucinous type and 10% of infiltrating lobular type? In our opinion, the approach to this problem as it relates to the histological classification of a single case is easy, in that it should be recorded as mammary carcinoma, NST, with small areas of mucinous and infiltrating lobular pattern. This accepts, for purposes of recording, the widely appreciated fact that breast cancers often exhibit diverse histological features, and allows more precise correlation of primary tumour with metastases. However, most classification schemes have failed to come to grips with this problem. This difficulty is minimized, or at least consistently dealt with, by the simple expedient of utilizing descriptive designations as noted above, recognizing that breast carcinoma occurs in both monomorphic histological types and in combinations of forms. Obviously, when describing lesions in a series of reported cancers, rules should be established for this problem and should be clearly stated. Simple rules such as

Table 13.2 Histological differentiation and biological behaviour of infiltrating carcinoma, common type (Japan Mammary Cancer Society).

Histological type	Mode of spread	Histological differentiation	Lymph node metastasis	Prognosis
Papillotubular	Predominantly intraductal	Good	Low	Good
Solid-tubular	Extraductal expansive	Moderate to poor	Intermediate	Intermediate
Scirrhous	Extraductal diffuse	Poor	High	Poor

predominantly or *over 50%* or *at least 90%* of dominant histological type will provide adequate guidelines for consistency in diagnosis.

This chapter will present the most common histological appearances of breast cancers, most of which have established prognostic significance. The following two chapters will present the less common and rare patterns seen in breast cancer, many of which have no proven prognostic implications.

Histological classification used in Japan

The histological classification of mammary cancer used in the Department of Pathology, Cancer Institute, Tokyo, has been adopted by the Japan Mammary Cancer Society (1975). This classification has been widely used throughout Japan and is fundamentally the same as the WHO classification (Azzopardi et al 1981) with the addition of a subclassification of the common or 'ductal' cancer group.

Infiltrating carcinoma is classified into common and special types. Infiltrating carcinoma of common type has three subgroups (Table 13.2): papillotubular carcinoma, solid-tubular carcinoma and scirrhous carcinoma (Sakamoto 1985, 1986). Papillotubular carcinoma is characterized by the projection of papillae into spaces (Fig. 13.1) and includes cribriform patterns (Fig. 13.2) and comedo patterns. Solid-tubular carcinoma is a solid tumour mass consisting of tubular or trabecular structures and reveals expansive growth compressing the surrounding tissue and forming a sharp border (Figs 13.3 and 13.4). Scirrhous carcinoma is characterized by cancer nests or cells accompanied by marked fibrosis. The subclassification of common type is based on the predomi-

nant one when there are two different histological types. When there are equal amounts of histological types, the one with the worse prognosis is the one chosen (Table 13.2). Special types include histological variants in concert with other classification schemes, particularly that adopted by the WHO: Mucinous, Medullary, Lobular, Adenoid Cystic, Squamous, Spindle Cell, Apocrine, with Sarcomatous Metaplasia, Tubular and Secretory (Sakamoto 1985).

Matched for extent of disease, survival of breast cancer in Japan is consistently better at 10 years than in Europe or the United States (Yonemoto 1980). This is largely accounted for by the greater incidence of the papillotubular and solid-tubular patterns. Rosen et al (1977) have documented the higher frequency of medullary and colloid cancers in Japan as well as the decreased incidence of lobular carcinomas. However, these differences appear to be decreasing (Sakamoto et al 1981).

REFERENCES

Anderson T J, Alexander F, Chetty U et al 1986 Comparative pathology of prevalent and incident cancers detected by breast screening. Lancet 1: 519–522

Azzopardi J G, Chepick O F, Hartmann W H and others 1981 Histologic typing of breast tumours, 2nd edn. World Health Organization, Geneva and Am J Clin Pathol 78: 806–816; and 1982 Tumori 68: 181–198

Dixon J M, Page D L, Anderson T J et al 1985 Long-term survivors after breast cancer. Br J Surg 72: 445–448

Fisher E R, Gregorio R M, Fisher B et al 1975 The pathology of invasive breast cancer. A syllabus derived from findings of the national surgical adjuvant breast project (protocol no 4). Cancer 36: 1–85

Fu Y S, Maksem J A, Hubay C A et al 1981 The relationship of breast cancer morphology and estrogen receptor protein status. In: Fenoglio C M, Wolff M (eds) Progress in surgical pathology, vol III. Masson New York p 65–76

Gallager H S 1984 Pathologic types of breast cancer: their prognoses. Cancer 53: 623–629

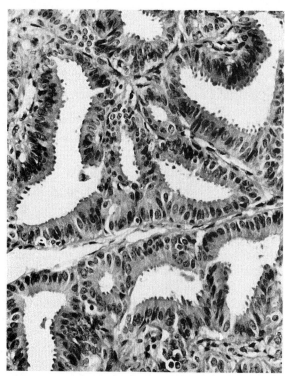

Fig. 13.1 Papillotubular carcinoma as recognized by the Japan Mammary Cancer Society. Note regular nuclei and pattern of cells (× 225).

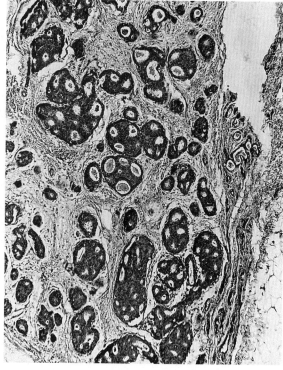

Fig. 13.2 Papillotubular carcinoma as recognized by the Japan Mammary Cancer Society. Note cribriform pattern and predominance of in situ disease (× 50).

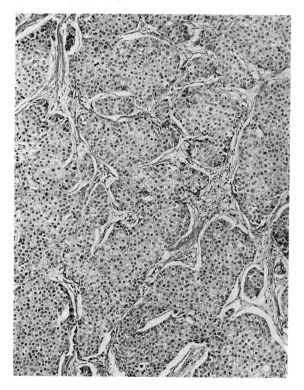

Fig. 13.3 Solid-tubular carcinoma as recognized by the Japan Mammary Cancer Society. This example is largely solid (× 50).

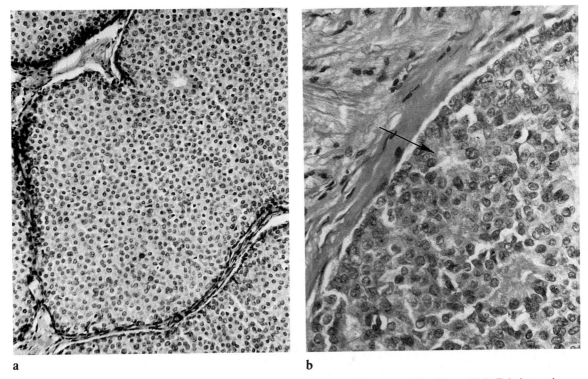

a   b

Fig. 13.4a,b The tubules of solid-tubular carcinoma are more apparent at higher power than Figure 13.3. Tubules are less crisp in (**b**), but many are present. Note that nuclei appear almost evenly arrayed about a central area (arrow) (**a** × 125; **b** × 275).

Japan Mammary Cancer Society 1975 General rule for clinical and histologic record of mammary cancer. Jpn J Surg 5: 118–131

McDivitt R W, Stewart F W, Berg J W 1968 Tumors of the breast. Atlas of tumor pathology, second series, fascicle 2. Armed Forces Institute of Pathology, Washington, D C

Rosen P P 1979 The pathological classification of human mammary carcinoma: past, present and future. Ann Clin Lab Sci 9: 144–156

Rosen P P, Ashikari R, Thaler H et al 1977 A comparative study of some pathologic features of mammary carcinoma in Tokyo, Japan and New York, USA. Cancer 39: 429–434

Sakamoto G 1985 Histological classification of the breast cancer. Jpn J Cancer Clin 31 (suppl 1): 105–113

Sakamoto G 1986 Histological classification of the breast cancer. Jpn J Cancer Clin 32 (suppl 1): 197–204

Sakamoto G, Sugano H, Hartmann W H 1981 Comparative pathological study of breast carcinoma among American and Japanese women. In : McGuire W L (ed) Breast cancer. Advances in research and treatment, vol 4 Plenum New York, p 211–231

Von Rosen A, Erhardt K, Hellstrom L, Somell A, Auer G 1985 Assessment of malignancy potential in so-called interval mammary carcinomas. Breast Cancer Res Treat 6: 221–227

Wallgren A, Silfversward C, Eklund G 1976 Prognostic factors in mammary carcinoma. Acta Radiol 15: 1–16

Yonemoto R H 1980 Breast cancer in Japan and United States. Epidemiology, hormone receptors, pathology and survival. Arch Surg 115: 1056–1062

NO SPECIAL TYPE (DUCTAL)

Terminology

This category is essentially a diagnosis of exclusion, comprising the majority of cases in any series of infiltrating mammary carcinomas. Largely because these cases do not have the lobular pattern discussed below, they have been termed ductal by many (see Table 13.1). As the site of origin is not proven in these cases and they are essentially defined as those remaining after the special types are removed (a diagnosis of exclusion), we prefer to term them *no special type* (NST). Fisher et al (1984) have retained the term ductal, but have added the phrase 'without special features or otherwise not specified type (NOS)'. Although such terminological considerations may seem trivial, we believe that calling attention to special types, even when absent, fosters the identification of special type cancers by both those generating reports and those receiving them. In a system of histological grading, these NST tumours would virtually all be within grade II or grade III (see Ch. 17), and may be so identified, e.g. mammary carcinoma of intermediate or high grade.

Anatomical pathology

No specific gross or microscopic features allow the recognition of no special type (NST) neoplasms for it is simply the lack of specific and consistent histological features of special type tumours which characterizes the NST cancers. For example, they regularly lack the uniformity of the mucinous and medullary carcinomas and often lack their sharp circumscription. Many of these neoplasms have a productive fibrosis within them, and other features that are discussed in Chapter 16.

Histologically, an extreme variety of patterns is seen, without the regularity and uniformity throughout the lesion which might characterize a tumour of special type. Features of single cell infiltration are often seen intermixed with poorly cohesive islands of infiltrating cells and occasional foci of poorly formed glands (Figs 13.5–13.9). Some suggestion of glandular formation is frequent, and may be a consistent pattern through most of the lesion (Figs 13.10–13.14). A mixture of these patterns is often seen, and may be considered to define this most common type of mammary carcinoma. Any of the patterns of special type cancers and any of the features noted in succeeding chapters may be seen focally or found in less than completely developed form (Figs 13.15–13.17). Nuclear patterns may be relatively orderly, or pleomorphic and bizarre.

There is one pattern, not reflected in special type cancers, which is sufficiently common to be helpful in suggesting the breast as the primary site from examination of metastases. This pattern has tightly cohesive islands of similar cells with rounded or irregular outer contours (Figs 13.18 and 13.19). Nuclei often demonstrate little atypicality.

Differential diagnosis

Lack of regular features of special tumour types throughout over 90% of an individual mammary neoplasm places it in the tumours of no special type category. The occasional tumours with 50–90% dominance of NST patterns should be regarded as NST cancers, but may be reported as containing other patterns. These tumours may present some features which give prognostic implication and, if these are predominant, their presence should be relayed in the final report. For example, as noted by Azzopardi (1979), gross formations demonstrating stellate, multinodular or circumscribed characters might be reported. As noted in Chapter 16 extensive necrosis within a neoplasm is a poor prognostic feature, and this should be documented. If the majority of a neoplasm is contained within preformed breast structures (in situ) this should be noted (see Ch. 16). These lesions may also be stratified on the basis of histological grades (see Ch. 17). The predominance of relatively well-formed glandular elements (moderately well-differentiated) has improved prognostic relevance over poorly differentiated tumours (Parl & Dupont 1982).

There are many benign histological patterns which may mimic invasive carcinoma to a greater

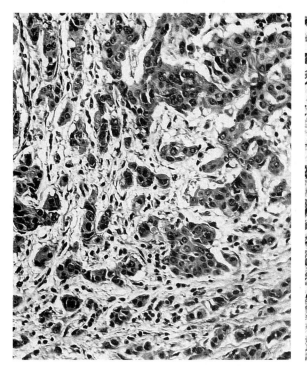

Fig. 13.5 Tightly cohesive islands have irregular shapes and sizes with occasional central lumina. Note at bottom, narrow strands and infiltration of single cells (× 225).

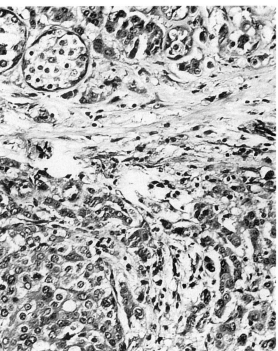

Fig. 13.6 Extreme variation of pattern in this infiltrating carcinoma of no special type has both large and small as well as tightly cohesive and loosely aggregated collections of cells (× 225).

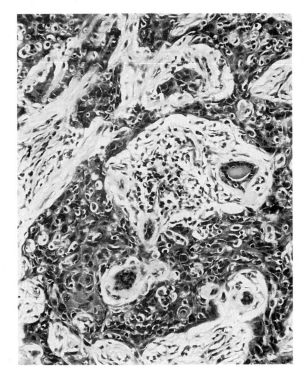

Fig. 13.7 This example of common type infiltrating mammary carcinoma has interlacing aggregates of frequently spindled carcinoma cells (× 225).

Fig. 13.8 Tightly cohesive islands of infiltrating carcinoma contrast with infiltration of small groups and individual cells above in this example of infiltrating carcinoma of common type (× 225).

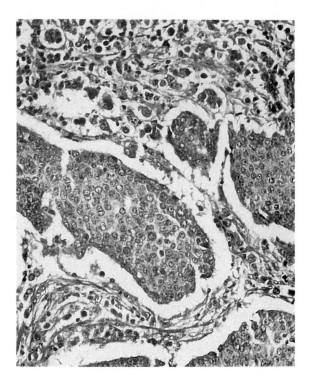

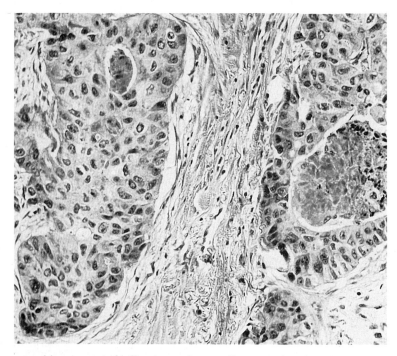

Fig. 13.9 Tightly aggregated large groups of infiltrating carcinoma cells suggest the orientation seen in squamous carcinoma. Note central necrosis much larger in the group at right than in the small necrotic focus in the upper part of group at left (× 225).

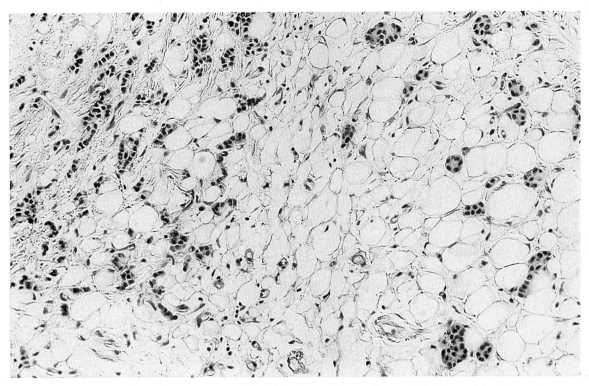

Fig. 13.10 Small groups of usually glandular-appearing infiltrating carcinoma cells are widely dispersed in this area of fatty tissue within the breast (× 225).

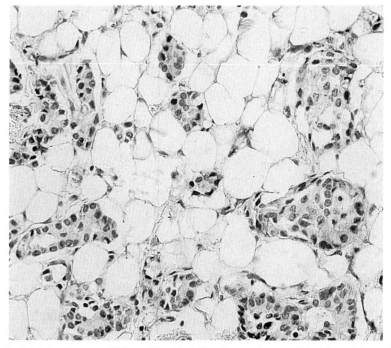

Fig. 13.11 Central glandular lumina are well formed in this infiltrating carcinoma. Although nuclei are of low grade, and this would be recognized as a low grade carcinoma, the regularity is insufficient to diagnose tubular carcinoma (× 225).

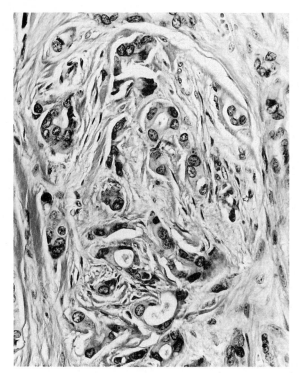

Fig. 13.12 Irregular gland formation with nuclei of intermediate grade is demonstrated in this no special type infiltrating carcinoma (× 450).

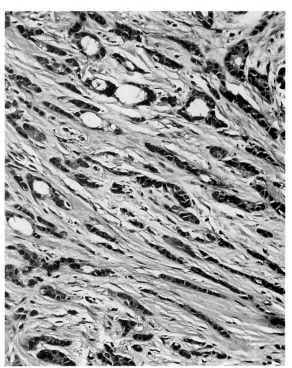

Fig. 13.13 Well-formed central lumina are occasionally present as well as tightly cohesive long, solid strands of infiltrating carcinoma cells (× 160).

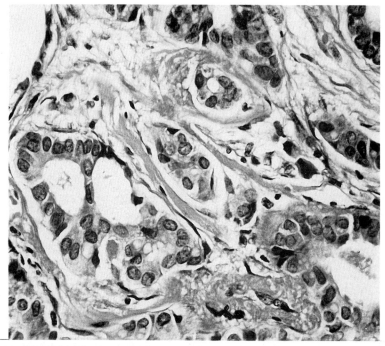

Fig. 13.14 Occasional well-formed lumina between cells are present as well as clear, rounded areas in the cytoplasm adjacent to nuclei which probably represent intracytoplasmic lumina (× 450).

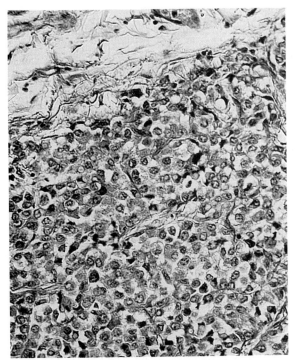

Fig. 13.15 This seeming solid mass of carcinoma cells mimics the solid variant of infiltrating lobular carcinoma; however, there are well-defined if subtle fibrovascular bands isolating somewhat rounded groups of tumour cells. The cells themselves are somewhat more pleomorphic than appropriate for a diagnosis of infiltrating lobular carcinoma (× 225).

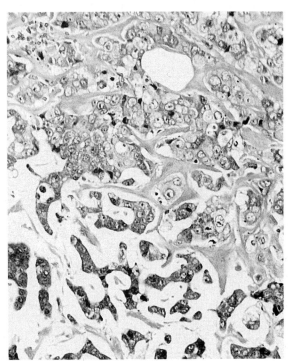

Fig. 13.16 Small islands of cancer cells float in pools of mucin at the lower part of this picture contrasting with the syncytial arrays of pleomorphic cells infiltrating in the upper portion of the picture. High grade infiltrating mammary carcinoma of no special type with focal mucinous differentiation is the appropriate diagnosis (× 225).

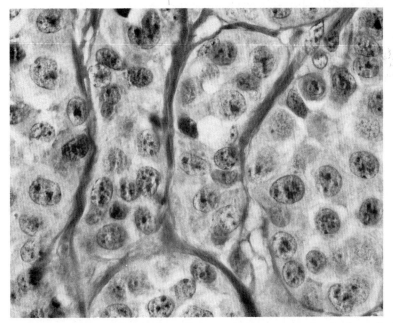

Fig. 13.17 These solid groupings of cancer cells, closely applied to each other, suggest the alveolar variant of infiltrating lobular carcinoma. However, the nuclear pattern is too pleomorphic, and this is better recognized as a no special type cancer (× 850).

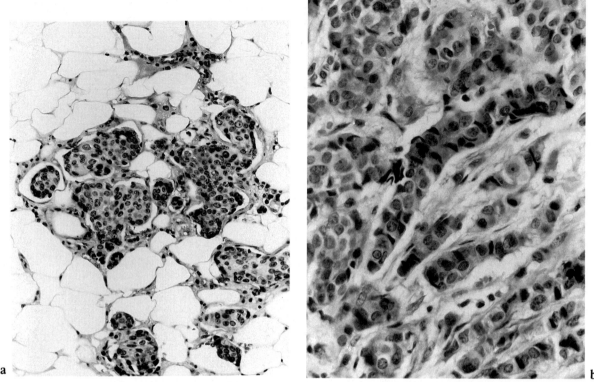

a   b

Fig. 13.18a,b Each of these examples of infiltrating carcinoma has tightly cohesive, usually rounded groupings of infiltrating cells with low grade nuclei (**a** × 225; **b** × 300).

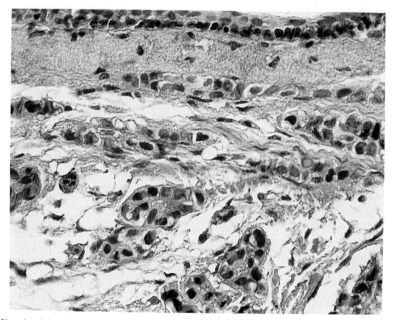

Fig. 13.19 These infiltrating islands are slightly irregular and occasionally linear as seen in the upper part of the picture. Linear cells at the very top are normal, ductal lining cells separated from a linear collection of carcinoma cells by an area of periductal elastosis (× 450).

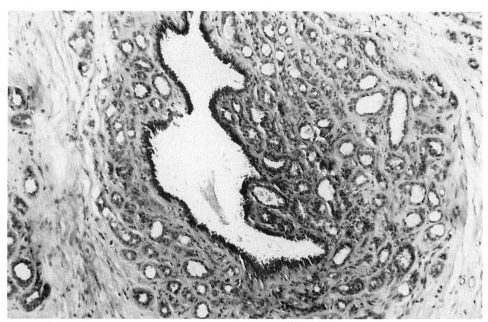

Fig. 13.20 These benign glands clustered about a central duct represent no diagnostic entity. However, infiltration by malignancy may be suggested. Note that there is a predictability in that gland size and orientation are somewhat similar in adjacent glands, and gradually change across the area. Note also that many of the cells appear flattened and perhaps atrophic, also not in keeping with a carcinoma diagnosis (× 160).

or lesser extent. Most of these are presented in the discussion of adenosis (Ch. 5) and adjacent chapters. One pattern reminiscent of adenosis has glands clustered about a duct (Fig. 13.20).

Clinical significance and prognostic implications

Neoplasms of no special type are recognized as having the poorest prognosis of any infiltrating carcinoma of the breast (Roses et al 1982). The many histological and cytological patterns seen within these neoplasms are of limited prognostic usefulness; rather, the prognosis of this tumour type rests largely upon other features such as size, lymph node status, and extent of necrosis within the neoplasm. Histological grading does provide a measure of prognostic stratification (see Ch. 16, 17 and 19). A report from a mammographic screening programme in Stockholm strongly supports the high grade NST cancer as the fastest growing ones by noting that almost all 'true' interval cancers (detected by clinical presentation between two-year screening intervals with no sign of tumour on review of previous mammogram)

were high grade and of no special type (von Rosen et al 1985). However, the interval cancers overall form a heterogeneous group and a different Swedish study indicates the overall survival and disease-free interval of those cases is similar to cancers diagnosed independent of screening (Holmberg et al 1986).

REFERENCES

Azzopardi J C 1979 Problems in breast pathology. Saunders, Philadelphia, p 245–274

Fisher E R, Sass R, Fisher B et al 1984 Pathological findings from the national surgical adjuvant project for breast cancers (protocol no 4). X. Discriminants for tenth year treatment failure. Cancer 53: 712–723

Holmberg L H, Tabar L, Adami H O, Bergstrom R 1986 Survival in breast cancer diagnosed between mammographic screening examination. Lancet 1: 579–522

Parl F F, Dupont W D 1982 A retrospective cohort study of histological risk factors in breast cancer patients. Cancer 50: 2410–2416

Roses D F, Bell D A, Flotte T J et al 1982 Pathological predictors of recurrence in stage 1 (TINOMO) breast cancer. Am J Clin Pathol 788: 817–820

Von Rosen A, Erhardt K, Hellstrom L, Somell A, Auer G 1985 Assessment of malignancy potential in so-called interval mammary carcinomas. Breast Cancer Res Treat 6: 221–227

MUCINOUS CARCINOMA

Anatomical pathology

This distinct type of invasive mammary carcinoma is usually 1–4 cm in diameter and is characterized grossly by smooth, rounded borders and a glistening cut surface as well as a soft consistency. The histological correlates of the gross appearance are a smooth, pushing border between the tumour and surrounding structures and a large proportion of the tumour mass composed of pools of mucinous material in which aggregates of tumour cells appear to be floating (Fig. 13.21). This carcinoma is synonymously designated as gelatinous, colloid or mucoid. The tumour cells are arranged most often in cohesive aggregates or islands with smooth borders and are consistently characterized by lack of bizarre features and nuclei with little atypia (Fig. 13.22). The islands of tumour cells frequently contain rounded or elongated spaces and thus may mimic a cribriform or even papillary pattern. Tumour nests may be extensively interconnected (Ferguson et al 1986), seemingly honey-combed by mucus producing a fenestrated appearance (Figs 13.23 and 13.24). The small amount of stroma associated with such tumours has little if any recognizable lymphoid or histiocytic infiltrate. Tumour nests may be most plentiful at the tumour margins where some may rest in stroma. Tumour necrosis and lymphatic invasion are regularly absent, and an associated in situ component is uncommon. Cytoplasmic argyrophilia, as seen in carcinoid tumours, may be demonstrable, and is discussed with carcinoid pattern in Chapter 15.

Differential diagnosis

Areas of tumour which are of no special type should remove such a tumour from the mucinous category. In other words, for a tumour to be designated a mucinous carcinoma it should demonstrate mucinous features in pure form throughout the entire lesion. The exception to this is small areas producing little mucin which have consistent cytology with the remainder of the tumour. Histological sampling of a tumour presenting grossly as mucinous should be specifically aimed towards identifying areas of firmness which may reveal a portion of the tumour to be of non-mucoid type. Reporting of such tumours should then relate this intermixture of types, producing a diagnosis such as 'mammary carcinoma with predominately mucinous features.' An accompanying explanatory comment should then relate the proportion composed of each element.

A loose and oedematous stroma is often seen in portions of a breast carcinoma of no special type. This loose stroma may mimic the mucin pools of a mucinous carcinoma. The presence of fibroblasts and vessels within these areas will identify them as stroma. Another histological feature occasionally suggesting a diagnosis of mucinous carcinoma is the presence of intracellular mucin. This feature is discussed extensively under the headings of lobular carcinoma and signet ring cell carcinoma and does not merit a diagnosis of mucinous mammary carcinoma. It is, then, the presence of pools of extracellular mucin which are the dominant histological and gross features of the mucinous carcinoma.

Blissfully rare is the finding of acellular mucin pools in stroma which must be noted as a point of differential diagnosis. Such benign interstitial mucin pools (Rosen 1986) present an obvious diagnostic dilemma because some portions of mucinous carcinomas may be remarkably paucicellular. Malignant cells must be present in an interstitial location in order to diagnose infiltrating carcinoma. The benign mucin pools are usually of 2–5 mm diameter maximally and are associated with benign local in situ epithelium although atypical hyperplasia may be present (Figs 13.25 and 13.26).

Prognosis and clinical features

Pure mucinous carcinomas comprise approximately 2% of most series of invasive breast cancer, and are associated with a rate of survival appreciably greater than that seen in the usual mammary carcinoma of no special type (Adair et al 1974). The survival figures at five and 10 years following mastectomy are intermediate between those of tubular carcinoma and carcinoma of no special type. In most series approximately 30% of

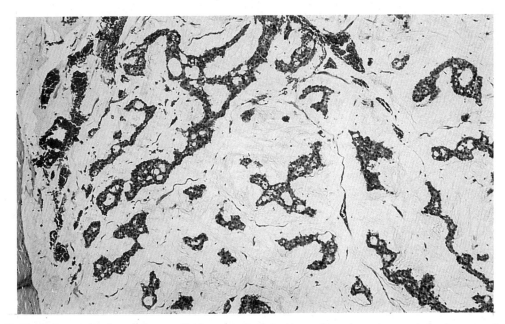

Fig. 13.21 Classical example of mucinous or colloid carcinoma of the breast. Note sharp circumscription by connective tissue at lower left (× 75).

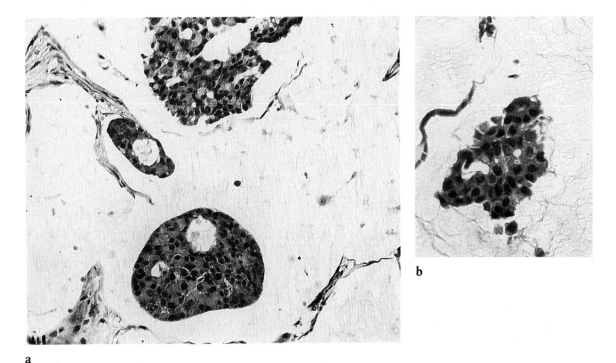

a

b

Fig. 13.22a,b These islands of carcinoma cells characteristically floating in pools of mucin have either smoothly irregular contours or sharp circumscription with well-defined internal rounded holes mimicking papillary and cribriform patterns (**a** × 225; **b** × 450).

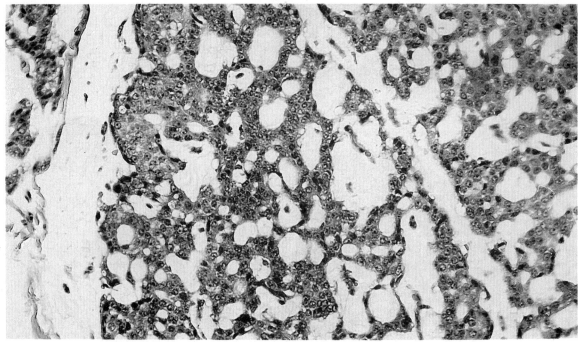

Fig. 13.23 Reticular or fenestrated pattern of mucinous carcinoma. Interconnecting masses of tumour cells still appear to float in mucin (× 250).

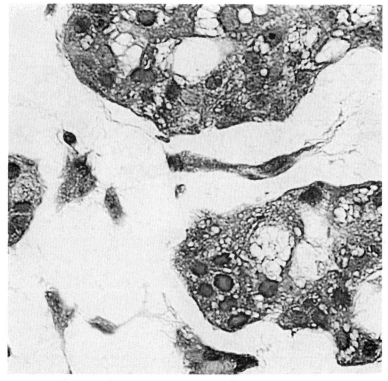

Fig. 13.24 Higher power of a case similar to Figure 13.23. Note delicate vessels placed centrally in mucinous pools between groups of carcinoma cells (× 800).

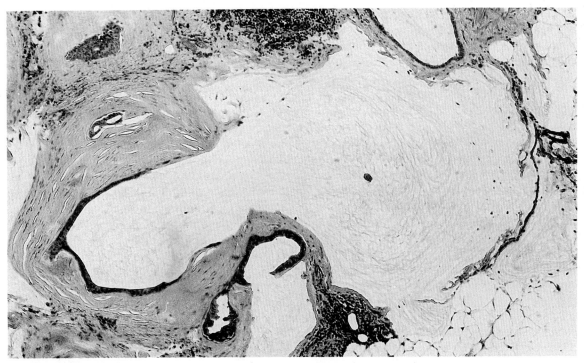

Fig. 13.25 Expanded epithelial space at left is continuous with mucin-filled stromal-lined space at right. This is benign and resembles a mucocele (× 80).

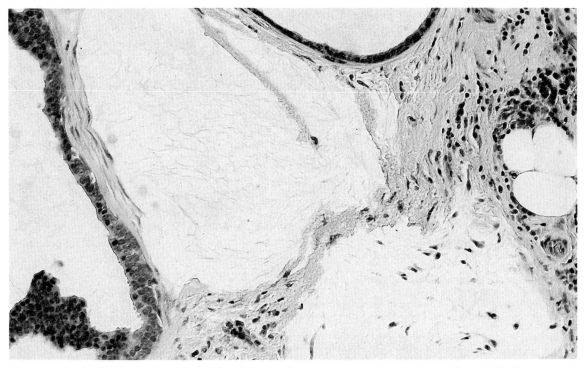

Fig. 13.26 Continuity of stromal and epithelial contained mucin pools are not evident here as in Figure 13.26. Note atypical hyperplasia at left and included histiocytes in mucin pool at lower right (× 250).

patients have metastases to axillary lymph nodes, although only 1 of 27 patients in the series of Norris & Taylor (1965) had metastases to lymph nodes. These 27 patients were carefully chosen as having pure mucinous carcinoma, and only 10% of the group died of disease. However, 29% of patients with 'mixed colloid carcinomas' died of carcinoma. This is the clearest evidence that excellent prognostic indications for this entity should be reserved for pure examples, while a better than average prognosis can be expected for cases with mixed histological features. Similarly, Rasmussen et al (1987) found that only 2 of 90 women with pure mucinous carcinomas presented with positive axillary nodes. The study of Silverberg et al (1971) corroborates this information as about 30% of women with 'mixed colloid' carcinoma were dead of disease in five years while only 14% of the pure cases died in the same time period.

Late recurrences are relatively common with one-half the deaths in two series of these cancers occurring more than 10 years after initial treatment (Rosen & Wang 1980; Clayton 1986).

Mucinous carcinoma is more common in older women than in young women, as Rosen et al (1985) found 1% of cancers to be mucinous type in women under 35 years of age and 7% of cancers to be of this type over the age of 75.

REFERENCES

Adair F, Berg J, Toubert L, Robbins GF 1974 Long-term follow-up of breast cancer patients: the 30 year report. Cancer 22: 1145–1150
Clayton F 1986 Pure mucinous carcinomas of breast. Hum Pathol 17: 34–38
Ferguson D J P, Anderson T J, Wells C A, Battersby S 1986 An ultrastructural study of mucoid carcinoma of the breast: variability of cytoplasmic features. Histopathology 10: 1219–1230
Norris H J, Taylor H B 1965 Prognosis of mucinous (gelatinous) carcinoma of the breast. Am J Clin Pathol 55: 355–363
Rasmussen B B, Rose C, Christensen I 1987 Prognostic factors in primary mucinous breast carcinoma. Am J Clin Path 87: 155–160
Rosen P P 1986 Mucocele-like tumours of the breast. Am J Surg Pathol 10: 464–469
Rosen P P, Wang T-Y 1980 Colloid carcinoma of the breast. Analysis of 64 patients with long-term follow-up. Am J Clin Pathol 73:304
Rosen P P, Lesser M L, Kinne D W 1985 Breast carcinoma at the extremes of age: a comparison of patients younger than 35 years and older than 75 years. J Surg Oncol 28: 90–96
Silverberg S G, Kay S, Chitale A R, Levitt S H 1971 Colloid carcinoma of the breast. Am J Clin Pathol 55: 355–363

TUBULAR CARCINOMA

Terminology and historical development

This special type of breast carcinoma has received general recognition only in the last 10 years. Because of the general orderliness of the histological pattern, and the well-formed character of the component parts, it has also been termed orderly or well-differentiated carcinoma. Most students of mammary histopathology prefer the term 'tubular carcinoma' because it is specifically descriptive. This type of carcinoma is more common in groups of cancers detected by mammography, largely explaining the increased interest in recent years (Patchefsky et al 1977)

Anatomical pathology

Grossly, the majority of these lesions are small, usually measuring about 1 cm in greatest dimension. Tubular cancers comprise a large percentage of very small invasive carcinomas, i.e. those of about 0.5 cm diameter. They are hard and fixed to the surrounding breast and on slicing may display a 'radial' appearance with pale streaks of elastosis centrally. Histologically, the tubular structures are characteristically oval or round, with an open central space lined by a single layer of orderly epithelium with cells appearing similar to one another (Figs 13.27–13.31). A frequent and almost characteristic feature is the bending or angulation of occasional spaces, producing the shape of a bent teardrop (Fig. 13.32). The tubules are fairly evenly and individually dispersed in a fibrous stroma which may be dense and hyalinized, particularly in the central part of the tumour, or loose and seemingly specially related to tumour elements. It is characteristic of these lesions to demonstrate infiltration of the adjacent fat without fibrous tissue separating tumour and fat. There is no relationship of the tubular elements to the local lobular architecture (Fig. 13.33). The cells have regular, round nuclei, usually without nucleoli. The luminal aspects of these cells often have bulbous projections from their apices (apical snouts). Foci of carcinoma in situ are usually intermingled with the invasive tumour. The CIS is usually centrally located and is most often of cribriform type, although mixture with micropapillary patterns is frequent. Often the in situ proliferation falls short of diagnostic criteria for CIS and is recognized as atypical hyperplasia of ductal pattern. A much smaller proportion of tubular carcinomas will be associated with carcinoma in situ of the lobular type (Oberman & Fidler 1979). Elastic tissue is frequently seen in stromal clumps or around ducts (Tremblay 1974).

Differential diagnosis

Separation of this entity from sclerosing adenosis and complex sclerosing lesion should be a constant concern of the diagnostic histopathologist. Features identifying this special type of breast cancer from other sclerosing lesions are listed in the accompanying Table 13.3. The differential diagnostic features with reference to complex sclerosing lesions are also discussed in Chapter 9.

Because tubular areas are found in many breast cancers, specific rules for the diagnosis of tubular cancer should be followed. Non-tubular areas should comprise less than 10% of the cancer in order to justify the diagnosis of tubular carcinoma, and even the non-tubular areas should have the same low grade nuclear features of the purely tubular areas. Some authors (Linell & Ljungberg 1980; Peters et al 1981) allow for histological patterns of breast cancer of no special type to make up 25% or more of the carcinoma diagnosed as tubular. Certainly, any breast cancer having more than one-quarter of its invasive component made up of non-tubular patterns should not be diagnosed as tubular, at least not without mention of the second pattern of invasive tumour. Thus a diagnosis of tubular carcinoma combined with less well-differentiated elements might be reported as: 'invasive mammary carcinoma with tubular and poorly differentiated elements'. Tumours of mixed tubular type with 75–90% tubular pattern have a good, but not excellent prognosis and should be reported as a mixed tubular or tubular variant carcinoma (Parl & Richardson 1983). Areas with the tubular pattern merging into less ordered glandular patterns are frequently found in carcinoma of no special type, and such cases should be diagnosed as NST cancers.

One feature that does not remove a case from the tubular category is the occasional presence of invasive tumour cell islands that have arches or smooth projections of tumour cells within tumour cell groups. This pattern is discussed in the section on invasive cribriform carcinoma. Because

Table 13.3 Histopathological differential diagnosis of tubular carcinoma.

Feature	Tubular carcinoma	Sclerosing adenosis	CSL*
Periphery	Infiltrative	Smooth circumscription	Radial arrangement of lobular units
Confinement to lobular units	No	Yes	Not applicable
In situ carcinoma	Usually present	Absent	Rare
Double cell layer	Absent, classically	Present	Usually present
Apical cytoplasmic 'snouts'	Often present	Seldom	Sometimes
Central spaces or lumens	Uniform, round or angulated	Most often, flattened, or oblong	Variable
Elastic tissue masses	Common	Insignificant	Common
Relation of glandular element to scar	Infiltrates beyond scar	Not applicable	Confined to central scar

*Complex sclerosing lesion/radial scar.

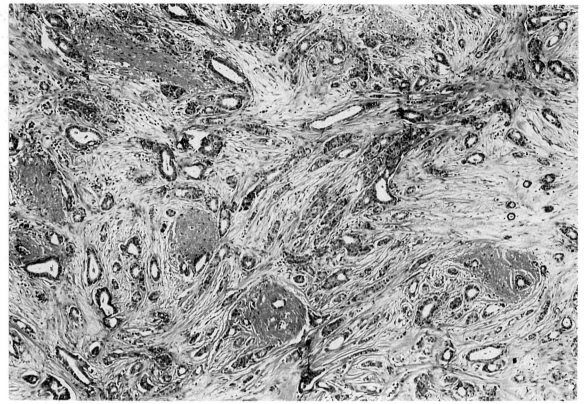

Fig. 13.27 At low power this classical tubular carcinoma has rounded and elongated infiltrating elements placed randomly over a large area. Note darkened clumps of hyaline, elastotic stromal material (× 75).

these tubular and cribriform patterns are regularly seen together, we have adopted an arbitrary rule that a tumour of 50% or greater tubular pattern with the remainder having the cribriform pattern will be reported as tubular. The invasive carcinoma designated 'tubulolobular' is described and discussed separately (Ch. 14).

Clinical features and prognosis

The excellent prognostic implications of a tubular carcinoma diagnosis makes the recognition and the careful recording of this special type of mammary carcinoma particularly important. Treatment of such a tumour by mastectomy is regularly followed by cure, and metastases and death following diagnosis of this tumour type is a distinctly unusual occurrence. When lymph node metastases are present (10–20% of cases in most series), they tend to be confined to one or two lymph nodes, and even these patients have excel-

lent prognosis. Multicentricity of carcinoma in the homolateral breast is recorded by Lagios et al (1981). They also report a 38% history of bilateral mammary carcinoma. This rate for contralateral cancer compares with 16% for Cooper et al (1978) and 18% for Taylor & Norris (1970).

When strictly defined, tubular carcinoma makes up approximately 2% of invasive mammary carcinomas. However, Patchefsky et al (1977) found a 9% incidence of strictly defined tubular cancers in the setting of screening by mammography. Predominantly tubular carcinomas containing 10–25% of other patterns will comprise an additional 3–8% of most current series. Although precise prognostic correlates of these tumours with mixed elements are not currently available, the important paper of Cooper et al (1978) indicates that the percentage of the tubular pattern as well as the size of the tumour may be important in identifying subgroups with a different prognosis. In their study with follow-up to 15 years or death,

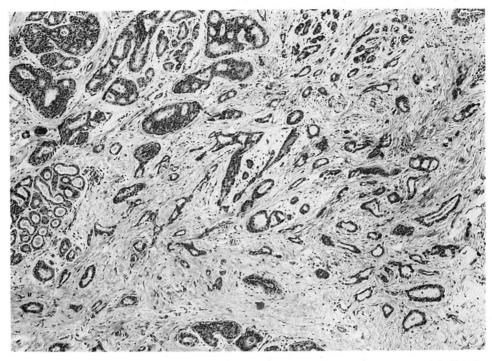

Fig. 13.28 Classic infiltrating tubular elements are intermixed with a few cribriform patterns at upper left. Tubular carcinoma is diagnosed as tubular elements predominate (× 75).

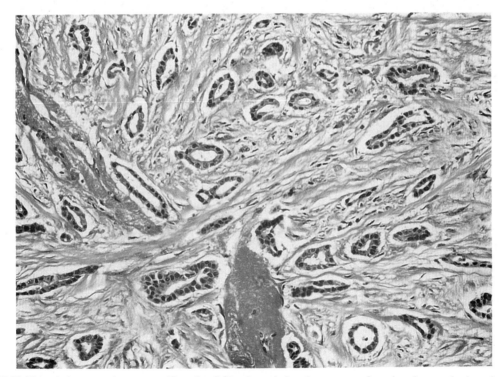

Fig. 13.29 Elastosis is seen at low centre. Note that infiltrating tubular elements are of varying shape and orientation (× 225).

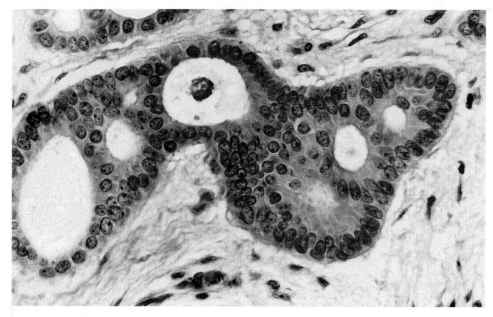

Fig. 13.30 Regular, low grade nuclei are present in this slightly cribriform pattern of tubular carcinoma (× 350).

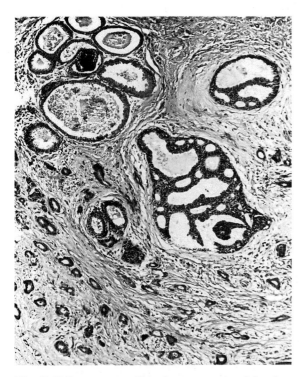

Fig. 13.31 Large spaces with arches are patterns of ductal carcinoma in situ surrounded, predominantly at left, by infiltrating tubular carcinoma (× 75).

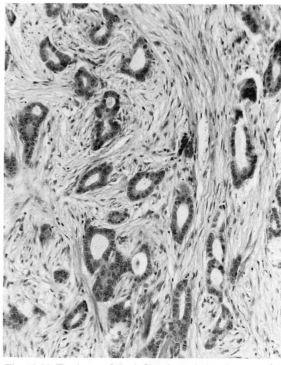

Fig. 13.32 Tendency of the infiltrating tubular elements of tubular carcinoma to form a single pointed contour is highlighted here (× 200).

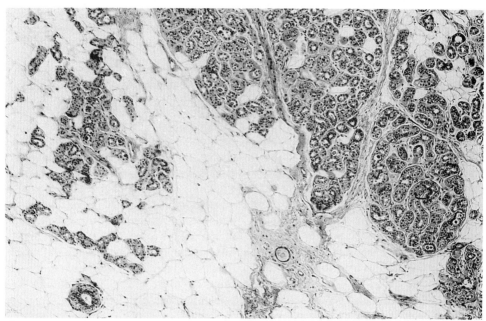

Fig. 13.33 Somewhat irregular lobular units resemble an infiltrating pattern at left. However, the haphazard array of elements seen in tubular carcinoma is absent. Note also, that fat is interspersed within a lobular unit at upper right. Thus, these are only mild and non-diagnostic alterations of lobular units (× 60).

no patient with pure tubular carcinoma died from the disease; and 72% were alive of those who had low grade tubular component of at least 90% admixed with no special type invasive carcinoma. Also, in that series, tumours of less than 1 cm in diameter intermixed with up to 50% carcinoma of no special type were associated with the same excellent prognosis found in the pure tubular carcinomas. Apparently, small tumour size and pure tubular patterns are independent variables indicating excellent prognosis (Peters et al 1981). There is also a relation between tumour size and purity of tubular pattern with pure being smaller than mixed tubular types (Linell & Ljungberg 1980). We can find no documentation of death from breast cancer after treatment for a pure tubular carcinoma of less than 1 cm diameter. The recent report from Columbia University (Peters et al 1981) records distant metastases only when the percentage of carcinoma of no special type constituted over 25% of the lesion. This approach of accepting 75% pure tubular component as identifying a more favourable prognosis is supported by Carstens et al (1985) and accepted as defining of tubular carcinomas by McDivitt et al (1982).

REFERENCES

Carstens P H B Greenberg R A, Francis D, Lyon H 1985 Tubular carcinoma of the breast. A long term follow-up. Histopathology 9: 271–280

Cooper H S, Patchefsky A S, Krall R A 1978 Tubular carcinoma of the breast. Cancer 42: 2334–2342

Lagios M D, Rose M R, Margolini F R 1981 Tubular carcinoma of the breast. Association with multicentricity, bilaterality and family history of mammary carcinoma. Am J Clin Pathol 73: 25–30

Linell F, Ljungberg O 1980 Breast carcinoma. Progression of tubular cancer and a new classification. Acta Pathol Microbiol Scand (A) 88: 59–60

McDivitt R W, Boyce W, Gersell D 1982 Tubular carcinoma of the breast. Am J Surg Pathol 6: 401–411

Oberman H A. Fidler W J Jr 1979 Tubular carcinoma of the breast. Am J Surg Pathol 3: 387–395

Parl F F, Richardson L D 1983 The histological and biological spectrum of tubular carcinoma of the breast. Hum Pathol 14: 694–698

Patchefsky A S, Shaber G S, Schwartz G J, Feig S A, Nerlinger R E 1977 The pathology of breast cancer detected by mass population screening. Cancer 40: 1659–1670

Peters G N Wolff M, Haagensen C D 1981 Tubular carcinoma of the breast — clinical pathological correlations based on 100 cases. Ann Surg 193: 138–149

Taylor H B, Norris H J 1970 Well-differentiated carcinoma of the breast. Cancer 25: 687–692

Tremblay G 1974 Elastasis in tubular carcinoma of the breast. Arch Pathol 98: 302–307

MEDULLARY CARCINOMA

Anatomical pathology

This well-recognized entity (Moore & Foote 1949; Richardson 1956) presents grossly as a smoothly rounded mass unfixed to the adjacent tissue. Sharp circumscription with a soft and uniform consistency are the grossly identifiable hallmarks of medullary carcinoma. Histologically, this cancer is characterized by tumour cells forming irregular bordered islands without sharp edges, which often interconnect. The tumour cells do not invade the adjacent breast tissue but rather seem to push against it, resulting in smooth borders and no apparent capsule (Fig. 13.34). Within the tumour there is a loose connective tissue stroma with a usually prominent lymphocytic and/or plasmacytic infiltrate (Figs 13.35 and 13.36). The lymphoid infiltrate does not become interspersed between the individual tumour cells. The cells of the tumour have large nuclei and copious cytoplasm. Nuclei have atypical or bizarre features, some clear areas and usually contain nucleoli. The cytoplasm is eosinophilic, occasionally granular, and the cytoplasmic borders are most often indistinct and may be irregular.

Differential diagnosis

The clumps of tumour cells with the characteristic cellular features should comprise at least three-quarters of the tumour. Development of glandular spaces or more tightly cohesive and regularly circumscribed islands, so commonly seen in tumours of no specific type, may be seen in a small proportion of the tumour. Regularly interconnecting trabeculae of tumour cells of only four to five cells wide do not qualify for this special histological type. The presence of more than one focus of invasion into the surrounding tissue should remove a tumour from this special type category. Squamous metaplasia may be seen in somewhat over 10% of these tumours. Tumour necrosis may be in small areas involving a few tumour cells. The presence of an in situ component does not exclude a case from this category, but if it is extensive it should introduce doubts, as in situ components are not prominent in medullary carcinomas. Bizarre tumour giant

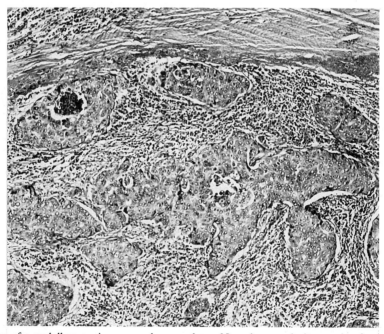

Fig. 13.34 Outer edge of a medullary carcinoma may be seen above. Note the smooth demarcation from surrounding stroma (× 75).

cells are found in pure examples in about 10% of cases (Ridolfi et al 1977).

Many carcinomas of no special type have a lymphocytic infiltrate, particularly at the advancing

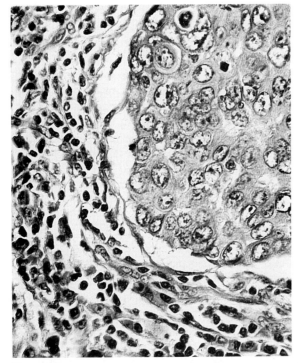

Fig. 13.35 Irregular placement of large vesicular nuclei is evident in this medullary carcinoma. Lymphocytes surround the island of tumour cells (× 450).

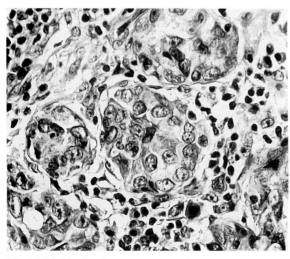

Fig. 13.36 Islands of tumour cells are quite irregular, but do not contain lymphocytes. Medullary carcinoma (× 450).

edge of the tumour, often interspersed with cancer cells. This finding without other features does not support a diagnosis of medullary carcinoma (Fig. 13.37). The diagnosis of medullary carcinoma should also be questioned when the characteristic lympho-plasmacytic infiltrate is sparse, i.e. is not readily identified in the loose stroma. Care must be taken to make certain that the characteristic cytological and histological features are present throughout the neoplasm. The stroma must be loose throughout the tumour, with only rare areas of dense collagen present.

Both Fisher et al (1975) and Ridolfi et al (1977) have identified a group of well-circumscribed breast cancers with some but not all of the features of medullary carcinoma. Such cases may be designated medullary variant cancers or atypical medullary carcinomas. These variant cases are more easily identified by the presence of atypical features rather than by the absence of classic criteria as noted above. A diagnosis of medullary

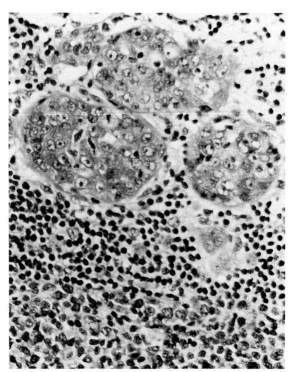

Fig. 13.37 This was an unusual focus in an otherwise ordinary, no special type, cancer demonstrating focal lymphocytic infiltration (× 300).

variant carcinoma is made when an otherwise well-circumscribed tumour with appropriate cytology presents several microscopic foci of 'invasion' into adjacent tissue. If a well-circumscribed carcinoma contains up to 25% of carcinoma of no special type with medullary type elsewhere, or demonstrates dense fibrous bands within the tumour, diagnosis of medullary variant cancer is appropriate.

In summary, the presence of sharp circumscription without infiltration beyond the well-defined border and the presence of the characteristic cytological features of medullary carcinoma are central to this diagnosis. If these features are not predominant, the cancer in question should not be considered a medullary carcinoma. The diagnosis of medullary variant carcinoma is useful to identify a group of cases with some but not all the features of medullary carcinoma.

Prognostic and clinical features

Characteristic medullary carcinomas may appear to be benign, both clinically and mammographically, because of their mobility, rounded contours and regular lack of calcification. This special type of mammary cancer is associated with a better than average survival rate at five years, 10 years, and beyond (Richardson 1956; McDivitt et al 1968; Ridolfi et al 1977). Whilst the precise definition of medullary carcinoma is best discussed by Ridolfi et al (1977), future studies will have to determine which of the several identifying features has the greatest prognostic utility. The practical usefulness of this diagnosis is that it does identify a group of women with a more favourable prognosis than the usual type of breast cancer, whether or not lymph node metastases are present (Ridolfi et al 1977). Histological grading would place medullary carcinoma in a poor prognosis category, where they obviously do not belong. Survival rate at 10 years for medullary carcinomas was 84% in the study of Ridolfi et al (1977) as opposed to 63% for breast carcinoma of no special type. The medullary variant carcinoma, or atypical medullary carcinoma, is a useful diagnostic category possibly associated with survival intermediate between that of medullary carcinoma and breast carcinoma of no special type (Ridolfi et al 1977).

REFERENCES

Fisher E R, Gregorio R M, Fisher B et al 1975 The pathology of invasive breast cancer. A syllabus derived from findings of the national surgical adjuvant breast project (protocol no 4). Cancer 36: 1–84
McDivitt R W, Stewart F W, Berg J W 1968 Tumours of the breast. Atlas of tumour pathology, second series, fascicle 2. Armed Forces Institute of Pathology, Washington, D C
Moore O S Jr, Foote F W Jr 1949 The relatively favourable prognosis of medullary carcinoma of the breast. Cancer 2: 635–642
Richardson R W 1956 Medullary carcinoma of the breast: a distinctive tumour type with a relatively good prognosis following radical mastectomy. Br J Cancer 10: 415–423
Ridolfi R L, Rosen P P, Post A, Kinne T, Mike V 11977 Medullary carcinoma of the breast. A clinical pathological study with 10 year follow-up. Cancer 40: 1365–1385

INFILTRATING LOBULAR CARCINOMA

Historical background

The first reports of infiltrating lobular carcinoma (ILC) (Foote & Stewart 1946) followed the recognition of lobular carcinoma in situ by these same pathologists (Foote & Stewart 1941). The classical pattern of single-filed, regular cells, diffusely infiltrating was associated with lobular carcinoma in situ in the same breast in over 60% of cases, leading to the nosological association of this type of infiltrating carcinoma with the previously described type of in situ carcinoma. The review by Wheeler & Enterline (1976) succinctly and completely covers confines of definition for the pure or classical forms of ILC. However, problems of definition are evident because different series of breast cancers contain percentages of ILC from 3–4% up to as much as 14% (Martinez & Azzopardi 1979). This probably led to the confusion with regard to prognostic implications which varied from somewhat worse to somewhat better than usual breast cancer. Variant patterns of invasive lobular carcinoma were carefully described in the late 1970s. Fechner (1975) reported ILC with a solid pattern and Martinez & Azzopardi (1979) described an alveolar pattern. Dixon et al (1982) separately analysed cytology and patterns of infiltration in a series of cases for which there was over a 10 year follow-up. The variations in lethality between the different types described in the latter report have not yet been confirmed by other studies, but their finding of improved survival in the classical type was strong.

Anatomical features

The gross presentation of invasive lobular carcinoma varies from a quite well-defined, scirrhous mass to a poorly defined area of induration. It is unique among infiltrating breast cancers in that it may be undetected by inspection as well as palpability in excised breast tissue.

Histologically, infiltrating lobular carcinoma must be understood to recognize or include two basic features which may occur together or singly. These two features are cytology and pattern of infiltration. When both appear together, a pure or classical type (Figs 13.38 and 13.39) is recognized (Table 13.4). Solid (Fig. 13.40) and alveolar (Fig. 13.41) variants are recognized when the appropriate cytological features are present, but the infiltration pattern is not classic. A mixed or pleomorphic group is recognized when the classical pattern of diffuse spread is present without the appropriate cytological features or when classical, solid, or alveolar patterns are intermixed (Figs 13.42–13.46). The concurrent presence of in situ changes of lobular carcinoma in situ or atypical lobular hyperplasia is more common in the classical form (approaching 90%) than in the other forms where it varies from approximately 40–60% (Dixon et al 1982).

Table 13.4 Criteria for separation of invasive lobular carcinoma into subgroups (modified from Dixon et al 1982).

Types	Pattern	Cell type
1. Classical	Single filing, targetoid peri-parenchymal distribution, diffuse multifocal invasion	
2. Solid variant	Sheet-like pattern or irregularly shaped nests of cells	Small, non-cohesive, regular cells with regular, round or oval nuclei
3. Alveolar variant	Globular aggregates of 20 or more cells	
4. Mixed group or	Mixture of above patterns	
Pleomorphic pattern or atypical group	Diffuse infiltration, often with irregular, small clumps of cells	Cohesive cells with nuclear pleomorphism

The histological appearance of the classical form is a diffusely infiltrating pattern of small, round and quite regular cells in single lines between collagen bundles. The alveolar variant has cell aggregates of uniform appearance and a solid

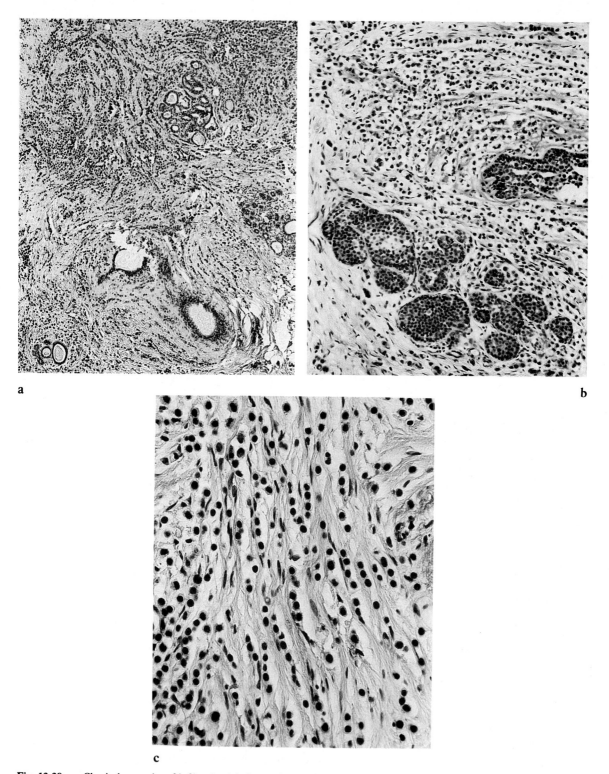

Fig. 13.38a–c Classical examples of infiltrating lobular carcinoma all have files of single cells diffusely infiltrating breast stroma. Note parallel arrays of single-filed cells often bordering parenchymal units (**a** × 50; **b** × 125; **c** × 320).

Fig. 13.39 High power view of a file of infiltrating lobular carcinoma of classical type shows that each tends to be related to its neighbour by opposed cell membranes (× 1200).

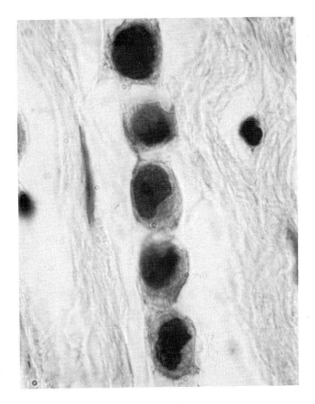

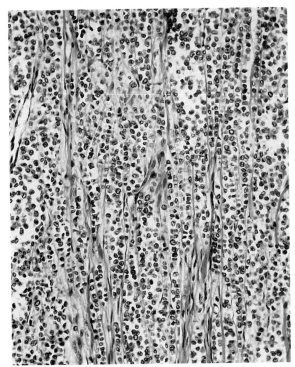

Fig. 13.40 Solid variant of ILC with tumour cells interspersed between delicate strands of fibrous tissue (× 160).

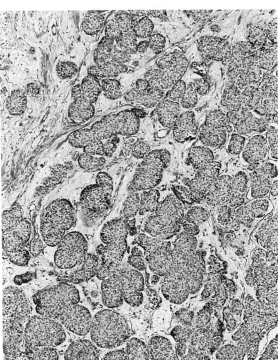

Fig. 13.41 Alveolar variant of ILC demonstrates rounded groups cells with characteristic, uniform cytology (× 50).

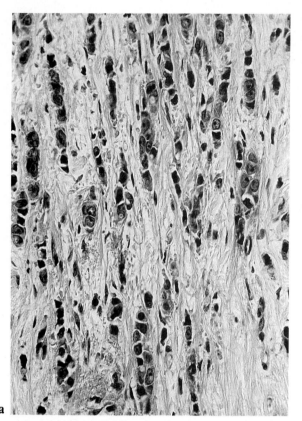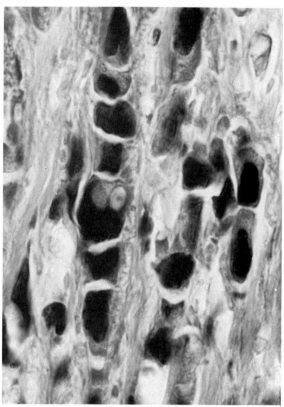

a b

Fig. 13.42a,b Pleomorphic variant of ILC demonstrates diffuse pattern of infiltration; however, nuclei are quite pleomorphic and there is a tendency for cells to aggregate. Note intracytoplasmic clear spaces, representing intracytoplasmic lumina (**a** × 320; **b** × 1200).

variant has sheets of cells. The mixed or atypical group was recognized by Dixon et al (1982) in order to provide confines of definition with regard to prognostic implication. This group contains several different histological patterns: mixtures of any of the classical, solid, or alveolar patterns or, a diffusely infiltrative pattern of more cytologically bizarre cells, often with some tendency for cell aggregation (Table 13.4).

Differential diagnosis

Most examples of classical ILC present little difficulty in diagnosis. Because improved prognosis may apply only to the classical type, the separate recognition of variant types is less important. Rigorous requirements for uniform presence of diffuse infiltrative pattern and regular cytological features facilitate the consistent recognition of the pure or classical type. The same

uniform nuclei should be present in the alveolar and solid variants.

The solid variant can present real problems in the differential diagnosis with lymphoma. Broad aggregates of poorly cohesive cells with slightly irregular margins describes most lymphoid neoplasms in soft tissue. Cytological features of various lymphocyte types will usually identify the presence of lymphoma (see Ch. 18). Special stains are indicated in this setting. An Alcian blue-PAS stain demonstrating a positive, rounded cytoplasmic area of vacuolar staining will prove the epithelial nature of neoplasm. Lymphoid cells may have clear spaces or solid, PAS-positive material. Electron microscopy is also useful. The packeting pattern of the alveolar variant allows reliable distinction from most lymphomas.

The most important differential diagnostic consideration is in the classical type. There may be few cells present, rendering diagnosis of carci-

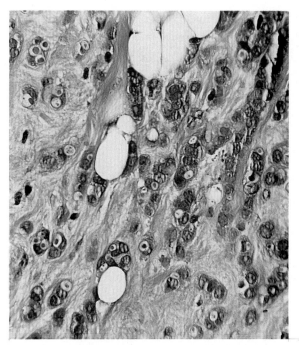

Fig. 13.43 Despite frequent intracytoplasmic lumina in a diffuse pattern of infiltration, this is a mixed or pleomorphic variant of ILC because of cellular aggregation (× 400).

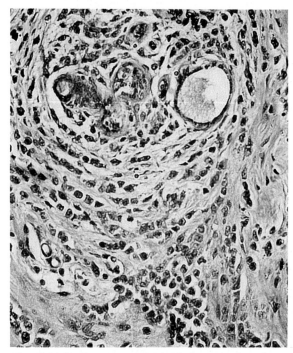

Fig. 13.44 Tendency to aggregation in lower portion of photograph should question appropriateness of pure ILC diagnosis. If extensive, the aggregated areas should indicate a mixed ILC diagnosis (× 225).

noma difficult both grossly and microscopically. This has long been known as a potential difficulty, and still remains so, accounting for several missed diagnoses. If there is any increase, or unusual grouping of small cells in stroma, the possibility of a paucicellular ILC of classical type should be considered. This possibility is particularly likely if in situ lobular disease (ALH/LCIS) is present. The Alcian blue-PAS stain without nuclear counterstain will be useful in recognizing cytoplasmic vacuoles in ILC cells (Fig. 13.47) because these are usually present in many cells in over 50% of cases. Some linear grouping of cells is necessary in order to recognize ILC. However, lymphocytes may be present in linear arrays (Fig. 13.48).

Many examples of ILC have some cells with enlarged, eccentric cytoplasmic compartments which resemble signet ring cells. While this is an important histological feature, the recognition of a special type of breast cancer with this designation is usually unwarranted. We are frequently careful to add the modifier 'with signet ring features' to a diagnosis. This will highlight the possible confusion of a later metastasis with a gastrointestinal primary tumour (see Ch. 19).

Infiltrating lobular carcinoma of any subtype may produce a confusing and easily misdiagnosed pattern of involvement of lymph nodes. The small size and regular cytological features produce a close mimicry of histiocytes, and they are easily confused with histiocytes in the subcapsular and intramedullary sinuses mimicking the familiar pattern of sinus histiocytosis (see Ch. 19). This is a particular problem when the cells appear adjacent to one another with an apparent lack of cohesion, thus closely mimicking the aggregations of sinus histiocytes as well as the cytology. Therefore, in a case of infiltrating lobular carcinoma of any type, the lymph nodes need to be examined with special care, keeping in mind this possible 'histiocytoid' appearance of metastatic carcinoma. Careful histological analysis of the 'internal control' appearance of histiocytes will usually clarify matters. Of course, when a great number of carcinoma cells are present with deformity of the lymph node, differential diagnosis is easily resolved. The utility of the Alcian blue-PAS stain is also apparent in this differential diagnostic situation.

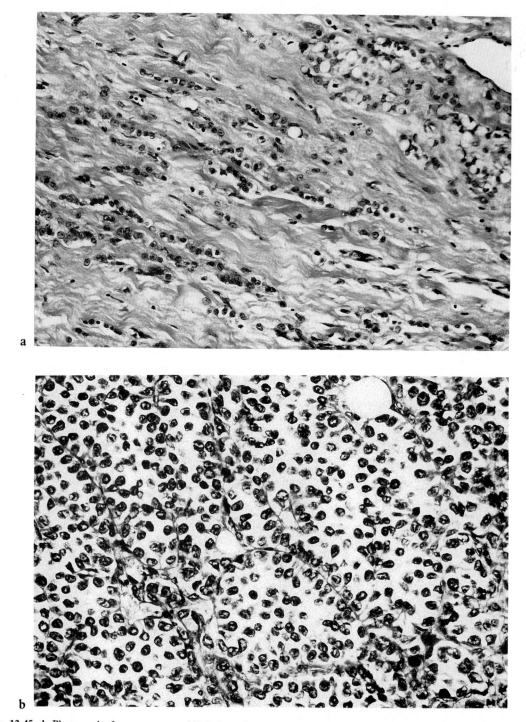

Fig. 13.45a,b Photographs from same case of ILC show classic pattern (left in **a**), aggregated cells with signet appearance (upper right in **a**) and a loose alveolar pattern in (**b**). Note also that the loose alveolar pattern if somewhat more compact, would be recognized as the solid pattern of ILC. Obviously, this case is reported as an example of mixed ILC (**a** × 225; **b** × 400).

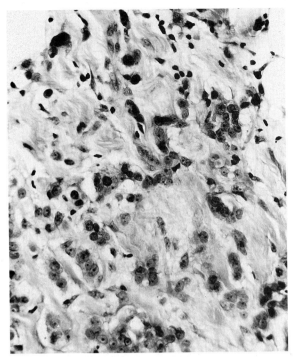

Fig. 13.46 Irregular small aggregates of diffusely infiltrating cancer cells suggest a pleomorphic lobular carcinoma. However, this could also be interpreted as poorly differentiated carcinoma of no special type. Fortunately, there is no proven prognostic difference between these diagnoses (× 320).

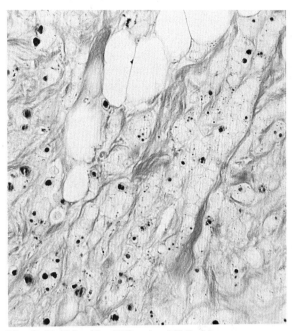

Fig. 13.47 Alcian blue-PAS stain of ILC without counterstain emphasizes cellular mucosubstances of intracytoplasmic lumina with the dark dots (× 400).

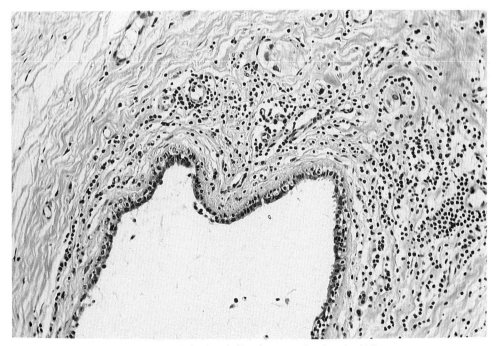

Fig. 13.48 Lymphocytes may simulate classic ILC when infiltrating around a duct (× 200).

Clinical and therapeutic implications

Prognostic implications of the diagnosis of ILC lie with greatest certainty in the pure or classical type. Papers of Haagensen et al (1978) as well as Dixon et al (1982) have supported the improved long-term prognosis for patients with classical examples of this special type of breast cancer. The prognosis lies somewhere intermediate between that for infiltrating breast carcinoma in general and the excellent prognosis attending tubular carcinoma (Dixon et al 1985). Future studies are required in order to clarify the association of this prognostic implication with other variables, such as clinical stage.

A diagnosis of ILC also has prognostic implications as regards the contralateral breast. It is likely that the incidence of cancer bilaterality is high in all types of infiltrating lobular carcinoma (Dixon et al 1983), and is probably highest for the mixed or pleomorphic type. Despite the increased risk of bilaterality, prognosis remains unaffected when the second tumour is not synchronous. Future studies seeking to clarify this association will need to subcategorize the types of infiltrating lobular carcinoma, as well as record the presence or absence of in situ disease in the initial breast with carcinoma, to make predictability more certain.

Infiltrating lobular carcinoma has implications with regard to mammographic detection of breast cancer. Although many cases of infiltrating lobular carcinoma will be detectable as a dominant mass, often with calcification present, a large proportion of these cases present difficulties in both mammographic and clinical detection because of the diffuse pattern of infiltration which may well not produce a dominant or well-defined mass lesion. Presentation of these areas of thickening and mammographically subtle or invisible areas of infiltration are usually seen in the pure and mixed or pleomorphic types.

Increased likelihood of oestrogen receptor positivity has been ascribed to the invasive lobular cancers, possibly particularly for the alveolar variant (Shousha et al 1986).

REFERENCES

Dixon J M, Anderson T J, Page D L, Lee D, Duffy S W 1982 Infiltrating lobular carcinoma of the breast. Histopathology 6: 149–161

Dixon J M, Anderson T J, Page D L, Lee D, Duffy S W, Stewart H J 1983 Infiltrating lobular carcinoma of the breast: an evaluation of the incidence and consequence of bilateral disease. Br J Surg 70: 513–516

Dixon J M, Lee D, Page D L et al 1985 Long term survivors after breast cancer. Br J Surg 72: 445–448

Fechner R E 1975 Histologic variants of infiltrating lobular carcinoma of the breast. Hum Pathol 6: 373–378

Foote F W Jr, Stewart F 1941 Lobular carcinoma in situ. A rare form of mammary cancer. Am J Pathol 7: 491–496

Foote F W Jr, Stewart F W 1946 A histologic classification of carcinoma in the breast. Surgery 19: 74–99

Haagensen C D, Lane N, Lattes R, Bodian C 1978 Lobular neoplasia (so-called lobular carcinoma in situ) of the breast. Cancer 42: 737–769

Martinez V, Azzopardi J G 1979 Invasive lobular carcinoma of the breast: incidence and variants. Histopathology 3: 467–488

Shousha S, Backhous C M, Alaghband-Zadeh J, Burn I 1986 Alveolar variant of invasive lobular carcinoma of the breast. Am J Clin Pathol 85: 1–5

Wheeler J E, Enterline H T 1976 Lobular carcinoma of the breast in situ and infiltrating. In: Sommers S C (ed) Pathol Annual pt 2: 161–188. Appleton Century Crofts, New York

INVASIVE CRIBRIFORM CARCINOMA

Historical background

Invasive cribriform carcinoma (ICC) has only recently received attention as a special type of breast carcinoma (Azzopardi 1979). The justification for acceptance of this type rests not only in a unique histological pattern but, most impellingly, in its excellent prognosis. Without specific categorization, the excellent prognosis will go unrecognized because these tumours may fall within the broad definition of carcinomas of no special type. Although grading will identify most cases as grade I or low grade carcinoma, some of them have more advanced nuclear atypia and might fall into grade II. Because ICC has an excellent prognosis, with distant metastases being as uncommon as those seen with pure tubular carcinoma, recognition of these ICC cases is of clinical importance, no matter what term might be used to relay this information. The long-term follow-up of a group of patients with ICC is presented in Page et al (1983).

Anatomical features

The gross appearance of these tumours is a firm mass with relatively smooth or occasionally stellate borders. Gross evidence of focal sclerosis is relatively common, but necrosis is unusual.

Histologically, these neoplasms demonstrate stromal invasion with islands of cells resembling those seen in cribriform carcinoma in situ. Individual islands have bars or arches of cells producing well-defined spaces between the cells (Figs 13.49–13.53). Areas of tubular differentiation characteristic of tubular carcinoma are intermixed in about 25% of cases, and both patterns may have apical cytoplasmic protrusions ('snouts') into the central spaces (Fig. 13.54). Adjacent in situ carcinoma of identical histological and usually cytological pattern is present in over three-quarters of cases. Some breast cancers associated with stromal giant cells have a related histological pattern (see Ch. 16). Occasional examples of ICC will have a two-cell population, the second population having clear cytoplasm found interspersed within islands of less rounded cells with coloured cytoplasm (Fig. 13.55).

As accepted in the related tubular carcinoma, ICC usually has quite regular nuclei, i.e. nuclear features of low grade (Fig. 13.56). However, with a regular and consistent histological pattern, intermediate grade nuclei (Figs 13.55 and 13.57) may be accepted as examples of ICC (Page et al 1983).

Analogous with tubular carcinoma, solid foci which maintain the same nuclear pattern as the majority of the tumour will not detract from a diagnosis of ICC (Fig. 13.58). Occasional examples of ICC will have cytoplasmic vacuoles representing intracytoplasmic lumina. Rarely, these will be so prominent as to suggest a signet cell pattern (Fig. 13.59).

Remarkably, the unusual lymph node metastases of ICC maintain the regularity of histological pattern characteristic of ICC (Fig. 13.60). This is apparently also true of regional recurrences (Fig. 13.61).

Differential diagnosis

Tubular carcinoma, cribriform carcinoma in situ, and adenoid cystic (adenocystic) carcinoma of the breast are the major contenders in a consideration of differential diagnosis. However, most of the cases of ICC that we have seen in consultation have not been recognized as of any special type, and have been called invasive ductal carcinoma, or carcinoma of no special type. Whatever term or approach might be used for these lesions of minimal threat to life, they should be so recognized and have their prognosis clearly understood by clinicians.

The invasive cell groups of invasive cribriform carcinoma have similar cytological and histological patterns to those seen with in situ disease of cribriform type. Occasionally these islands of ICC will have fewer atypical features than found in cribriform CIS. Considering that lobular units and ducts may be greatly deformed by pre-existing scarring process as well as expansion and distortion by neoplastic cells, it is easy to see that differentiating ICC from in situ carcinoma may be very difficult. The same diagnostic approach detailed in microinvasive cancer is used, except

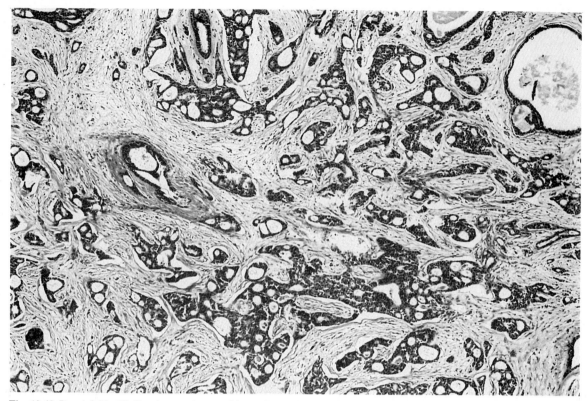

Fig. 13.49 Broad field of infiltrating carcinoma with a quite uniform cribriform pattern predominating. Focally, tubular elements are apparent. Invasive cribriform carcinoma (× 75).

that variation in cytology between the in situ and invasive components is of no aid. Apart from identifying cribriform tumour clearly within supporting connective tissue or fat, and therefore clearly beyond the confines of lobular units, the irregular clustering of tumour cell groups (a hallmark of invasive disease in any organ) suffices to qualify a lesion as invasive. Another histological feature of most ICCs is that the invasive islands tend to be evenly spaced and of similar size to each other. A striking variant of this uniformity is gradual gradations in island size as viewed under low power. Larger tumour islands are most often found within the centre with smaller ones at the periphery.

Differentiation of ICC from adenoid cystic carcinoma of the breast (ACCB) may be difficult or impossible, indeed we believe that many cases reported as ACCB may be better understood as ICC, but with the ACCB having a more crisp definition to the rounded spaces within the cellular islands and having other defining features (see adenoid cystic carcinoma). In any case, the prognostic implication of each diagnosis is the same. Fisher et al (1975) and Fisher (1977) have proposed the term 'adenocystic carcinoma' for these lesions, less strictly defined than adenoid cystic, indicating that the confining diagnostic features of adenoid cystic carcinoma recognize only a small number of similar neoplasms. They also suggested that the adenocystic configuration represents a variation of the tubular structures of tubular carcinoma.

Many students of breast cancer include some cases of ICC in the tubular category. This will serve to identify the excellent prognosis; however, many cases which are predominantly cribriform will not be recognized. We have arbitrarily chosen over 50% dominance of pattern to decide between diagnoses of tubular or invasive cribriform cancer when the two patterns are present.

As noted above, intermediate grade nuclei may

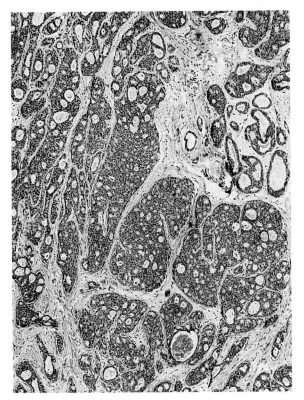

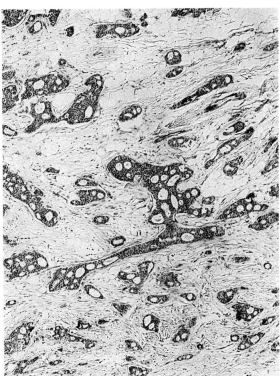

Fig. 13.50 Larger islands of invasive cribriform carcinoma than usual for the entity are present (× 50).

Fig. 13.51 Thin strands of ICC predominate. Occasional tubular elements are present as well (× 50).

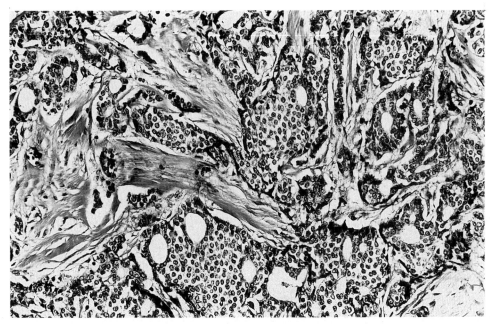

Fig. 13.52 Occasional interlacing islands of invasive carcinoma are apparent in this example of ICC (× 200).

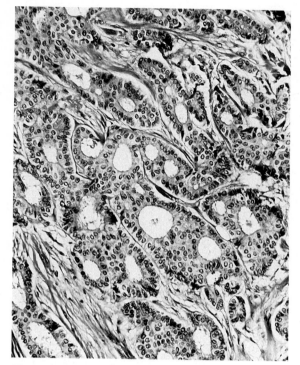

Fig. 13.53 Islands of ICC are closely packed (× 255).

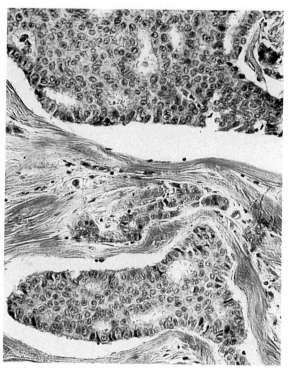

Fig. 13.54 Apical cytoplasmic protrusions into intercellular spaces are present. Note variation in size of cell groups in this ICC (× 225).

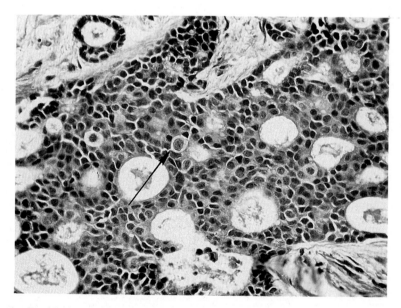

Fig. 13.55 Occasional cells with clear cytoplasm are present in this ICC with moderate grade nuclei. One clear cell is indicated by the arrow, and one is present to left and right of arrowed cell (× 320).

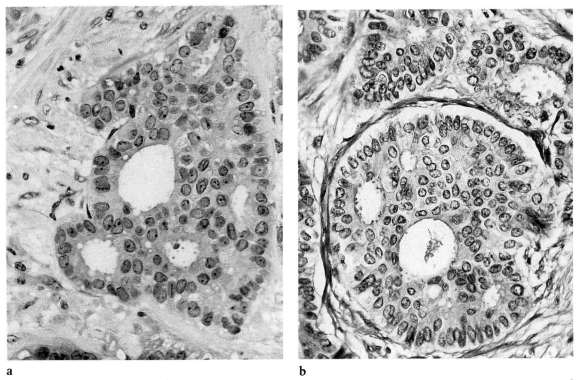

a   b

Fig. 13.56a,b Low grade, quite uniform nuclei are evident in these examples of ICC (**a, b** × 320).

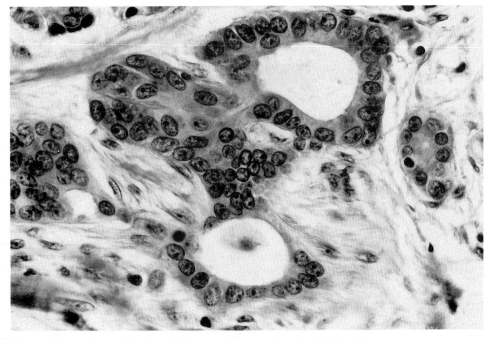

Fig. 13.57 Intermediate grade nuclei with mild pleomorphism populate this ICC (× 450).

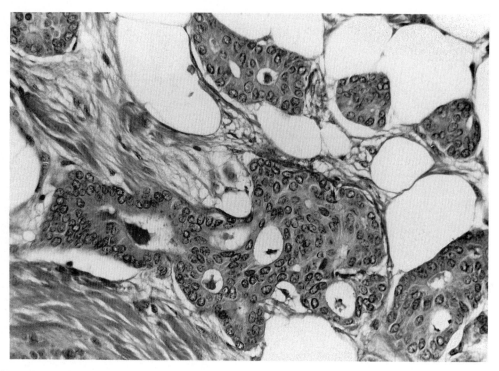

Fig. 13.58 Small, solid islands of ICC are in fat at upper right. Because their cytology and cellular placement are similar to the more characteristic portions of tumour, this is still ICC (× 330).

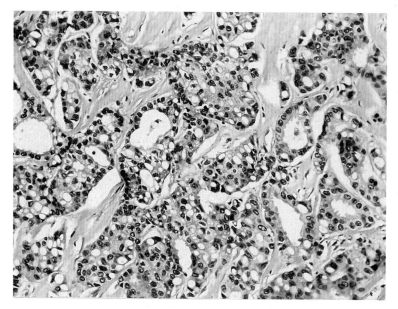

Fig. 13.59 This case of ICC has the unusual cytoplasmic feature of vacuolization. The vacuoles are intracytoplasmic lumina, some large enough to displace the nuclei (× 160).

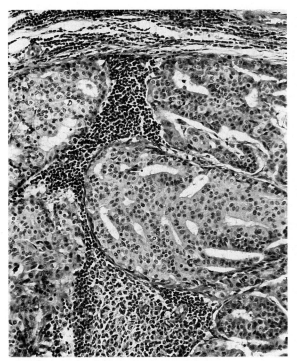

Fig. 13.60 The even pattern of ICC is maintained in this metastasis in an axillary lymph node (× 125).

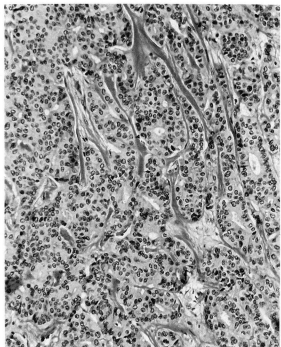

Fig. 13.61 This local recurrence of ICC occurred 14 years after mastectomy (× 125).

be accepted within the ICC category, but high grade nuclei should place a tumour into no special type (Fig. 13.62). Such tumours usually have more irregular intercellular spaces and cellular placement than ICC as well.

Occasional low grade carcinomas will suggest a diagnosis of ICC, but without a well-developed cribriform pattern, are best left recognized as low grade no special type tumours (Fig. 13.63).

Clinical features and prognosis

The clinical presentation of these tumours is no different from usual invasive breast cancer, although they tend to be relatively small and probably often lack calcifications. Average diameter of the classic type of ICC was over 3 cm in our own series (Page et al 1983); however, case recruitment preceded frequent clinical use of mammography.

It is in prognosis that these tumours are special. Patients with pure ICC comprised 3.5% of invasive breast cancers and follow-up of 35 patients at 10–21 years after diagnosis revealed no distant metastases, despite documentation of local nodal metastases in 14% of these patients. Local recurrence many years after initial diagnosis was also followed by no evidence of distant metastasis. Excellent prognosis was also accorded this pattern by Dawson et al (1986).

ICC as well as tubular carcinomas are more common in groups of women screened for breast cancer by mammography. Anderson et al (1986) found 12% of detected invasive carcinomas at first mammogram to be of tubular or cribriform type; variant tubular or ICC (defined as having 50–90% of such a component) comprised 23% of invasive carcinomas. The percentage was reduced at incident screens to 7% and 14% respectively.

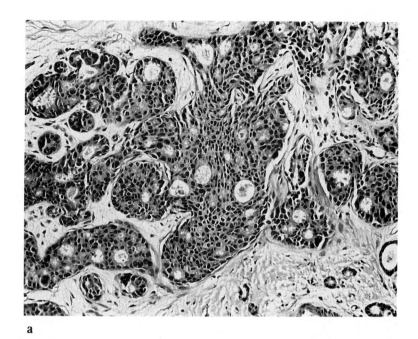

a

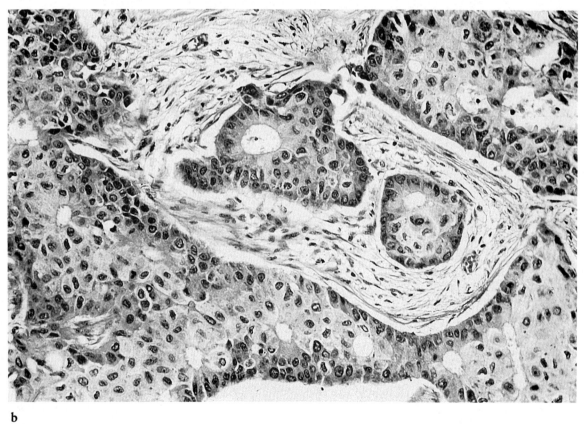

b

Fig. 13.62a,b Although reminiscent of ICC, these carcinomas are better regarded as of no special type because of high grade nuclei and irregular cell placement (**a** × 320; **b** × 225).

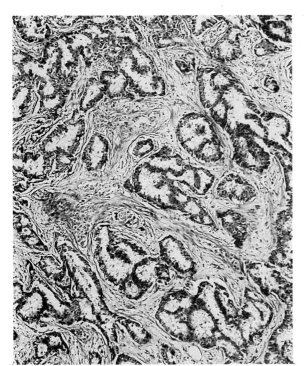

Fig. 13.63 Regularity of pattern and resemblance to ductal carcinoma in situ may suggest ICC in this invasive tumour. However, the pattern is not cribriform. It is best recognized as a low grade carcinoma. The Japan Mammary Cancer Society would recognize it as a papillotubular carcinoma, also recognizing a relatively good prognosis ($\times$ 50).

REFERENCES

Anderson T J, Lamb J, Alexander F et al 1986 Comparative pathology of prevalent and incident cancers detected by breast screening. Lancet 1: 519–522

Azzopardi J C 1979 Problems in breast pathology. Saunders, Philadelphia, p 241–274

Dawson P J, Karrison T, Ferguson D J 1986 Histologic features associated with long-term survival in breast cancer. Hum Pathol 17: 1015–1021

Fisher E R 1977 Pathology of breast cancer. In: McGuire W L (ed) Breast cancer. Advances in research and treatment. Plenum New York, p 43–123

Fisher E R, Gregorio R M, Fisher B 1975 The pathology of invasive breast cancer. A syllabus derived from findings of the national surgical adjuvant breast project (protocol no 4). Cancer 36: 1–85

Page D L, Dixon J M, Anderson T J, Lee D, Stewart H J 1983 Invasive cribriform carcinoma of the breast. Histopathology 7: 525–536

Uncommon types of invasive carcinoma

Entities presented in this chapter are characterized by their rarity. No cancer type included here comprises more than 1% of any breast cancer series, and indeed, only one is encountered that often. In sum, these tumours will be found in somewhat less than 2% of invasive breast cancers. In spite of their infrequent occurrence, they should be recognized as special types of cancer. The diagnostic terms may be used in clinical reporting without further clarification as each has intrinsic clinical correlates. Carcinoma with spindle cell metaplasia is included here more because of the importance of avoiding a sarcoma diagnosis than because of known clinical or prognostic implications. In essence, then, these nine special types of breast cancer are to be contrasted with those patterns and features enumerated in the succeeding two chapters which cannot stand alone as entities with intrinsic clinical relevance.

SECRETORY CARCINOMA

Background

This acknowledged special type of carcinoma is both rare and of little threat to life in the majority of cases. Our current ability to predict which of these lesions is biologically malignant is not an uncharted sea, but is analogous to knowledge of the North Atlantic after the second voyage of Columbus. This is not a totally frivolous analogy, but relates to the rarity of this lesion and current lack of certainty as to which histological features guarantee only local growth potential.

In 1966, McDivitt & Stewart (1966) described an uncommon variety mammary carcinoma in children which they designated 'juvenile carcinoma'. Since that time the histological pattern described has been found in adults, and the descriptive term 'secretory carcinoma' has been widely accepted.

Anatomical pathology

Secretory carcinomas are characteristically well circumscribed and often small, many examples measuring less than 2 cm in greatest diameter. Gross circumscription has characterized most reported examples, and as focal invasion into surrounding tissue may be present in some cases, it is useful to examine the margins with some care in order to demonstrate this phenomenon. Histologically, most will have a well-delimited border often with a layer of connective tissue between the neoplasm and the surrounding tissues. The delimiting fibrous tissue may be discontinuous, but when it is, the tumour cell groups are usually adjacent (Figs 14.1 and 14.2). Prominent collections of fibrous tissue are often present within the lesion (Figs 14.3 and 14.4). Abundant intra- and extracellular rounded partially clear areas of various size with secretions are the major defining features of secretory carcinoma (Figs 14.5–14.7). Intracytoplasmic vacuolization may, but does not usually, seem to push the nucleus to one side. Abundant intercellular lumina containing secretory material (usually similar in appearance to that seen intracellularly) are also frequent in most examples. The non-vacuolated cytoplasm is characteristically finally granular. Secretory material both within the cells and in intercellular

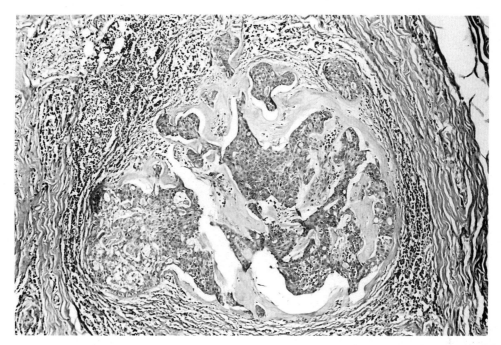

Fig. 14.1 Island of secretory carcinoma. Nowhere in this tumour did groups of cancer cells lose contact with specialized, hyaline stroma. Same case as Figure 14.4 (× 60).

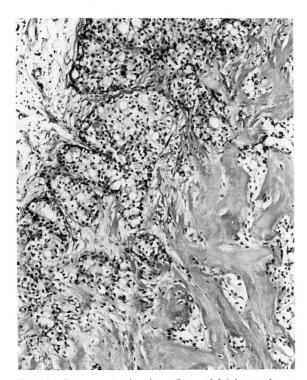

Fig. 14.2 Dense connective tissue (lower right) is prominent in central portion of this secretory carcinoma. Note quite sharp border at upper left (× 125). (Courtesy of H. A. Oberman, University of Michigan.)

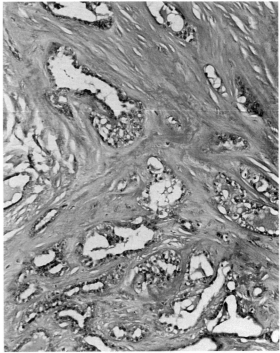

Fig. 14.3 Relatively few neoplastic cells are present in dense stroma. Focally, follicular spaces with central secretory material are evident (× 125). (Courtesy of H. A. Oberman, University of Michigan.)

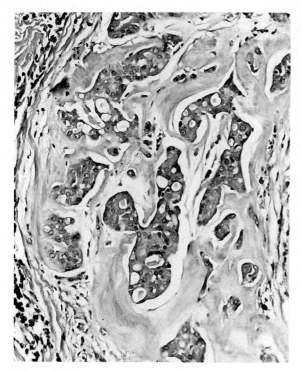

Fig. 14.4 Higher power of same tumour as Figure 14.1. Note better developed secretory spaces (× 225).

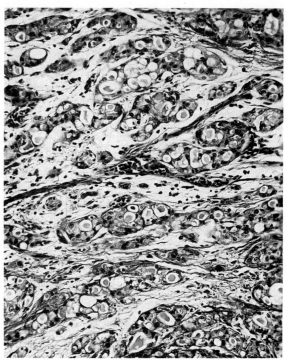

Fig. 14.5 A more evidently infiltrative pattern than in other examples of secretory carcinoma is seen here (× 160). (Courtesy of H.J. Norris, Washington, D C.)

spaces stains variably with virtually all stains for mucosubstances particularly PAS (not removed by diastase) and Alcian blue. Mucicarmine staining is usually positive in at least a few cells (Tavassoli & Norris 1980).

Clinical features and prognosis

Although originally thought confined to a juvenile population, it is clear that these neoplasms may occur in women into the seventh decade (Oberman 1980). An excellent prognosis seems to attend virtually all women reported under the age of 20; however, this is not true for older women (Tavassoli & Norris 1980). It may well be, then, that such tumours in juveniles may occasion a low expectation of malignant behaviour. The six examples in adults reported by Oberman (1980) were all followed by benign behaviour. Also, all of the six described by Oberman (1980) were 2.1 cm or less in greatest dimension. Of the 19 examples reported by Tavassoli & Norris (1980), four of the 11 with axillary node dissections had nodal

metastases and a single patient, 24 years old at presentation, died of disseminated tumour. Three of these four cases with nodal metastases had focal areas of infiltration with an irregular extension of tumour cells into the stroma, and this finding of invasion was present in only four of the 19 cases. In their series, none of the five neoplasms of less than 2 cm in diameter metastasized, and the four tumours having axillary metastases were from 2–6 cm in largest size. It will take a much larger experience with this unusual neoplasm in order to be more certain with regard to prognostication. However, it does seem that lesions in children, less than 2 cm in size, and without stromal invasion at the periphery may be regarded as having a very low possibility of malignant behaviour.

It should also be noted that not all carcinomas occurring in children are of this secretory pattern. Standard issue and highly malignant mammary carcinomas do occur in this age group (Nichini et al 1972), although they are of great rarity. Only 2% of breast carcinomas appear under the age of

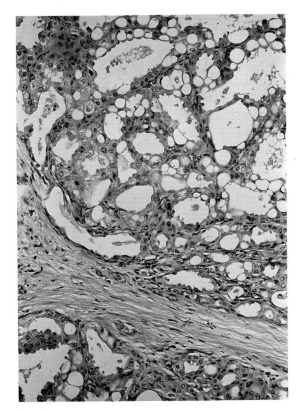

Fig. 14.6 Intra and extracellular spaces are abundant in this secretory carcinoma (× 200). (Courtesy of H. A. Oberman, University of Michigan.)

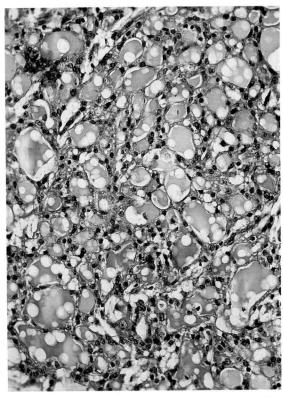

Fig. 14.7 A follicular pattern is evident from this region of a secretory carcinoma (× 210). (Courtesy of H. J. Norris, Washington, D C.)

30 and the great majority of these occur over the age of 20. These aggressive carcinomas occurring in children and juveniles should be evaluated as for older patients (Oberman 1979).

It is notable that a recent presentation of secretory carcinoma in adults (Akhtar et al 1983) details one of three patients who had five positive lymph nodes and focal infiltration into surrounding breast tissue and adipose tissue from a tumour of 5 cm in greatest dimension. This observation supports the suggestion above, that size and stromal invasion are determinants of metastatic capacity. Oberman & Stephens (1972) have presented a case of secretory carcinoma presenting intially at the age of 4 when a 1 cm mass was locally excised with local recurrences four and 21 years later.

REFERENCES

Akhtar M, Robinson C, Ali A M, Godwin J T 1983 Secretory carcinoma of the breast in adults. Light and electron microscopic study of three cases with review of the literature. Cancer 51: 2245–2254

McDivitt R W, Stewart F W 1966 Breast carcinoma in children. J A 195: 388–390

Nichini F M, Goldman L, Lapayowker M S, Levy W M, Maier W, Rosemond G P 1972 Inflammatory carcinoma of the breast in a 12-year-old girl. Arch Surg 105: 505–508

Oberman H A, Stephens P J 1972 Carcinoma of the breast in childhood. Cancer 30: 470–474

Oberman H A 1979 Breast lesions in the adolescent female. Pathol Annu 14 (1): 175–201

Oberman H A 1980 Secretory carcinoma of the breast in adults. Am J Surg Pathol 4: 465–470

Tavassoli F A, Norris H J 1980 Secretory carcinoma of the breast. Cancer 45: 2404–2413

SQUAMOUS CELL CARCINOMA

Squamous cell carcinoma of the breast parenchyma is exceedingly rare. It must be carefully separated from lesions involving the epidermis and/or nipple region which must be considered as squamous carcinoma of the skin or dermal appendages. The well-known features of squamous differentiation in malignant neoplasms should be present throughout the lesion if acceptance as a primary breast squamous cancer is appropriate. If the features of sharp cytoplasmic borders with desmosomes and keratin formation, which characterize squamous differentiation, are present in more than half of the neoplasm mixed with some other pattern, both patterns should be diagnosed. Cases have been described in which a squamous cell carcinoma is mixed with neoplasms having a mesenchymal element resembling fibroadenoma (Fisher et al 1983). Squamous metaplasia within an otherwise typical mammary carcinoma of no special type is relatively common and is discussed with miscellaneous features of breast cancer (Ch. 16). The possible confusion of squamous differentiation with the presence of apocrine-like cells in carcinoma is also discussed there.

Many of the purely squamous cell carcinomas within the breast are partially or largely cystic (Hasleton et al 1978). Cystic spaces or a major cystic space may be filled with keratin debris. Other lesions acceptable as squamous cell carcinoma will have infiltrating islands of poorly differentiated cells demonstrating squamous differentiation and keratinization centrally (Shousha et al 1984). Note that the latter appearance would be readily accepted as squamous cell cancer in the lung, but in the breast would often be accepted as poorly differentiated, usual mammary carcinoma with extensive squamous metaplasia. There is no known prognostic significance available to favour one stance over the other. In any case, it is prudent to document the prominent squamous features in the reporting of such cases so that later metastases will be better understood and not assumed to come from organs more frequently birthing squamous tumours. Least often, acceptable squamous cell carcinomas of breast will be solid and uniformly have keratinizing features. Only a handful of such cases have been reported (Eggers & Chesney 1984).

Purely squamous neoplasms may rarely arise in phyllodal tumours (Cornog et al 1971; Azzopardi 1979) and spindle cell metaplastic tumours, discussed below, may often be considered as examples of squamous metaplasia.

Although Toikkanen (1981) considered pure squamous differentiation a sign of poor prognosis, Eggers & Chesney (1984) found their two cases to have good prognoses. Reported cases are too few to be definitive regarding prognosis, and it is prudent to regard both pure and mixed squamous carcinomas the same as the ordinary, intermediate to high grade carcinoma of no special type (Azzopardi 1979). Recognition of a pure acantholytic variant may indicate a poor prognosis (Eusebi et al 1986).

REFERENCES

Azzopardi J 1979 Problems in breast pathology. Saunders, Philadelphia, p 297–300
Cornog J L, Mobini J, Steiger E, Enterline H T 1971 Squamous carcinoma of the breast. Am J Clin Pathol 55: 410–417
Eggers J W, Chesney T McC 1984 Squamous cell carcinoma of the breast: a clinicopathologic analysis of eight cases and review of the literature. Hum Pathol 15: 526–531
Eusebi V, Lamovec J, Cattani M G et al 1986 Acantholytic variant of squamous cell carcinoma of the breast. Am J Surg Pathol 10: 855–861
Fisher E R, Gregorio R M, Palekar A S, Paulson J I 1983 Mucoepidermoid and squamous cell carcinomas of the breast with reference to squamous metaplasia and giant cell formation. Am J Surg Pathol 7: 15–27
Hasleton P S, Misch K A, Vasudev K S, George D 1978 Squamous carcinoma of the breast. J Clin Pathol 31: 116–124
Toikkanen S 1981 Primary squamous cell carcinoma of the breast. Cancer 48: 1629–1632
Shousha S, James A H, Fernandez M D, Bull T B 1984 Squamous cell carcinoma of the breast. Arch Pathol Lab Med 108: 893–896

SALIVARY GLAND TYPES

These very unusual patterns or types of breast carcinoma are recognized because they resemble well-accepted tumours of salivary gland origin. They are rare with less than 100 cases recorded.

Adenoid cystic carcinoma of the breast has been discussed frequently in published reports. The justification for this term rests on the histological resemblance between rare breast tumours and the classic and well-accepted adenoid cystic carcinoma of salivary glands (Perzin et al 1978). Unfortunately, the confines of definition have had to be drawn so stringently that only one in 1000 breast carcinomas may be reliably so identified (Azzopardi 1979). Stringency is necessary because of the gradual merging of the precise histology with similar histological patterns of other breast tumours. A potential source of confusion is that the prognostic implications in breast and salivary gland are disparate. The lesions in the salivary gland are characterized by a great degree of infiltrative capacity and frequently kill, despite prolonged clinical evolution (Thackray & Lucas 1974), while adenoid cystic carcinoma of the breast is associated with an excellent prognosis (Peters & Wolff 1982). The use of the same diagnostic term for such different clinical prophecies may perplex some, but the application of the term to breast tumours is well embedded in histopathological practice. The breast lesions have the same superb prognosis as lesions with a histological resemblance to the adenoid cystic pattern, presented in Chapter 13 as *invasive cribriform carcinoma*. Local metastases are unusual, and only one carefully studied case of adenoid cystic carcinoma has documented lymph node metastases (Wells et al 1986). Apparently local recurrences do not alter the favourable prognosis (Anthony & James 1975; Qizilbash et al 1977). Adenoid cystic carcinoma of the breast usually presents with a sharply defined, smoothly bordered lesion which may be painful (Jaworski et al 1983).

A diagnostic pattern of adenoid cystic carcinoma requires very crisply defined circular spaces in evenly defined, oval or pointed islands of cells (Fig. 14.8). This even definition of spaces within the islands does not allow for apical cytoplasmic protrusions into the spaces. The cells have low grade nuclei and often form narrow, delicate arches. It has further been suggested that the mucus-filled intercellular cystic spaces demonstrate neutral as well as acidic mucosubstances by special stains. While this may be true, this criterion is met in many proliferative lesions and is not a specific criterion. Two diagnostic requirements restrict the recognition of adenoid cystic carcinoma of the breast to rare examples: (1) intercellular cystic spaces lined by basement membrane material, and (2) biphasic cellularity with myoepithelial cells intermixed with another cell type (Koss et al 1970; Anthony & James 1975; Gould et al 1975). The status of hormone receptors in these tumours is not clear, but some have been negative (Zaloudek et al 1984).

Mucoepidermoid carcinoma, analogous to lesions of salivary gland, has been described in the breast. However, considering that both mucin production and squamous differentiation are so common in breast cancers, it is difficult to obtain precise limits of histological definition for this diagnosis in the breast. It is nonetheless valuable to recognize that mucin production and keratinizing cytology may coexist in breast carcinomas. This knowledge may be particularly useful in the low grade lesions which have probable, good prognosis as first reported by Patchefsky et al (1979) and supported by Fisher et al (1983). There is less utility in attempting to recognize the higher grade lesions as a special mammary tumour type. First, there is no known prognostic significance beyond that of cancers of no special type with similar cytology and, second, these high grade lesions differ from high grade mucoepidermoid carcinoma of salivary gland in having a preponderance of mucus-secreting cells relative to epidermoid components (Kovi et al 1981). Hanna & Kahn (1985) have demonstrated mixtures of mucin-secreting, squamous, intermediate and myoepithelial cells in these tumours. Note that in a setting in which one must differentiate a primary breast cancer from other possibilities, the included myoepithelial cells of these tumours are S-100 protein positive (Hanna & Kahn 1985). The S-100 protein, first described in the central nervous system, is a marker for neuroepithelial differentiation, as well as others (Kahn et al 1983).

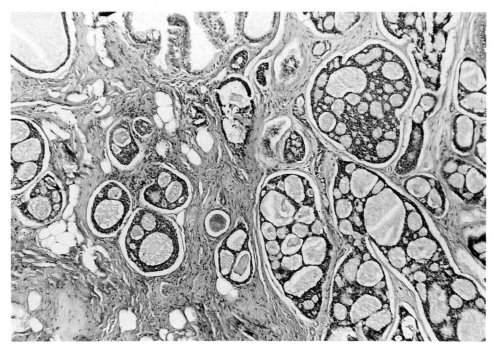

Fig. 14.8 Adenoid cystic carcinoma of breast with orderly islands of neoplastic cells containing rounded spaces filled with hyaline material (× 50).

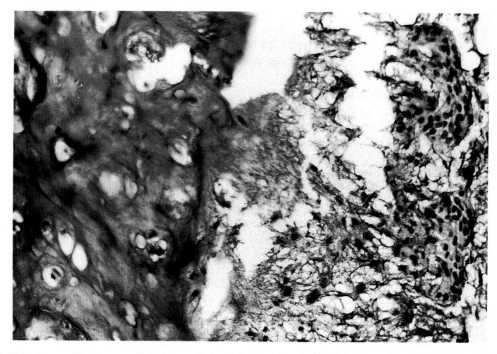

Fig. 14.9 This pleomorphic adenoma of the breast displays islands of bland epithelial cells at right and cartilage at left (× 225).

Pleomorphic adenoma or *mixed tumour* of the breast is discussed here, despite its benignancy, because of its relation to tumours classically found in the salivary glands. The salivary gland lesions are well described (Thackray & Lucas 1974), and are characterized by bosselated but sharply demarcated margins and a mixed cell population of epithelial and stromal cells (Fig. 14.9). The stroma frequently resembles cartilage. Such neoplasms are rare in the human breast with less than 20 cases reported since the seminal series of Smith & Taylor (1969). Bone formation is found in over 50% of cases (van der Walt & Rohlova 1982), a finding which is unusual in similar lesions of dogs in which the tumour type is relatively common.

Pleomorphic adenoma is relatively easily recognized histologically because of the distinctiveness of a myxoid and chondroid stroma with foci of epithelial cells. Many of these tumours have a clear intraductal component (Smith & Taylor 1969). No pleomorphic adenoma has demonstrated a malignant clinical evolution in women, and even recurrence is unusual. However, similar lesions in dogs may act in a malignant fashion when they usually demonstrate a monomorphic malignant component (Moulton 1977), so that careful histological evaluation for malignant foci is indicated.

REFERENCES

Anthony P P, James P D 1975 Adenoid cystic carcinoma of the breast: prevalence, diagnostic criteria, and histogenesis. J Clin Pathol 28: 647–655

Azzopardi J G 1979 Problems in breast pathology. Saunders, Philadelphia, p 335–339

Fisher E R, Gregorio R M, Palekar A S, Paulson J D 1983 Mucoepidermoid and squamous cell carcinomas of the breast with reference to squamous metaplasia and giant cell tumors. Am J Surg Pathol 7: 15–27

Gould V E, Miller J, Wellington J 1975 Ultrastructure of medullary, intraductal, tubular, and adenocystic breast cancers. Comparative patterns of myoepithelial differentiation and basal lamina deposition. Am J Pathol 78: 401–416

Hanna W, Kahn H J 1985 Ultrastructural and immunohistochemical characteristics of mucoepidermoid carcinoma of the breast. Hum Pathol 16: 941–946

Jaworski R C, Kneale K L, Smith R C 1983 Adenoid cystic carcinoma of the breast. Postgrad Med J 59: 48–51

Kahn H J, Marks A, Thom H, Baumal R 1983 Role of antibody to S100 protein in diagnostic pathology. Am J Clin Pathol 79: 341–347

Koss L C, Brannan C D, Ashikari R 1970 Histologic and ultrastructural features of adenoid cystic carcinoma of the breast. Cancer 26: 1271–1279

Kovi J, Duong H D, Leffall Jr L D 1981 High grade mucoepidermoid carcinoma of the breast. Arch Pathol Lab Med 105: 612–614

Moulton J E 1977 Tumors in domestic animals, 2nd edn. University of California Press, Berkeley, p 365–366

Patchefsky A S, Frauenhoffer C M, Krall R A, Cooper H S 1979 Low grade mucoepidermoid carcinoma of the breast. Arch Pathol Lab Med 103: 196–198

Perzin K H, Gullane P, Clairmont A C 1978 Adenoid cystic carcinoma arising in salivary glands. Cancer 42: 265–282

Peters G N, Wolff M 1982 Adenoid cystic carcinoma of the breast. Report of 11 new cases: review of the literature and discussion of biological behavior. Cancer 52: 680–686

Qizilbash A H, Patterson M C, Oliveira K F 1977 Adenoid cystic carcinoma of the breast. Arch Pathol Lab Med 101: 302–306

Smith B H, Taylor H B 1969 The occurrence of bone and cartilage in mammary tumors. Am J Clin Pathol 51: 610–65

Thackray A C, Lucas R B 1974 Adenoid cystic carcinoma. In: tumors of major salivary glands. Atlas of tumour pathology, second series, fascicle 10. Armed Forces Institute of Pathology, Washington, D C, p 91–99

van der Walt J D, Rohlova B 1982 Pleomorphic adenoma of the human breast. A report of a benign tumor closely mimicking a carcinoma clinically. Clin Oncol 8: 361–365

Wells C A, Nicoll S, Ferguson D J P 1986 Adenoid cystic carcinoma of the breast: a case with axillary lymph node metastasis. Histopathology 10: 415–424

Zaloudek C, Oertel Y C, Orenstein J M 1984 Adenoid cystic carcinoma of the breast. Am J Clin Pathol 81: 297–307

TUBULOLOBULAR

Background

This special type of breast carcinoma was recognized by Fisher et al (1977). Azzopardi (1979) also recognizes the presence of tubules in invasive lobular carcinoma (ILC) and records it as a variant of ILC.

Anatomical pathology

Grossly, tubulolobular carcinomas are usually firm and have irregular borders. They tend to be small, averaging less than 1 cm in diameter. Histologically, single strands of tumour cells are seen in a variable and diffuse distribution intermixed with tubular arrangements containing well-formed, central lumina (Figs 14.10 and 14.11). The other pattern of infiltration is often linear or 'targetoid' around parenchyma and arranged between collagen bundles (Fig. 14.12). Tubular elements, in situ disease and elastosis, occur as in classical tubular cancer. Nuclei are of low grade.

Differential diagnosis

These cases are easily recognized as carcinoma because of their diffusely infiltrative pattern. The mixture of single strands and tubular formations of tumour cells both defines the tumour type and immediately suggests the only relevant differential diagnostic problem: differentiation from the tubular and lobular types of invasive carcinoma. We feel that nuclear features are also important and that severely atypical nuclei should introduce doubt about inclusion in this category. We have found this to be of little practical difficulty as nuclear pleomorphism tends to be associated with poorly formed tubular formations which favour categorizing a lesion as no special type.

Clinical and prognostic features

No formal studies have yet defined the full range of clinical correlates associated with these

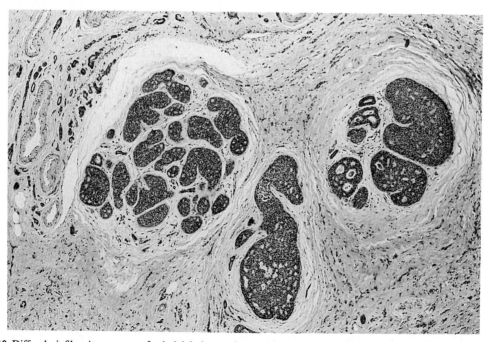

Fig. 14.10 Diffusely infiltrating pattern of tubulolobular carcinoma. Note in situ cribriform carcinoma in a duct at lower centre and lobular unit to either side of duct. Most dark cells in stroma are cancer cells, singly or in narrow file. Tubules are present at left upper area (× 50).

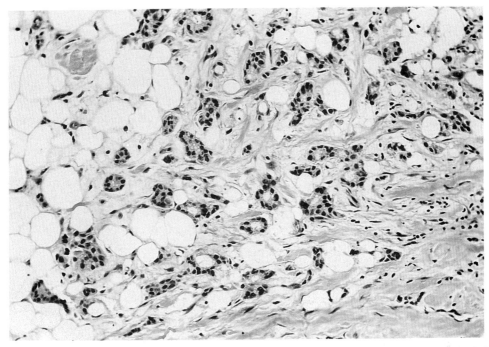

Fig. 14.11 Slightly dishevelled infiltrating tubular elements dominate in this focus of a tubulolobular carcinoma. Lobular elements with singly filed cells are present in fat at left, and elsewhere (× 200).

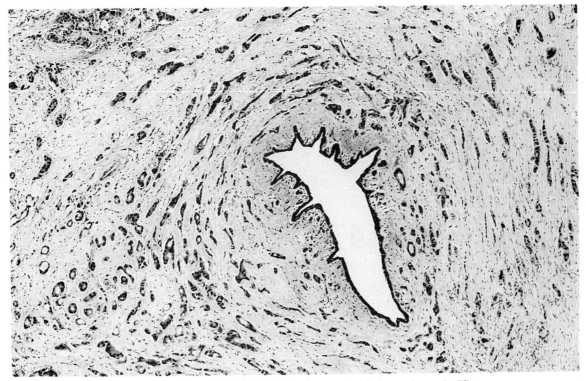

Fig. 14.12 'Targetoid' pattern of infiltration around a large duct by a tubulolobular carcinoma (× 75).

tumours. However, the difficulty of setting precise limits for their histopathological definition will probably inhibit their general acceptance as a specific carcinoma type. Using the approach of Fisher et al (1977) we identified 1% of 1000 breast carcinomas as of this type. The prognosis at 10–20 years was, in agreement with Fisher et al (1977), intermediate between that of invasive lobular and tubular carcinomas. Even though it is difficult to be enthusiastic about accepting this pattern as a special tumour type, the coexistence of two patterns of infiltration will engender difficulties in interpretation, and it is well to be forewarned that this problem exists. We recognize several different approaches to this dilemma that each have clinically relevant merit: the tumour may be placed in the no special type category and graded (usually as grade II); alternatively, it may be regarded as a variant of the tubular or lobular special types recording the variant feature. Each of these three possibilities should be amended by a comment regarding prognosis: somewhat worse than classical tubular, or somewhat better than the usual or no special type cancer.

REFERENCES

Azzopardi J 1979 Problems in breast pathology. Saunders, Philadelphia, p 243
Fisher E R, Gregorio R M, Redmond, C, Fisher B 1977 Tubulolobular invasive breast cancer: a variant of lobular invasive cancer. Hum Pathol 8: 679–683

INFLAMMATORY CARCINOMA

Inflammatory carcinoma of the breast is a clinical concept and a diagnostic term. The diagnosis is made when there is redness, oedema and warmth of the breast which contains carcinoma.

The concept of this clinical presentation, indicating a dismal prognosis, is 100 years old. However, controversy has been associated with whether anatomical demonstration of dermal lymphatic involvement by tumour is defining. At least 80% of women presenting the clinical signs of inflammatory carcinoma (about 1% of breast cancers) have demonstrable tumour emboli in dermal lymphatics. These patients represent complete, or definite examples of the entity. Questions have been raised about patients with one feature, but not the other, i.e. inflammatory signs without lymphatic tumour emboli and vice versa (Saltzstein 1974). Ellis & Teitelbaum (1974) pointed out that rare, long-term survivors with clinical signs of inflammation lacked lymphatic tumour emboli, and suggested that 'dermal lymphatic carcinomatosis of the breast' become the term and concept to replace 'inflammatory carcinoma'. This approach was strongly challenged by Lucas & Perez-Mesa (1978) who found that patients with the clinical picture alone had as poor survival as those with the inflammatory signs and histological lymphatic involvement. The familiar term and concept continues to be favoured for the clinical presentation with or without lymphatic involvement (Sherry et al 1985), although some have demanded both features (Hagelberg et al 1984)

The clinical signs of inflammation are not appreciated in the gross or microscopic examination of removed tissue, except for subtle changes of vascular dilatation and stromal oedema. The carcinoma associated with the clinical picture of inflammation is most frequently poorly differentiated, with high nuclear grade. Lymphatic involvement is discussed in Chapter 16.

Five-year survivors following a diagnosis of inflammatory carcinoma are rare, although aggressive chemotherapy improves this picture

(Sherry et al 1985). It is probable that women with either dermal involvement or inflammatory signs have a somewhat better prognosis than women with both, but this difference is slight. However, those patients with one sign without the other may be viewed differently from patients with both signs with regard to therapy, i.e. with regard to mastectomy.

Women with inflammatory carcinoma and a determinant mass may have a better prognosis than the remainder (Hagelberg et al 1984). It is also interesting that any woman with dermal oedema, usually in lower or outer quadrant without inflammation, is liable to have a worse prognosis (Shukla et al 1979).

REFERENCES

Ellis D L, Teitelbaum S L 1974 Inflammatory carcinoma of the breast: a pathologic definition. Cancer 33: 1045–1047
Hagelberg R S, Jolly P C, Anderson R P 1984 Role of surgery in the treatment of inflammatory breast carcinoma. Am J Surg 148: 115–131
Lucas F V, Perez-Mesa C 1978 Inflammatory carcinoma of the breast. Cancer 41: 1595–1605
Saltzstein S I 1974 Clinically occult inflammatory carcinoma of the breast. Cancer 34: 382–388
Sherry M M, Johnson D H, Page D L, Greco F A, Hainsworth J D 1985 Inflammatory carcinoma of the breast. Am J Med 79: 355–364
Shukla H S, Hughes L E, Gravelle I H, Satir A 1979 The significance of mammary skin edema in noninflammatory breast cancer. Ann Surg 189: 53–57

INVASIVE PAPILLARY CARCINOMA

Background and definitions

The clear separation of papillary carcinoma into invasive and non-invasive kinds has recently been championed by Fisher et al (1980), using the rich resource of the National Surgical Adjuvant Breast Project in the USA. They designated 35 of a total of 1603 cancers (2.1%) as 'invasive papillary mammary cancers', and clearly separated these cases from non-invasive papillary carcinoma. Prior to this publication, the term 'papillary carcinoma' was in common use indicating largely, but not exclusively, those lesions without stromal invasion and including cribriform and micropapillary carcinoma in situ. It is now mandatory to modify the diagnostic term 'papillary carcinoma' with the terms *invasive* or *non-invasive* (see 'Non-invasive papillary carcinoma', Ch. 12) — a requirement which we espouse.

Anatomical pathology and differential diagnosis

Gross appearances of these carcinomas are quite varied, but many are well circumscribed. Most are soft, but foci of sclerosis are frequent. Papillary formations within stroma are the defining feature, and most cases present fibrovascular cores within these formations (Fig. 14.13). Many examples have the microscopic appearances of papillary ovarian carcinomas (Fig. 14.14) or mammary mucinous tumours. In the latter instance papillary clusters float in mucin and the separation from mucinous carcinomas is arbitrary (Fisher et al 1980). Some mucin was present in approximately two-thirds of tumours in the Fisher et al series (1980). Differentiation from invasive cribriform and non-invasive cancer in deformed parenchymal units is important. Cytoplasmic characteristics are greatly varied and include well-developed apocrine appearances and apocrine-like apical protrusions. Nuclei are of intermediate or anaplastic grade. Many cases have adjacent in situ ductal carcinoma, usually of papillary or cribriform type.

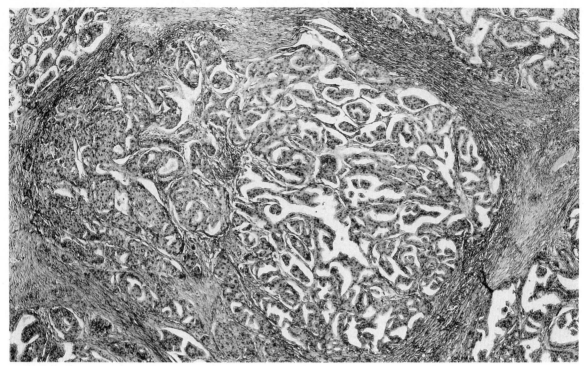

Fig. 14.13 Complex pattern of invasive breast cancer with papillary features. Focal pools of extracellular mucin are present (× 50).

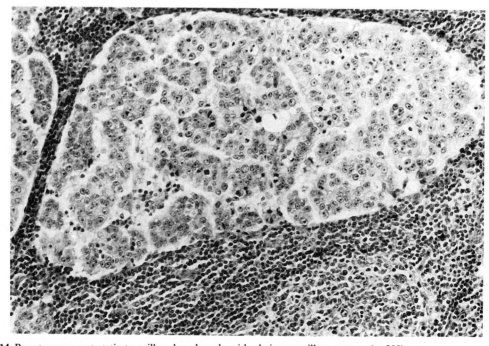

Fig. 14.14 Breast cancer metastatic to axillary lymph node with obvious papillary pattern (× 200).

Clinical correlation and prognostic considerations

Fisher et al (1980) found these cases most often in older and non-Caucasian women. Although 32% of cases with nodal dissection had nodal involvement, only 2 of 22 (9%) such cases had four or more lymph nodes with metastases. Overall, five-year disease-free survival was in the range of 90%, approximately that of mucinous carcinoma. Furthermore, only one of the total of three patients with recurrence had died of cancer; thus giving further evidence of the minimal threat to life of these lesions when treated by mastectomy.

It is not clear what the enhanced predictability of prognosis might be if these lesions were further stratified by tumour size, nuclear grade or nodal status. Such important considerations will involve the study of many more cases.

REFERENCES

Fisher E R, Palekar A S, Redmond C, Barton B, Fisher B 1980 Pathologic findings from the national surgical adjuvant breast project (protocol no. 4). VI. Invasive papillary cancer. Am J Clin Pathol 73: 313–322

CARCINOMA WITH SARCOMATOUS METAPLASIA

Most dramatic of the breast carcinomas demonstrating metaplasia are those with intermixed sarcomatous elements. These latter elements may be: (1) bone; (2) cartilage; (3) myxoid stroma; (4) loose spindle and fibromyxoid stroma; (5) dense spindle and fibrosarcomatoid stroma; and (6) anaplastic stroma with giant cell features. It is now generally accepted that these cases represent a metaplastic alteration of carcinoma cells, and this contention is supported by the ultrastructural demonstration of a sequence of change from epithelial to mesenchymal differentiation (Kaufman et al 1984) and also the retention of epithelial features in metaplastic elements (Gonzalez-Licea et al 1967). However, induction of deviant differentiation in tumour stroma as an explanation for bone and cartilage in breast cancer is espoused by some (Teisa et al 1983). It is quite possible that either event may occur.

The true rarity of these malignant tumours is highlighted by a recent series from the M.D. Anderson Hospital (Kaufman et al 1984) which reported a 0.2% incidence of carcinoma with sarcomatous metaplasia. Because patients with unusual lesions are selected for appearance in referral centres such as that one, this figure must be viewed as a maximal one. These tumours will include those which have been referred to as carcinosarcomas, and will not include malignant phyllodes tumours (see Ch. 20).

Grossly, these tumours are firm, nodular and relatively large, averaging about 5 cm in diameter. Fixation to skin and/or underlying fascia is common. Histologically, the sarcomatous element varies from 10–95% of the mass. The carcinomatous element is regularly a poorly differentiated one of no special type. The six sarcomatous elements noted above may be solitary or mixed (Figs 14.15 and 14.16). A dense spindle and fibrosarcomatous stroma, as well as bone and cartilage, are the most frequent; and these metaplastic elements usually have intrinsically malignant histological features. The loose, fibrous and myxoid elements are uncommon as the dominant

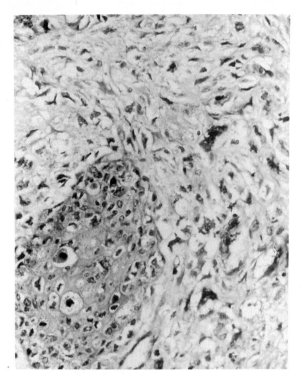

Fig. 14.15 Carcinoma with sarcomatous metaplasia. Note island of squamous cells at lower left (× 225).

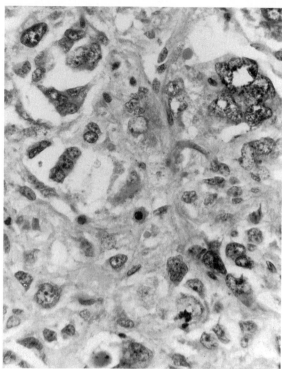

Fig. 14.16 Area of sarcomatous metaplasia in a breast cancer with giant cell features predominating (× 400).

element in these tumours. An anaplastic sarcomatous pattern with giant cells dominated in only one of Kaufman et al's 26 cases (1984), and differs from the stromal giant cell pattern described below (see Ch. 16). Frequently an undifferentiated element (not recognizable as epithelial or mesenchymal) is interposed between foci of carcinoma and heterologous mesenchymal elements such as cartilage or bone.

Prognosis is related to several definable elements but is considerably worse, controlled for clinical stage, than usual breast cancers. Larger tumours have a poorer prognosis. Most defining is the predominance of epithelial v. sarcomatous elements. Women with predominantly epithelial tumours had a 62% five-year actuarial survival, while those with predominantly sarcomatous malignancies had only a 28% survival experience (Kaufman et al 1984). Nodal metastases, present in only 25% of cases in this recent series, have no

influence or prognostication. Smith & Taylor (1969) reported a 38% five-year survival in patients with osseous and cartilaginous metaplasia in carcinoma. While regional metastases are regularly epithelial, distant metastases may have any combination of elements, pure or mixed.

REFERENCES

Gonzalez-Licea A, Yardley J H, Hartmann W H 1967 Malignant tumour of the breast with bone formation studies of light and electron microscopy. Cancer 20: 1234–1247

Kaufman M W, Maerti J R, Gallager H S, Hoehn J I 1984 Carcinoma of the breast with pseudosarcomatous metaplasia. Cancer 53: 1908–1917

Smith B H, Taylor H B 1969 The occurrence of bone and cartilage in mammary tumours. Am J Clin Pathol 51: 610–618

Teisa A N, Grathwohl M, Frable W J 1984 Breast carcinoma with osseous metaplasia: an electron microscopic study. Am J Clin Pathol 81: 127–132

CARCINOMA WITH SPINDLE CELL METAPLASIA

Well-documented examples of this unusual entity number less than 50 (Bauer, et al 1984). The dominant feature of these cases is the presence of a spindle cell 'pseudosarcomatous' stroma and, frequently, a population of squamous carcinoma. Regions of squamous carcinoma tend to be surrounded by a striking spindle cell population of cells which are usually relatively bland in appearance and often have a storiform pattern suggestive of fibrous histiocytoma (Figs 14.17 and 14.18). Occasionally, squamous or undifferentiated carcinoma cells or small groups may be found in the spindled areas. These lesions are analogous to similar tumours of the head and neck (Bauer et al 1984). The squamous features of spindle cells have been demonstrated by electron microscopy (Battifora 1976; Gersell & Katzenstein 1981).

There is no indication currently that these unusual tumours differ in gross presentation or in prognostic implication from usual breast carcinomas of intermediate malignancy (Bauer et al 1984). It is important to note that upon occasion the squamous element may be inapparent, and differentiation of these tumours from sarcomas can be difficult and may necessitate special studies by immunocytochemistry and ultrastructural analysis.

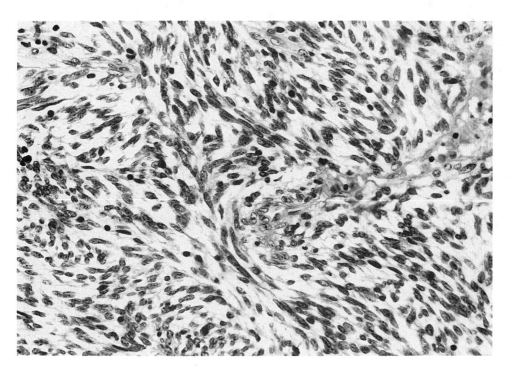

Fig. 14.17 Spindle cell metaplasia in a breast cancer. Note intersecting bundles of spindled cells. Carcinoma elements were rare in this example (× 300).

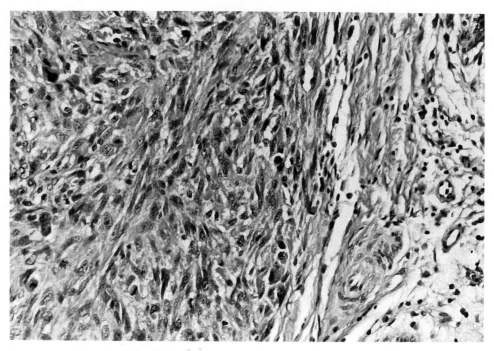

Fig. 14.18 Spindle cell metaplasia with somewhat more atypical nuclei than Figure 14.17. Note occasional somewhat rounded cells, resembling epithelial cells (× 300).

REFERENCES

Bauer T W, Rostock R A, Eggleston J C, Baral E 1984
Spindle cell carcinoma of the breast: four cases and review
of the literature. Hum Pathol 15: 147–152

Battifora H 1976 Spindle cell carcinoma. Cancer
37: 2275–2282
Gersell D J, Katzenstein A A 1981 Spindle cell carcinoma of
the breast: a clinicopathologic and ultrastructural study.
Hum Pathol 12: 550–560

Rare patterns of invasive carcinoma

The patterns of carcinoma discussed in this chapter are not regarded as integrated disease entities. Many of these patterns or features have been proposed as types of breast carcinoma, but none is associated with adequate knowledge concerning incidence, prognosis and even histological confines to be accepted as specific disease entities. In general, we feel that the profusion of different 'types' of breast tumours has been confusing and has led to feelings on the part of many that these fine distinctions lack relevance. This has fostered the diagnosis of invasive ductal carcinoma of no special type as a way to escape from the conflict as to which of many subtypes are to be diagnosed. Consequently, the clinical significance of many of these diagnoses is unclear. Whilst there is undoubted validity in the recognition of histopathological patterns discussed in this chapter, we do not issue clinical reports specifying these types (or proposed types) without detailing the information available concerning them. Rather, the identification of features discussed in this chapter may be noted as ancillary, i.e. existing within another cancer type which has known clinical prognostic relevance. Nothing, however, is so clear cut in the nosology of unusual breast cancer patterns. The reader will discover below that we suggest signet ring carcinoma may be diagnosed when the pattern is prominent. Unfortunately we must accept the fact that just how prominent, qualitatively or quantitatively, the feature must be to guarantee a profoundly unfavourable prognosis, is unknown. So also with cystic carcinomas, which have relevant clinical correlates, but their association with varied cancer types necessitates that the diagnostic term must not stand alone without further specification.

SIGNET RING CARCINOMA

Prominent presence of signet ring cells in breast carcinomas is a rare but important phenomenon. This importance derives from: (1) possible misinterpretation of metastatic deposits as a primary lesion of the organ to which such cancers may metastasize (particularly the stomach) and, (2) prominent signet ring cytology in a breast cancer indicates a high likelihood of metastasis.

Grossly, lesions with prominent signet ring cells are often poorly defined and diffusely infiltrative. Histologically, the confines of definition of signet ring carcinoma have varied. Hull et al (1980), following the approach of Steinbrecher & Silverberg (1976), accepted cases with discrete, mucicarminophilic, or PAS-positive, diastase-resistant cytoplastic vacuoles in the cytoplasm when present with more than 20 neoplastic cells containing these vacuoles per high power field. They found 24 examples (4%) in 535 cases of surgically treated breast cancer. Merino & Li Volsi (1981) found 2% of breast cancers to qualify for their stricter criteria in a larger series of breast cancers. Most of these cases produced firm, solid masses and they accepted cases if clear, vacuolated cytoplasm and a compressed nucleus were elements comprising at least 20% of the tumour. They included Alcian blue positivity as well as the two stains noted above. They found a marked overlap with infiltrating lobular carcinoma and 46% of their cases had lobular carcinoma in situ also. In a review of 1050 breast cancers from Edinburgh, we found two examples of pure signet ring cell carcinoma with compressed nucleus and a central clear vacuole largely filling the cytoplasm present in over 90% of cells. However defined, both the series of Hull et al (1979) and the series of Merino & LiVolsi (1981) demonstrated poor prognosis in lesions in which signet ring cells were prominent.

The overlap with patterns of infiltrating lobular carcinoma will present difficulties in differential diagnosis as many of these latter cases present small cytoplasmic vacuoles (see Ch. 13). These are crisply defined and although they may displace the nucleus to one side of the cell when large, they do not usually indent the nucleus. These small vacuoles of lobular carcinoma stain deeply for mucin materials at their margins corresponding to the glycocalyx of the limiting membranes which resemble cell luminal borders by ultrastructure. The larger mucin globules of signet ring cancer cells may stain uniformly for mucin and are often less sharply demarcated at the edges than intra-cytoplasmic lumina (Battifora 1975). Although precise separation of intracytoplasmic lumina from

globules of membrane-bound mucin material in the cytoplasm by light microscopy cannot be accomplished, it is clear that in many of the marked examples of signet ring change, when the nucleus is actually compressed, that the cytoplasm is largely filled with membrane-bound mucin material rather than intracytoplasmic lumina (Harris et al 1978; Al-Hariri 1980). We feel that very few breast cancers will qualify for the primary diagnostic term of 'signet ring carcinoma', but that any carcinoma with pronounced cytoplasmic mucin globules, particularly if the nuclei are often indented, should be noted to have signet ring features. Most of these cases with either predominant or marked signet ring elements will have the diffuse pattern of invasion with non-cohesive cells so characteristic of infiltrating lobular carcinoma (Fig. 15.1), and should have that as the primary diagnosis. However, some cases with marked cytoplasmic vacuolization and even nuclear compression will have pronounced packeting of tumour cells indicating a primary

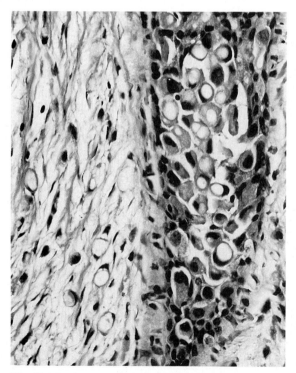

Fig. 15.1 In situ carcinoma with signet ring cytology is present in well-defined area at right. This is mirrored in a diffuse infiltration of frequently similar cells in stroma (× 500).

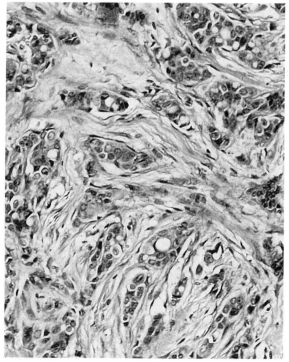

Fig. 15.2 Breast carcinoma of no special type with occasional signet ring cells (× 225).

Fig. 15.3 Only occasional cells suggest signet ring cytology in this carcinoma of no special type, poorly differentiated (× 800).

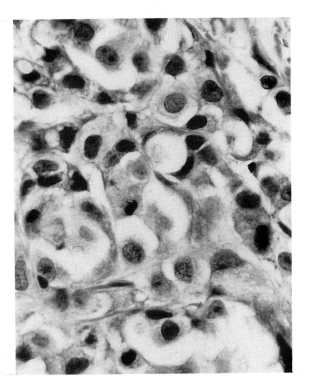

diagnosis of no special type cancer (Figs 15.2–15.4) or pleomorphic infiltrating lobular carcinoma (Fig. 15.5).

A predominant presence of signet ring cells in breast cancer is associated with a poor prognosis, as documented by Hull et al (1980) who found development of distant metastases in all four of their patients with a predominant signet ring cell pattern. This poor prognostic experience was mirrored in the study of Merino & LiVolsi (1981) who also demonstrated an unusual metastatic pattern for these carcinomas with a propensity to involve the gastrointestinal tract and serosal surfaces. There was also a tendency for this serosal infiltration to extend so that ureters might be blocked in a pattern similar to that of retro-peritoneal fibrosis without the formation of a domi-nant mass (see Ch. 19). Metastases of mammary

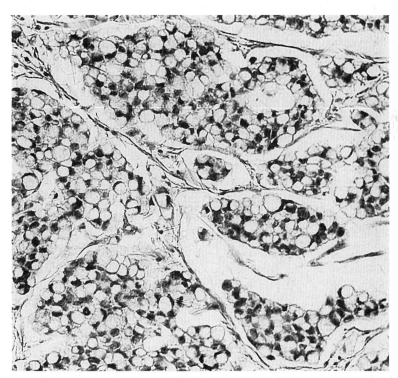

Fig. 15.4 Dominant signet ring cytological features in a tumour suggesting mucinous type because clear intercellular regions separating islands from stroma are mucus. Without extracellular mucus and with more irregular mucin collections, secretory cancer would be suggested (× 225).

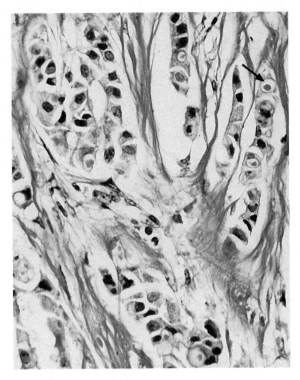

Fig. 15.5 Exemplifying the problem of overlapping features, this carcinoma of no special type has cytoplasmic vacuoles with central staining (arrow) indicating intracytoplasmic lumina of lobular carcinoma. Signet ring cytology is also suggested. Pleomorphic lobular carcinoma could also be diagnosed (× 450).

cancer with signet ring cells can present in a submucosal location in the stomach (Kondo et al 1984) and bladder, presenting obvious differential diagnostic problems.

REFERENCES

Al-Hariri J A 1980 Primary signet ring cell carcinoma of the breast. Virchows Arch (A) 388: 105–111
Battifora H 1975 Intracytoplasmic lumina in breast carcinoma. Arch Pathol 99: 614–617
Harris M, Vasudev K S, Anfield C, Wells S 1978 Mucin-producing carcinomas of the breast: ultrastructural observations. Histopathology 2: 177–188
Hull M T, Seo I S, Battersby J S, Csicski J F 1980 Signet-ring cell carcinoma of the breast: a clinicopathologic study of 24 cases. Am J Clin Pathol 73: 31–35
Kondo Y, Akita T, Sugano I, Isono K 1984 Signet ring cell carcinoma of the breast. Acta Pathol Jpn 34: 875–880
Merino M J, LiVolsi V A 1981 Signet ring carcinoma of the female breast: a clinicopathologic analysis of 24 cases. Cancer 48: 1830–1837
Steinbrecher J S, Silverberg S G 1976 Signet ring cell carcinoma of the breast. Cancer 37: 828–840

LIPID RICH

The production of fat, a major component of milk, is an obvious capability of breast epithelium. Therefore, the presence in breast cancers of a foamy, lipid-rich cytoplasm resembling that of lactation is no more surprising than the finding of other milk products.

Histologically, such lesions have predominantly clear cytoplasm, foamy or diffusely vacuolated, in which neutral lipid may be documented by the oil red O stain in undehydrated tissue. The nuclei are usually markedly irregular and atypical, and the histological pattern is usually poorly formed without glandular formations or regular orientations of cellular groups (Fisher et al 1977). The stroma is scant and loose.

Unlike van Bogaert & Maldague (1977), who sought specific morphological patterns and then documented the presence of neutral lipids, Fisher et al (1977) examined 87 consecutive breast cancers for the occurrence of these substances. Their study revealed that 30% of the tumours possessed moderate to marked amounts of neutral lipid. Furthermore, strikingly positive staining for lipids was identified in 6% of all cases, and these lesions demonstrated no particular histological pattern.

As this feature is present in tumours of many different histological patterns, and its definition requires use of staining for neutral lipid, this presence of extensive cytoplasmic lipid cannot be recommended as establishing a definite type of breast carcinoma. The presence of extensive cytoplasmic lipid may be a useful histological discriminant in identifying tumours with poor prognosis (Azzopardi 1979), but as the nuclear and histological features are also markedly anaplastic, these elements are as prognostically useful as is the presence of lipid. Thus breast carcinomas with a striking amount of cytoplasmic lipid are usually of high grade, and there is no evidence that the presence of cytoplasmic lipid adds to the poor prognostic implication recognized by grading.

REFERENCES

Azzopardi J C 1979 Problems in breast pathology. Saunders, Philadelphia, p 301–305

Fisher E R, Gregorio R, Kim W S, Redmond C 1977 Lipid in invasive cancer of the breast. Am J Clin Pathol 68: 558–561

van Bogaert L J, Maldague P 1977 Histologic variants of lipid secreting carcinoma of the breast. Virchows Arch (A) 375: 345–353

CLEAR CELL

Breast carcinomas do not have the expanded, clear cytoplasm with haematoxylin and eosin stains which is characteristic of clear cell carcinomas of the kidney. However, many cases have some cells with cytoplasm that is largely clear (Figs 15.6 and 15.7). These clear areas may be stainable as mucin, fat or glycogen. Clear areas may also not be stainable for these elements.

Mucosubstance staining is discussed with infiltrating lobular carcinoma and signet ring patterns. Mucin may also be found in cancers of no special type in which it is usually focal and has no known association with histological grade or prognosis. Mucin positivity may be demonstrated by any of the stains for mucosubstances.

Intracellular fat, as either a dominant or a minor histological feature in breast cancer, is discussed in lipid-rich pattern.

Glycogen as the basis for clear areas in cytoplasm of carcinomas is relatively uncommon and of no diagnostic or prognostic significance. Foraker (1956) found glycogen most commonly in benign lesions; however, some may also be found in many carcinomas. Therefore its absence or presence is of no defining or clinical significance. Foci of squamous metaplasia often contain cytoplasmic glycogen as defined by diastase-labile PAS positivity.

Mention should be made of two possibly unique case reports of breast neoplasms with clear cytoplasm containing glycogen as a dominant feature. One was largely papillary and resembled fetal breast (Hull et al 1981) and the other was more solid, but also had thin fibrous septae separating sheets of tumour cells (Benisch et al 1983). Neither tumour had axillary nodal metastases nor staining positivity for mucosubstances or fat. A very orderly growth pattern and little invasive tendency would identify each as of little biological aggressiveness, particularly in the case of Hull et al (1981) in whom the mass had been slowly enlarging for 20 years. Fisher et al (1985) have commented that this case appears analogous to benign, eccrine-related mammary neoplasms. The tumour with a more solid growth pattern

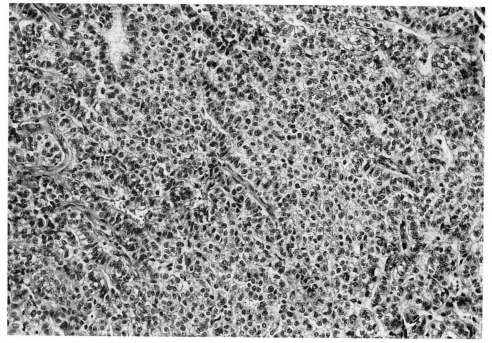

Fig. 15.6 Orderly pattern and low grade nuclei predict a good prognosis for this breast cancer. Clear cytoplasm which contains glycogen may be considered a secondary feature (× 200).

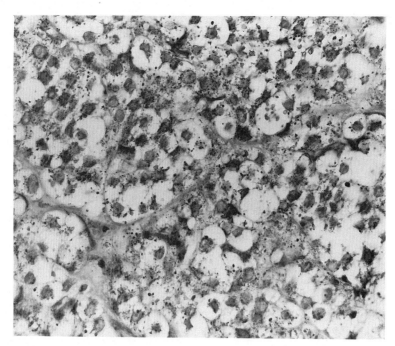

Fig. 15.7 Dark cytoplasmic granules are PAS positive, and were removed by diastase. Thus this is a clear cell pattern of a no special type cancer which contains glycogen (× 400).

resembled the myoepithelial tumours which are also of low malignant potential and rich in glycogen.

Fisher et al (1985) have reported a 3% incidence of breast carcinomas with over 50% of cells containing optically clear cytoplasm and, usually, a centrally placed nucleus. PAS positivity, removed by diastase, proved the presence of glycogen in each case. There was no favoured association with any histological type and only a mild association with higher grade neoplasms and nodal metastases. They concluded that clear cell cytological features were variants of well-established histological types of breast cancer and lacked significant independent influence on survival. It is evident that neither clear cytoplasm nor cytoplasmic glycogen may be used as determinants of tumour classification in the breast.

REFERENCES

Benisch B, Peison B, Newman R, Sobel H J, Marquet E 1983 Solid glycogen-rich clear cell carcinoma of the breast. Am J Clin Pathol 79: 243–245

Fisher E R, Tavares J, Bulatao I S et al 1985 Glycogen-rich, clear cell breast cancer: with comments concerning other clear cell variants. Hum Pathol 16: 1085–1090

Foraker A G 1956 A histochemical study of breast carcinoma. Surg Gynecol Obstet 102: 1–8

Hull M T, Priest J B, Broadie T A, Ransburg R C, McCarthy L J 1981 Glycogen-rich clear cell carcinoma of the breast. Cancer 48: 2003–2009

MYOEPITHELIOMA

Spindle cell neoplasms with mixed myoid and epithelial differentiation are rare indeed, with seven well-documented cases recorded (Thorner et al 1986; Bigotti & DiGiorgio 1986). They are potentially malignant with lymph nodal metastases reported in two cases, but distant metastases remain to be noted.

Glandular elements attesting to epithelial differentiation may be present, surrounded by spindled myoepithelial cells, often with nodules of pure myoepithelial cells (Toth 1977). One remarkable case (Fig. 15.8) only had pure nodules of myoid cells in a local recurrence (Cameron et al 1974). This experience indicates that malignant behaviour may develop in any of these tumours, but that complete removal of the more orderly examples should be curative.

Histologically, the neoplastic myoepithelial element resembles leiomyoma or leiomyosarcoma with bundles of often interlacing spindled cells. Cytoplasm is at least focally eosinophilic and may appear filamentous even by light microscopy. Although these lesions may probably be reliably identified by light microscopy, electron microscopy and immunocytochemistry for actin and cytokeratin are defining (Thorner et al 1986). Note that although these special studies may show mixed differentiation in many breast neoplasms (keratin indicating epithelial, and actin marking myoid), it is only when smooth muscle differentiation and growth pattern are dominant over purely epithelial that the diagnosis of myoepithelioma is appropriate. Resemblance to similar tumours of salivary glands was noted by Zarbo & Oberman (1983).

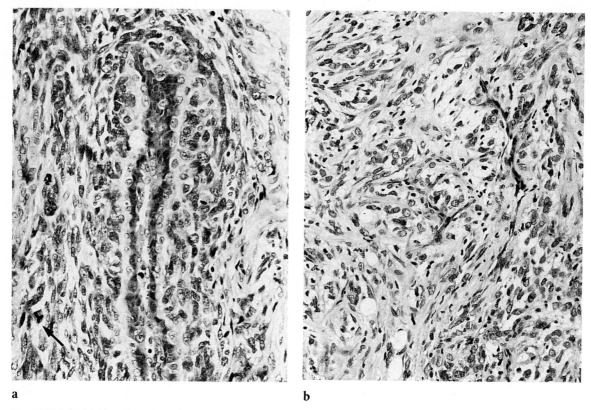

a   b

Fig. 15.8(a) Initial biopsy showing longitudinally cut duct, surrounded by spindle-shaped cells blending with stromal cells and exhibiting variable nuclear morphology. Note tripolar mitosis (arrow). (**b**) Recurrence at 18 months with leiomyosarcomatous features and effacement of epithelial structures (**a** × 180; **b** × 160). (Courtesy Dr H. Cameron.)

REFERENCES

Bigotti G, DiGiorgio C G 1986 Myoepithelioma of the breast: histologic, imunologic, and electronmicroscopic appearance. J Surg Oncol 32: 58–64

Cameron H M, Hamperl H, Warambo W 1974 Leiomyosarcoma of the breast originating from myothelium (myoepithelium). J Pathol 114: 89–92

Thorner P S, Kahn H J, Baumal R, Lee K, Moffatt W 1986 Malignant myoepithelioma of the breast. An immunohistochemical study by light and electron microscopy. Cancer 57: 745–750

Toth J 1977 Benign human mammary myoepithelioma. Virchows Arch (A) 374: 263–269

Zarbo R J, Oberman H A 1983 Cellular adenomyoepithelioma of the breast. Am J Surg Pathol 7: 863–870

CARCINOID FEATURES

Terminology and historical development

Feyrter & Hartmann (1963) reported the first examples of breast tissue which morphologically resembled carcinoid tumours of the intestine. Several authors have since reported carcinoid tumours of the breast but because of inconsistent definition and because the various studies present a relatively small sample size, controversy has arisen over terminology.

Traditionally, pathologists diagnosed typical carcinoids on the basis of histological pattern, nuclear morphology, stromal characteristics and demonstration of cytoplasmic granules by histochemical or ultrastructural techniques. However, identification of composite tumours possessing both typical carcinoid and non-carcinoid neoplastic elements, together with the growing realization that non-carcinoid tumours may produce neurosecretory type granules and contain numerous endocrine-like cells, led to complexity and confusion over the question of what characteristics warrant a diagnosis of carcinoid tumour. The classical descriptions of intestinal carcinoids (Williams & Sandler 1963; Soga & Tazawa 1971) identify nodular, trabecular and glandular patterns with uniformity of cell type, but leave latitude for interpretation, and also comment on the highly vascularized fibrous stroma. Functional properties were defined according to histochemistry (silver impregnation), electron microscopy, biochemistry and clinical manifestations.

Over the past 10 years, beginning with Cubilla & Woodruff (1977), there have been several reports of breast tumours with carcinoid characteristics, but opinions have differed in their interpretation either as variants of conventional breast cancer (Taxy et al 1981) or as distinctive lesions with specific morphological and immunocytochemical features (Cross et al 1985). In accordance with Pearse's theory of a diffuse endocrine system (Pearse 1969) such endocrine cells were believed to migrate to various epithelial tissues from the embryological neural crest. Whilst there is ample evidence of these endocrine cells in the intestinal epithelium, the natural presence of similar cells in normal mammary duct epithelium is a question still to be resolved, although evidence for this has been published (Bussolati et al 1985). Indeed, mucoid tumours of breast were the earliest types to be associated with carcinoid features (Fisher et al 1979; Capella et al 1980) because argyrophilia and ultrastructural dense core granule features were presented as proof of carcinoid nature and histogenesis. However, these proposals have not been uniformly accepted. Neither, it must be added, has an alternative explanation that such granules contain lactalbumin (Clayton et al 1982) been generally acknowledged or verified. Indeed, such immunoreactivity has been reported to be related to a contaminant (Bussolati et al 1987). Furthermore, the inconsistency in that series of 20 cases in reaction for argyrophilia and of immunocytochemical markers for endocrine differentiation (including chromogranin) is a further inhibition to accepting this evidence as support for the occurrence of true carcinoids of the breast. The finding of typical dense core granules in a broad range of breast tissues (Ferguson & Anderson 1985) has been a further obstacle to definition of the characteristics of breast carcinoids.

Another approach to account for these observations in breast tumours is that cells with histochemical and ultrastructural features of carcinoids could emerge as part of the neoplastic transformation. This would involve deregulation of gene sequences responsible for neuroendocrine function, and evidence for this has been presented (Vuitch & Mendelsohn 1981; Woodward et al 1981). The problem of identifying tumours with carcinoid characteristics is not confined to the breast and a practical approach to the terminology of such tumours in all situations has been given by DeLellis et al (1984). An excellent discussion of the situation is provided, with emphasis on the hormone profile identification by immunohistochemistry as an aid to improved classification. However, present indications are that this will prove difficult in the breast (Bussolati et al 1985; Nesland et al 1986). The issue of breast carcinoids is likely to remain controversial despite current appreciation of the wide latitude of cellular differentiation within tumours (Gould 1986).

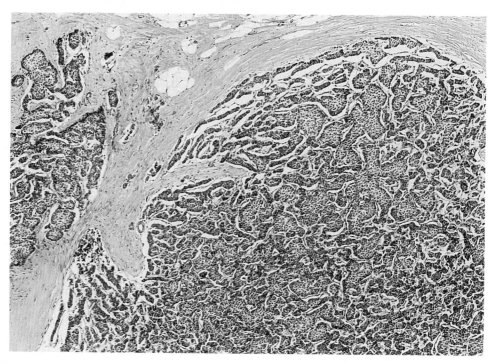

Fig. 15.9 Small islands of breast cancer cells have apparent palisading of peripheral cells simulating a carcinoid tumour (× 60).

Anatomical pathology

Tumours of the breast with carcinoid features usually present as well-circumscribed, non-encapsulated masses. The lesions range from 1–4 cm in greatest dimension, with the average being approximately 2 cm (Cubilla & Woodruff 1977). These tan tumours generally possess a firm, rubbery texture and a solid, cut surface, although a cystic appearance has been described.

Microscopically, breast carcinoids, by definition, demonstrate features classically associated with carcinoids derived from the primitive gut. The histological pattern represents the most obvious clue to the diagnosis; patterns identified include nests of cells (Figs 15.9 and 15.10), cords of cells, acinar arrangement of cells, and mixtures of these patterns. On haematoxylin and eosin stained sections, these tumours possess a uniform population of cells having pale, eosinophilic cytoplasm and round or oval nuclei. These nuclei contain one or two small nucleoli and demonstrate a finely stippled chromatin. The cells reside in a characteristic fibrovascular stroma. These three features — morphological pattern, cytological detail and stromal characteristics — are most useful in evaluating the possibility of a breast carcinoid at the time of frozen section. If a frozen section of a breast lesion illustrates these characteristics, a sample of the mass should be fixed for diagnostic electron microscopy, and histochemistry for endocrine differentiation carried out. In this regard, formalin fixatives are not optimal, improvements being gained with Bouin's fixation. The Grimelius argyrophil method (Grimelius 1968) is most commonly used (Fig. 15.11) but a modification of this (Churukian & Schenk 1979) is claimed to give superior results (Smith & Haggitt 1983). Immunohistochemical identification of hormone products has proved difficult (Bussolati et al 1985; Nesland et al 1986) but attempts to do so are to be encouraged.

The reporting of such breast tumours can be guided by the proportion of the lesion with the carcinoid characteristics. When these occur in more than 50% of a well-sampled tumour, which also has non-carcinoid areas, then the term carci-

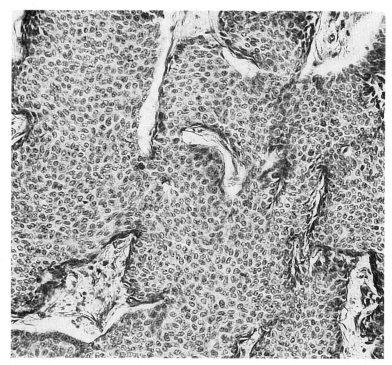

Fig. 15.10 Broad islands of quite uniform infiltrating cancer cells in a primary breast cancer mimic a carcinoid tumour (× 225).

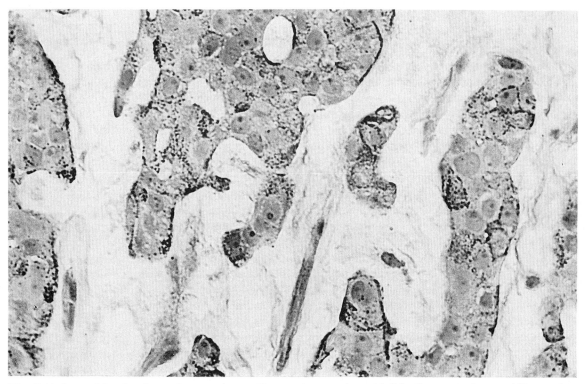

Fig. 15.11 Argyrophil stain of a mucinous carcinoma. Note mucin separating epithelial cell groups and argyrophilic granules in cytoplasm. Obviously, argyrophil positivity cannot be accepted as defining of carcinoid tumours in the breast (× 800).

noid is appropriate with the qualification of a non-carcinoid component suitably described. When the carcinoid features affect less than half then the tumour should be diagnosed according to the predominant characteristics, with a note that the carcinoid component was also identified. Possession of argyrophilia or abundance of ultrastructural neurosecretory granules alone is not adequate grounds to designate a tumour as carcinoid whilst the significance of these features is presently not known.

Differential diagnosis

The differential diagnosis of a primary breast tumour with carcinoid features primarily includes medullary carcinoma, mucinous carcinoma and lobular carcinoma; metastasis from a carcinoid involving another organ also has to be considered. It must also be remembered that each of these primary breast tumours probably has the potential to coexist with carcinoid elements, a fact which necessitates, as discussed above, a descriptive diagnosis of the relative proportions of each histological type identified. It is thus apparent that attention to light microscopic criteria of the tumours included in the differential diagnosis may help rule out the presence of a breast carcinoid. For example, medullary carcinoma usually exhibits a low power morphological similarity yet, at higher power, the cells tend to possess more pleomorphism, coarser clumping of nuclear chromatin, and more prominent nucleoli than the cells of carcinoid tumours. Also, the distinct lymphocytic and plasmacellular infiltrate and loose stromal elements of medullary carcinomas present a clear contrast to the minimal inflammatory response and prominent fibrovascular stroma of carcinoids.

The diagnosis of a mucinous variety of carcinoid is now less likely in view of the awareness that argyrophilia and dense core granule content are not unusual characteristics of mucinous carcinomas (Ferguson et al 1986); argyrophilia has also been reported in 25% of an unselected series of carcinomas, occurring not only in mucinous, but also tubular and those of no special type histology (McCutcheon & Walker, 1987). It is thus apparent

that the pathologist must interpret the results of silver stains and of electron microscopy applied to mucinous tumours with some degree of caution.

Because of its tendency to grow in circumscribed nests and bundles and because of its monomorphic cell population characterized by bland nuclei, lobular carcinoma in situ may resemble breast carcinoid. Invasive lobular carcinomas may possess histochemical and ultrastructural features suggesting carcinoids (Taxy et al 1981; Nesland et al 1986). However, the typical carcinoid fibrovascular stroma is lacking and the pattern of single cell and peri-parenchymal infiltration in multiple diffuse foci will usually allow the pathologist to identify the carcinoma type correctly.

Metastatic carcinoid may occasionally present as a primary breast lesion (Warner & Seo 1980), and the pathologist may not have the clinical data needed in order to make this decision. To distinguish between a primary breast cancer with carcinoid features and a metastatic lesion, one must obviously conduct a thorough search of the gastrointestinal tract and lung in order to rule out primary lesions in these areas (Ahlman et al 1986).

Clinical features and prognosis

Breast 'carcinoids' possess no clinical features to distinguish them from other mammary carcinomas (Cubilla & Woodruff 1977; Chen 1981; Azzopardi et al 1982; Nesland et al 1985). The currently available data indicates that these lesions present clinically and behave biologically as other primary breast carcinomas of no special type. Generally, the patient presents with a painless breast mass at an average age (54 years) similar to that for routine breast cancers (Cubilla & Woodruff 1977). These facts suggest that therapy decisions should conform to those recommended for other mammary carcinomas, including the nature of oestrogen responsiveness (Cubilla & Woodruff 1977; Woodward et al 1981).

Comments on prognosis are not presently appropriate, but must await improved understanding of the significance of carcinoid features occurring in breast tumours. Inconsistencies in the use of the term carcinoid will only serve to confuse both the diagnostic pathologist and the clinician, but can be avoided if the guidelines above are followed.

REFERENCES

Ahlman H, Larsson I, Gronstad K et al 1986 A case of midgut carcinoid with breast metastasis and cellular localization of serotonin and substance. P J Surg Oncol 31: 170–173

Azzopardi J, Muretto P, Goddeeris V, Lauweryns J 1982 Carcinoid tumours of the breast: the morphological spectrum of argyrophil carcinomas. Histopathology 6: 549–569

Bussolati G, Gugliotta P, Sapino A, Eusebi V, Lloyd R V 1985 Chromogramin-reactive endocrine cells in argyrophilic carcinomas ('carcinoids') and normal tissue of the breast. Am J Pathol 120: 186–192

Bussolati G, Papotti M, Sapino A et al 1987 Endocrine markers in argyrophilic carcinomas of the breast. Am J Surg Pathol 11: 248–256

Capella C, Eusebi V, Mann B, Azzopardi J G 1980 Endocrine differentiation in mucoid carcinoma of the breast. Histopathology 4: 613–630

Chen K T K 1981 Breast carcinomas with carcinoid features. Breast 7: 2–5

Churukian C J, Schenk E A 1979 A modification of Pascual's argyrophil method. J Histotechnol 2: 102–103

Clayton F, Ordonez N G, Sibley P K, Haussen G 1982 Argyrophilic breast carcinomas. Evidence of lactational differentiation. Am J Surg Pathol 6: 323–333

Cross A S, Azzopardi J G, Krausz T, Van Noorden S, Polak J M 1985 A morphological and immunocytochemical study of a distinctive variant of ductal carcinoma in situ of the breast. Histopathology 9: 21–37

Cubilla A L, Woodruff J M 1977 Primary carcinoid tumour of the breast. A report of eight patients. Am J Surg Pathol 1: 283–292

DeLellis R, Dayal Y, Wolfe H 1984 Carcinoid tumors: changing concepts and new perspectives. Am J Surg Pathol 8: 295–300

Ferguson D J P, Anderson T J 1985 Distribution of dense core granules in normal, benign and malignant breast tissue. J Pathol 147: 59–65

Ferguson D J P, Anderson T J, Wells C, Battersby S 1986 An ultrastructural study of mucoid carcinoma of the breast. Histopathology 10: 1219–1230

Feyrter F, Hartmann G 1963 Uber die carcinoide Wuchsform des carcinoma mammae, insbesondere das carcinoma solidum (gelatinosum) mammae. Frankf Z Pathol 73: 24–35

Fisher E R, Palekar A S and NSABP collaborators 1979 Solid and mucinous varieties of so-called mammary carcinoid tumour. Am J Clin Pathol 72: 909–916

Gould V E 1986 Histogenesis and differentiation: a re-evaluation of these concepts as criteria for the classification of tumours. Hum Pathol 17: 212–215

Grimelius L 1968 A silver nitrate stain for alpha-2 cells in human pancreatic islets. Acta Soc Med (Upsala) 73:243

McCutchson J, Walker R A 1987 The significance of argyrophilia in human breast carcinomas. Virch Arch (A) 410: 369–374

Nesland J M, Menoli V A, Holm R, Gould V E, Johannessen J V 1985 Breast carcinomas with neuroendocrine differentiation. Ultrastruct Pathol 8: 225–240

Nesland J M, Holm R, Johannessen J V, Gould V E 1986 Neurone specific enolase immunostaining in the diagnosis of breast carcinomas with neuroendocrine differentiation. Its usefulness and limitations. J Pathol 148: 35–43

Pearse A G E 1969 The cytochemistry and ultrastructure of polypeptide hormone-producing cells of the APUD series and the embryologic, physiologic and pathologic implications of the concept. J Histochem Cytochem 17: 303–313

Smith D M Jr, Haggitt R C 1983 A comparative study of generic stains for carcinoid secretory granules. Am J Surg Pathol 7: 61–68

Soga J, Tazawa K 1971 Pathologic analysis of carcinoids. Cancer 28: 990–998

Taxy J B, Tischler A S, Insalaco S J, Battifora H 1981 Carcinoid tumor of the breast: a variant of conventional breast cancer. Hum Pathol 12: 170–179

Vuitch M F, Mendelsohn G 1981 Relationship of ectopic ACTH production of tumor differentiation. A morphologic and immunohistochemical study of prostatic carcinoma with Cushing's syndrome. Cancer 47: 296–299

Warner T, Seo I S 1980 Bronchial carcinoid appearing as a breast mass. Arch Pathol Lab Med 104: 531–534

Williams E D, Sandler M 1963 The classification of carcinoid tumors. Lancet 1: 238–239

Woodward B H, Eisenbarth G, Wallace N R, Mossler J A, McCarty K S 1981 Adrenocorticotrophic production by a mammary carcinoma. Cancer 47: 1823–1827

INTRACYSTIC CARCINOMA

'Intracystic carcinoma' is a descriptive term referring to rare tumours which should be considered variants of other carcinoma types. Formation of a cyst should be considered secondary to the definition of type and extent of disease, with care being given to the presence or absence of stromal invasion as well as the presence of in situ carcinoma beyond the cyst. Thus, the diagnostic term 'intracystic carcinoma' should always be modified by the type and component character of the invasive carcinoma. Azzopardi (1979) considered intracystic carcinoma only in his discussion of carcinoma in situ of ductal type suggesting that these be classified as *DCIS (intracystic)*. These special in situ cancers are discussed as 'non-invasive papillary carcinomas' in Chapter 12. While non-invasive carcinoma accounts for many

of these cases (Carter et al 1983), cystic masses with carcinoma may contain other tumour patterns, and have special problems in adequate anatomical analysis and diagnosis. They also exhibit some consistent clinical associations.

Most seemingly encysted tumours diagnosed as carcinoma will be intracystic or non-invasive papillary carcinomas (see Ch. 12). Others will have more fluid (usually bloody) than tissue within the cyst and will be larger, often over 10 cm in diameter. A well-defined fibrous wall delimits the cyst and should be carefully examined for nodules of tumour which may be confined to the inner aspect of wall, (non-invasive), or found to invade beyond the wall (Fig. 15.12). In the latter situation, invasive carcinoma of whatever histological pattern should be considered the primary diagnosis. As presented with the discussion of squamous cell carcinomas of the breast, many are cystic.

It is certainly not clear how many of these cases

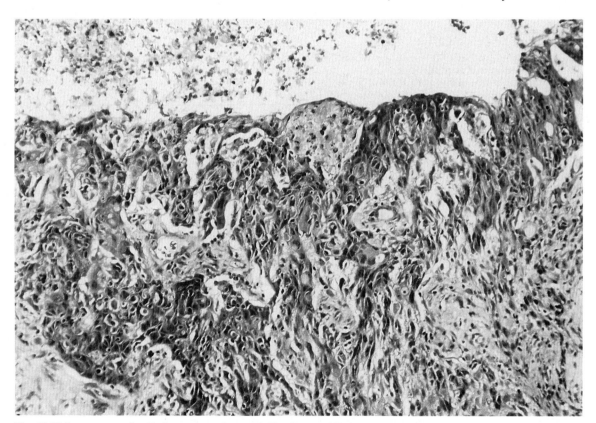

Fig. 15.12 Inner aspect of wall of a cystic carcinoma. Infiltrating, undifferentiated carcinoma has appearance approaching that of squamous differentiation. Note necrotic cells floating in central fluid above (× 200).

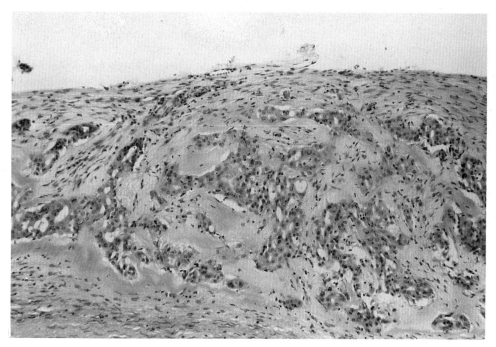

a

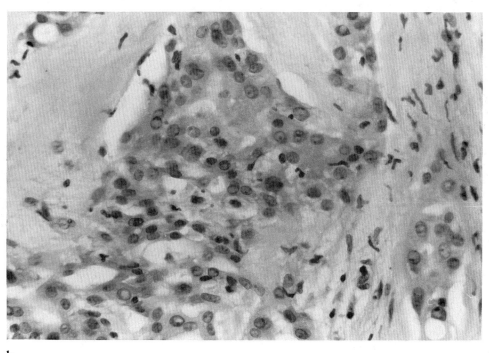

b

Fig. 15.13 (a) The central cyst above contained a papilloma with proliferated epithelium of the same pattern present here as pseudoinfiltrating epithelial nests in the cyst wall. Note outer fibrous limit of this lesion at lower left. (b) Higher power of epithelium in wall delimiting a papilloma. Note bland nuclei and spacing which characterizes usual hyperplasia (a × 1500; b × 400).

evolve as intraductal lesions that become encysted (or pseudoencapsulated) and how many represent invasion of a cyst by carcinoma, but the latter seems unlikely. For the purpose of adequate differential diagnosis, supposition as to histogenesis is immaterial.

Differential diagnostic considerations include benign epidermal cysts occasionally reaching 9 cm in size (Kowand et al 1984). This may have atypia in the squamous lining cells (Roth et al 1977). Other cystic masses may have pseudoinvasion of the fibrous wall (Fig. 15.13). The cytological features of pseudoinvasive epithelium will mirror that of benign epithelium within the cyst and be inconsistent with carcinoma.

Reported cases of so-called intracystic carcinoma do show a definite predilection for older women, those with prolonged clinical history and black women (Czernobilsky 1967; Squires & Betsill 1981). These cases are accepted as having a relatively good prognosis despite the fact that many reported lesions have not been adequately characterized as to presence or absence of invasion. We are confident that the infrequent presence of extension beyond the fibrous wall is largely if not exclusively responsible for the relatively good prognosis. Cystic change may be more common in cancers of males (5–7.5% of male cancer; Ramos et al 1985) than in females (0.5%, approximately; Hunter & Sawyers 1980).

The problem of occurrence of multiple histological cancer types in cystic masses is nicely demonstrated by the second case presented by Dalla Palma & Parenti (1983). This large, cystic mass was lined largely by atypical squamous epithelium, but had papillary areas and foci of invasive glandular carcinoma. Although it was presented as a case of squamous breast cancer, it is clear that other diagnoses are creditable. It is perhaps notable that the patient had a bleeding intraductal papilloma removed from the same breast 12 years previously.

We also echo the comments of Knight (1985) that the rarity of cystic carcinoma does not justify the routine submission of cyst fluid for cytological examination for its exclusion. Such a policy is inefficient at best and better replaced by alertness to other signs, such as residual mass or blood-containing fluid, which give an adequate measure of suspicion in the provisional recognition of malignancy in cystic masses (Devitt & Barr 1984). This is particularly true in perimenopausal or younger women in whom benign cysts are so common, and cystic carcinomas so rare.

REFERENCES

Azzopardi J G 1979 Problems in breast pathology. Saunders, Philadelphia, p 244

Carter D, Orr S L, Merino M J 1983 Intracystic papillary carcinoma of the breast. After mastectomy, radiotherapy or excisional biopsy alone. Cancer 52: 14–19

Czernobilsky B 1967 Intracystic carcinoma of the female breast. Surg Gynecol Obstet 124: 93–98

Dalla Palma P, Parenti A 1983 Squamous breast cancer: Report of two cases and review of the literature. Appl Pathol 1: 14–24

Devitt J E, Barr J R 1984 The clinical recognition of cystic carcinoma of the breast. Surg Gynecol Obstet 159: 130–132

Hunter C E Jr, Sawyers J J 1980 Intracystic papillary carcinoma of the breast. South Med J 73: 1484–1486

Knight I A 1985 Early detection of breast cancer (letters). J A M A 253: 2194–2195

Kowand L M, Verhulst L A, Copeland C M, Bose B 1984 Epidermal cyst of the breast. Can Med Assoc J 131: 217–219

Ramos C V, Boeshart C, Restrepo G L 1985 Intracystic papillary carcinoma of the male breast. Arch Pathol Lab Med 109: 858–861

Roth J A, Feinberg M, McAvoy J M 1977 Carcinoma arising in the wall of a breast cyst during pregnancy. Ann Surg 185: 247–250

Squires J E, Betsill Jr W L 1981 Intracystic carcinoma of the breast. A correlation of cytomorphology, gross pathology, microscopic pathology and clinical data. Acta Cytol 25: 267–271

Miscellaneous features of carcinoma

While breast cancers in which there is a predominant component of ductal carcinoma in situ (DCIS) may have a better prognosis than those with little or no associated intraductal carcinoma (Silverberg & Chitale 1973), the recent increased use of radiotherapy after local cancer excision in the treatment of early stage breast carcinoma has further highlighted the importance of recognizing the extent of CIS of ductal type in infiltrating NST ductal carcinomas. The extent of associated ductal CIS appears to be an important predictor of breast recurrence after local excision and radiotherapy. In an update of a series of 356 patients with infiltrating ductal (NST) carcinoma treated by total gross excision of the palpable tumour along with a surrounding rim of grossly normal breast tissue (usually 1 cm or less) followed by radiation therapy, the only significant risk factor for breast relapse was the presence of an extensive intraductal component (EIC) in the excision specimen (Schnitt et al 1984, 1985). EIC was defined as the combination of intraductal carcinoma comprising 25% or more of the area defined by the borders of the infiltrating tumour, and intraductal carcinoma in the adjacent tissue (either in sections free of infiltrating tumour or extending clearly beyond the infiltrating margins of the tumour). Also included in this group were tumours that were primarily DCIS with focal or multifocal invasion.

The group of 223 patients whose tumours lacked EIC had a five-year actuarial risk of breast recurrence of only 2%. In contrast, among the 133 patients whose tumours showed EIC, the risk of developing a breast recurrence at five years was 24%. The number of patients at 10 years was relatively small but the actuarial risk of local failure was 40% for patients with EIC and only 3% for patients whose tumour lacked EIC.

It is important to note that among the factors found not to be significant in predicting breast failure were the size of the tumour (T1 v. T2), lymph node status, tumour differentiation, and radiation dose to the primary within the therapeutic dose range (5000–7000 rad).

It must also be emphasized that most patients with infiltrating carcinoma have some associated intraductal component and it was only the patients with EIC, as defined above, in whom a high risk of breast failure was observed. Even the group of patients who had DCIS in the tissue adjacent to the infiltrating tumour were at low risk for breast recurrence provided that their tumours had little DCIS within them.

In an attempt to determine why a subset of patients who had undergone a complete gross excision of their tumour were at high risk for developing a breast relapse after radiotherapy, Schnitt et al (1987) studied the frequency, type, and extent of residual carcinoma at the tumour site following a complete gross removal of the primary and related these findings to the histological features of the primary excision specimen. They examined pathological material in 71 patients with infiltrating carcinoma of no special type treated with gross excision of the tumour and then selected for re-excision of the tumour site prior to radiotherapy because of the presence of EIC in the primary excision specimen or microscopic tumour at or close to margins in the initial excision. Residual carcinoma (infiltrating or intraductal) was seen in 62% of all patients but was more frequent among patients with EIC than among those without it (88% v. 48%). The nature of the residual carcinoma was different for patients with and without EIC in the primary excision specimens. Residual tumour in patients without EIC was usually limited in quantity and usually consisted of scattered microscopic foci of either infiltrating or intraductal carcinoma. In contrast, residual carcinoma in patients with EIC was often widespread and composed predominantly of intraductal carcinoma. 44% of patients with EIC in the primary excision specimen had extensive residual DCIS in the re-excision specimens compared with only 2% for patients without EIC. This figure is strikingly similar to their projected 10-year actuarial risk of breast failure for patients with EIC (40%). The finding of EIC in the primary excision specimen, therefore, appears to be a marker for a lesion which is prone to more extensive local involvement of the breast than can be appreciated by the surgeon at the time of the lumpectomy. It should also be noted that the vast majority of the breast recurrences in these patients are seen at or adjacent to the initial excision site and therefore appear to represent failures to control the primary tumour, rather than evolution of multicentric foci of carcinoma.

The importance of EIC in predicting breast recurrence may be dependent upon the initial size of the surgical excision. For example, in contrast to the results obtained at the Joint Center for Radiation Therapy in Boston, where breast surgery prior to irradiation is typically very limited, the extent of in situ disease has not been reported to be predictive of breast recurrence at institutions in which the initial breast operation is a wide excision of the tumours, with a generous margin of surrounding normal tissue (Clarke et al 1985; Calle et al 1986; Fisher et al 1986). However, the data of Calle et al (1986) indicate that even with a wide excision prior to irradiation the breast recurrence rate is greater among tumours categorized as intraductal with micro-invasion than for infiltrating carcinomas NST (17% v. 8%), although these differences were not statistically significant. Finally, the extent of DCIS within a tumour is not predictive of local

(chest wall) recurrences after mastectomy (Rosen et al 1986).

While it is difficult to compare series from different institutions utilizing widely different surgical techniques, it appears that the importance of the intraductal component in predicting local recurrence in the breast may be dependent upon the extent of surgical resection of the primary, with the greatest effect observed in patients who undergo the most limited types of local excision.

Conversely, the extent of the surgical excision which is necessary to achieve optimal local tumour control may be best determined by the pathological features of the primary tumour (Harris et al 1985). The majority of patients, whose tumours lack EIC, may require only limited breast surgery with a simple gross excison of the tumour. Patients whose biopsies reveal EIC may be best treated by local excision followed by a re-excision to evaluate the extent of the residual intraductal carcinoma. If intraductal carcinoma appears to be limited and adequately resected, these patients may be good candidates for radiotherapy. If, on re-excision, intraductal carcinoma is extensive and involves new margins, a mastectomy may be advisable.

Two studies attempting to relate the extent of DCIS to prognosis are also worthy of note. Silverberg & Chitale (1973) quantitated the relative amount of ductal carcinoma in situ (DCIS) in mastectomy specimens and found about 40% cancer deaths in five years in women with 10% or less of the tumour mass consisting of DCIS and no deaths in five years if over 90% of the tumour mass was DCIS. An intermediate survival was found in women when 10–89% of the tumour consisted of intraductal carcinoma. The quantity of DCIS was inversely related to nodal involvement. Somewhat surprisingly, smaller tumours did not have an increased DCIS component over larger ones. There was a slight tendency for tumours with a larger invasive component to be of higher grade.

In another series, the presence of concurrent ductal carcinoma in situ (DCIS) within or adjacent to an invasive carcinoma was found not to be predictive of improved survival after mastectomy (Rosen et al 1986). Systemic recurrence within five years of mastectomy averaged 27% in women without concurrent DCIS and 19% in women with DCIS within and/or adjacent to the major invasive mass. However, in a multivariate analysis, nodal status and grade were more predictive of survival. Rosen et al (1986) found no difference in survival between patterns of DCIS, i.e. within or outside the tumour. There was a higher incidence of DCIS in other breast quadrants in cases with DCIS adjacent to the main cancer mass, but there was no difference in multicentricity of invasive disease in other quadrants.

Thus, the cited studies support the usefulness of documenting the presence, extent, and distribution of in situ disease of ductal type in the reporting of invasive breast cancers (Rosen et al 1986), particularly if conservation therapy is envisioned.

It is also useful to report the presence of LCIS in a resected specimen containing invasive carcinoma. It is probable that concurrent lobular carcinoma in situ will predict a greater incidence of bilateral cancer no matter what the type of the infiltrating cancer (see 'Multicentricity'). The precise magnitude of this risk is unknown because of small numbers in studies formally examining this association (Davis & Baird 1981).

REFERENCES

Calle R, Vilcoq J R, Zafrani B, Vielh P, Fourquet A 1986 Local control and survival of breast cancer treated by limited surgery followed by irradiation. Int J Radiat Oncol Biol Phys 12: 873–878

Clarke D H, Le M G, Sarrazin P, Lacombe M J, Fontaine F 1985 Analysis of local regional relapses in patients with early breast cancers treated by excision and radiotherapy: experience of the Institue Gustave Roussy. Int J Radiat Oncol Biol Phys 11: 137–145

Davis N, Baird R M 1984 Breast cancer in association with lobular carcinoma in situ: clinicopathologic review and treatment recommendation. Am J Surg 147: 641–645

Fisher B, Bauer M, Margolese R et al 1985 Five-year results of a randomized clinical trial comparing total mastectomy and segmental mastectomy with or without radiation in the treatment of breast cancer. N Engl J Med 312: 665–673

Harris J R, Connolly J L, Schnitt S J et al 1985 The use of pathologic features in selecting the extent of surgical resection necessary for breast cancer patients treated by primary radiation therapy. Ann Surg 201(2): 164–169

Rosen P P, Kinne D W, Lesser M, Hellman S 1986 Are prognostic factors for local control of breast cancer treated by primary radiotherapy significant for patients treated by mastectomy? Cancer 57: 1415–1420

Schnitt S J, Connolly J L, Harris J R, Hellman S, Cohen R B 1984 Pathologic predictors of early local recurrence in stage I and stage II breast cancer treated by primary radiation therapy. Cancer 53: 1049–1057

Schnitt S J, Connolly J L, Silver B, Recht A, Harris J R 1985 Updated results of the influence of pathologic features on treatment outcome in stage I and II breast cancer patients treated by primary radiation therapy. Int J Radiat Oncol Biol Phys II (suppl 1): 104

Schnitt S J, Connolly J L, Khettry U et al 1987 Pathologic findings on re-excision of the primary site in breast cancer patients considered for treatment by primary radiation therapy. Cancer 59: 675–681

Silverberg S G, Chitale A R 1973 Assessment of significance of proportions of intraductal and infiltrating tumour growth in ductal carcinoma of the breast. Cancer 32: 830–837

MULTICENTRICITY AND BILATERALITY

Many studies have been devoted to the determination of multicentric occurrence of breast carcinoma both in the breast with cancer and in the contralateral breast. Although these studies have varied in methodology as well as in diagnostic criteria for acceptance of the diagnosis of carcinoma separate from a primarily diagnosed site, critical review of this data by McDivitt (1984) led him to conclude that the overall rate of breast cancer multicentricity in the index breast was in the range of 25–50% but that the incidence of invasive foci in the multicentric areas was only 5–10%. Carter (1986) supports a general figure of one-third of breasts containing foci of cancer after local resection of a carcinoma. These multicentric foci are not limited to the breast quadrant containing the primary indexed tumour (indeed, most studies define multicentricity as occurrence in a separate quadrant), and they frequently involve the breast in the region of the nipple. Multicentricity appears increased when the index breast cancer is of large size, involves the nipple, or is accompanied by in situ carcinoma (Fisher et al 1975). However, two studies (Schwartz et al 1980; Lagios et al 1981) suggest that small primary invasive tumours may be associated with a greater incidence of multicentricity than larger ones. This disagreement with Fisher et al (1975) may well be due to differences in size (larger in the Fisher study) and method of detection as the later two studies had more cases detected by mammography. The Lagios et al (1981) study is also notable in that in situ ductal carcinomas less than 25 mm in dimension were not found to have foci of occult invasion in the remainder of the breast. Gump et al (1986) found ninety per cent of secondary foci to be in close proximity to the primary.

Holland et al (1985) have presented a very careful analysis of many aspects of the multiple foci phenomenon including correlation of mammographical and anatomical size determinations. They found no difference between carcinomas of less than 2 cm and those of 2–4 cm in terms of presence or absence of distant tumour foci or distance of tumour foci from the reference tumour. If the 264 invasive cancers of 4 cm or less in diameter had been removed with a margin of 3–4 cm, about 8% would have had invasive foci remaining in the breast and 4–9% would have had foci of non-invasive carcinoma left in the remaining breast tissue.

Rosen et al (1975) found a 26% incidence of carcinoma in quadrants distant from that containing the primary cancer, equally divided between invasive and non-invasive. This incidence rose somewhat in tumours over 2 cm in diameter. This study also reported no apparent increase of multicentricity for women with a positive family history. However, the risk for breast cancer in the contralateral breast is apparently doubled for breast cancer patients with a strong family history (Hislop et al 1984; Anderson & Badzioch 1985), and Lagios (1977) found a greater likelihood of a family history of breast cancer in patients with multicentric tumours.

All the above studies have considered the histological identification of concurrent lesions within the cancerous breast. It is also relevant to record the experience of Crile et al (1980) who followed women after partial mastectomy for breast cancers of 2 cm or less in diameter. Some indication of the clinical relevance of multicentric lesions is obtained by such longitudinal observations. Follow-up was at least five years; only 0.6% of patients had in situ disease alone and one-third received radiotherapy. 12% experienced local recurrence and another 3% developed cancer in another region of the same breast. The occurrence of a second primary cancer in the contralateral breast was also 3%.

The clinical importance of these observations lies in their implications for conservation therapy for breast cancer, i.e. conserving the breast by avoiding mastectomy. It has been assumed that multicentricity would indicate that local resection would be contraindicated as cancerous areas would remain in the breast. However, the clinical outcome of local resection of cancer combined with radiotherapy as a primary treatment is comparable to that obtained with mastectomy (Harris et al 1985). The extent of ductal carcinoma in situ is indicative of local treatment failure in this therapeutic setting (see above).

There may also be prognostic clinical relevance in the evaluation of multicentricity as Egan & McSweeney (1984) have suggested that women with multicentric cancers may have a worse prognosis than those with unicentric tumours.

The occurrence of malignancy in the contralateral breast either synchronously with a cancer or during a follow-up period (metachronous) is a special and clinically relevant example of multicentricity (Wanebo et al 1985). The classical study of Robbins & Berg (1964) has been largely supported by subsequent studies. The 1964 study reported a risk of 1% per year for the development of cancer in the remaining breast after mastectomy. Chaudary et al (1984) found an incidence of second cancers in 0.76% of patients at risk per year. This was independent of the detection of simultaneous bilateral cancers in 3% of patients. Detectability of the synchronous bilateral tumours was enhanced five-fold by the use of mammography. Thus the slight discrepancy with the 1964 study of Robbins & Berg (1964) is largely explained by a difference in the simultaneously diagnosed cases. Also of practical importance is that the risk of subsequent carcinoma in the contralateral breast is age dependent, with women initially diagnosed at less than 40 years of age having a three times risk of bilaterality when compared to older women. The relative risk of a second non-simultaneous primary was 5.9 times higher than that of the risk of breast cancer in the general population (Chaudary et al 1984). Leis (1980) found an analogous rate of subsequent contralateral cancer development in 10 years of 9.3%. Survival figures when calculated from second cancer diagnosis are similar to women with unilateral cancer (Burns et al 1984). At least during the first 10 years after initial diagnosis, the risk of contralateral cancer remains relatively constant (at somewhat less than 1% per year) although Fisher et al (1984) reported a peak of 1.75% absolute risk in the second postmastectomy year. This percentage risk falls in subsequent years.

Histological assessment of both the initially diagnosed breast cancer as well as the subsequent, contralateral breast cancer has clinical relevance.

Fisher et al (1984) reported that lobular carcinoma in situ in the vicinity of the dominant mass of the initial breast cancer was statistically significantly associated with bilateral disease. Also, when the initial breast cancer was of lobular invasive or tubular types, the incidence of bilateral disease was significantly elevated. However, the degree of risk of these discriminants was no greater than 2 to 3:1. The assessment of invasive lobular carcinoma (ILC) as an indicator of bilateral breast cancer risk is also discussed in Chapter 13, where it is noted that all histological variants of ILC are associated with increased risk of bilaterality.

Histological assessment of a carcinoma occurring in the second breast is of importance with regard to differentiating an intramammary metastasis from a second primary neoplasm. When such metastases occur they are usually within the fat of the medial aspect of the breast. True intramammary parenchymal metastases from a contralateral breast primary in the absence of concurrent distant metastases are extremely rare. Certainty that the second lesion is a primary lesion is confirmed if it is of a different histological pattern than the first breast cancer or, if both are of no special type, when the second cancer is of a lesser grade. The association of a putative second primary with adjacent in situ disease is also strong evidence of a second primary neoplasm. Note, however, that a metastasis within the breast may grow within ducts. Despite the evident difficulty this may present in differentiating primary from metastatic tumours, ductal growth in a metastasis is regularly identical with the stromal component. The intraductal component of a primary cancer is often histologically different from the invasive component. This difference is more likely to be reflected in intercellular patterns and cytoplasm than in nuclear features.

REFERENCES

Anderson D E, Badzioch M D 1985 Bilaterality in familial breast cancer patients. Cancer 56: 2090–2098

Burns P E, Dabbs K, May C et al 1984 Bilateral breast cancer in northern Alberta: risk factors and survival patterns. Can Med Assoc J 130: 881–886

Carter D 1986 Margins of 'lumpectomy' for breast cancer. Hum Pathol 17: 330–332

Chaudary M A, Millis R R, Hoskins E O L et al 1984 Bilateral primary breast cancer: a prospective study of disease incidence. Br J Surg 71: 711–714

Crile G Jr, Cooperman A, Esselstyn C B Jr, Hermann R E
1980 Results of partial mastectomy in 1973 patients
followed for from five to ten years. Surg Gynecol Obstet
150: 563–566

Egan R L, McSweeney M B 1984 Multicentric breast
carcinoma. Recent Results Cancer Res 90: 28–35

Fisher E R, Gregorio R, Redmond C, Vellios F, Sommers
S C, Fisher B 1975 Pathologic findings from the national
surgical adjuvant breast project (protocol no 4). I.
Observations concerning the multicentricity of mammary
cancer. Cancer 35: 247–254

Fisher E R, Fisher B, Sass R et al 1984 Pathologic findings
from the national surgical adjuvant breast project (protocol
no 4). XI. Bilateral breast cancer. Cancer 54: 3002–3011

Gump F E, Habit D V, Logerto P et al 1986 The extent and
distribution of cancer in breasts with palpable primary
tumors. Ann Surg 204: 384–390

Harris J R, Hellman S, Kinne D W 1985 Limited surgery
and radiotherapy for early breast cancer. N Engl J Med
313: 1365–1368

Hislop T G, Elwood J M, Coldman A J, Spinelli J J, Worth
A J, Ellison L G 1984 Second primary cancers of the
breast: incidence and risk factors. Br J Cancer 49: 79–85

Holland R, Veling Solke H J, Mravunac M, Hendriks
J H C L 1985 Histologic multifocality of TIS, T1–2
breast carcinomas. Implications for clinical trials of breast-
conserving surgery. Cancer 56: 979–990

Lagios M D 1977 Multicentricity of breast carcinoma
demonstrated by routine correlated serial subgross and
radiographic examination. Cancer 40: 1726–1734

Lagios M D, Westdahl P R, Rose M R 1981 The concept
and implications of multicentricity in breast carcinoma.
Pathol Annu 16(2): 83–102

Leis P H Jr 1980 Managing the remaining breast. Cancer
46: 1026–1030

McDivitt R W 1984 Breast cancer multicentricity. In:
McDivitt R W, Obermann H A, Ozzello L, Kaufman N
(eds) The breast. Williams and Wilkins, Baltimore,
p 139–148

Robbins G F, Berg J W 1964 Bilateral primary breast
cancer: a prospective clinocopathological study. Cancer
17: 1501–1527

Rosen P P, Fracchia A A, Urban J A, Schottenfeld D,
Robbins G F 1975 'Residual' mammary carcinoma
following simulated partial mastectomy. Cancer
35: 739–747

Schwartz G F, Patchesfsky A S, Feig S A, Shaber G S,
Schwartz A B 1980 Multicentricity of non-palpable breast
cancer. Cancer 45: 2913–2916

Wanebo H J, Senofsky G M, Fechner R E, Kaiser D, Lynn
S, Paradies J 1985 Bilateral breast cancer. Ann Surg
201: 667–677

PATHOLOGY OF THE THERAPEUTICALLY IRRADIATED BREAST

A small proportion of breast cancer patients treated by breast-conserving surgery and radiotherapy (primary radiation therapy) require biopsy of the treated breast at some point following irradiation because of the development of a new abnormality on physical examination or mammography. The surgical pathologist must, therefore, be familiar with the pathological alterations which may be observed in the breast following tumoricidal doses of ionizing radiation.

Radiation-induced changes in the skin of the breast are identical to those previously described in irradiated skin from other sites (Fajardo 1982). The nature of these changes is, in part, dependent upon the interval between irradiation and histological examination.

Morphological changes in breast carcinomas which have been treated by radiotherapy without prior excision have also been well described and include stromal fibrosis and hyalinization with entrapment of tumour cells, increased necrosis, cytoplasmic vacuolization, and increased nuclear pleomorphism (Haagensen 1986).

Patients treated by radiation therapy following local excision of the tumour occasionally develop areas of fat necrosis in the vicinity of the primary. These lesions may clinically, mammographically and macroscopically resemble carcinoma (Stefanik et al 1982; Clarke et al 1983). Surgical excision and histological examination are the best means by which the correct diagnosis can be made in such patients.

A characteristic constellation of histological changes has been observed in non-neoplastic irradiated breast tissue of patients treated by primary radiation therapy (Schnitt et al 1984). The most frequent finding is that of scattered atypical epithelial cells in the terminal duct-lobular unit (TDLU), usually associated with variable degrees of lobular sclerosis and atrophy (Fig. 16.1). These atypical cells are large, with enlarged, diffusely hyperchromatic nuclei, small or inconspicuous nucleoli and finely vacuolated eosinophilic cyto-

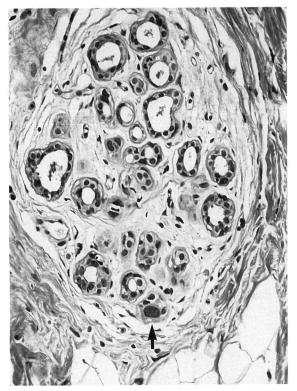

Fig. 16.1 Radiation-induced changes in a terminal duct-lobular unit. There is a mild degree of acinar atrophy. A few enlarged epithelial cells with large, diffusely hyperchromatic nuclei are evident (e.g. arrow) but there is no evidence of cellular proliferation (× 230).

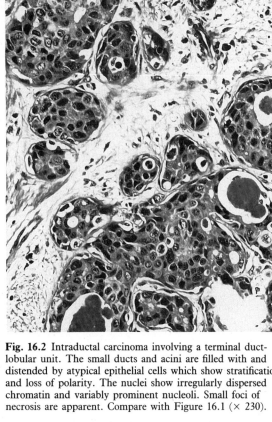

Fig. 16.2 Intraductal carcinoma involving a terminal duct-lobular unit. The small ducts and acini are filled with and distended by atypical epithelial cells which show stratification and loss of polarity. The nuclei show irregularly dispersed chromatin and variably prominent nucleoli. Small foci of necrosis are apparent. Compare with Figure 16.1 (× 230).

plasm. The cells often protrude into the lumen of the involved duct or acinus but do not show evidence of proliferation, such as cellular stratification, loss of polarity or mitotic activity. These TDLU changes have been observed in varying degrees in virtually all breast tissue excised from patients who have been treated by primary radiation therapy and do not appear to be related to the presence or absence of recurrent cancer elsewhere in the breast, patient age, interval between the end of therapy and the post-irradiation biopsy, use of adjuvant chemotherapy or radiation dose within the therapeutic dose range (i.e. 4500–5000 rad whole breast irradiation plus 1500–2000 rad supplemental dose (boost) to the primary site). Radiation effects on the TDLU must be distinguished from carcinoma to prevent an incorrect diagnosis of tumour recurrence. The distinction between radiation change and lobular

carcinoma in situ is not difficult because of the characteristic histological appearance of the latter, i.e. a monotonous population of relatively small cells which fill and distend ductules and acini. The differentiation of radiation-induced changes from intraductal carcinoma extending into the TDLU (cancerization of lobules) may be more difficult. However, when intraductal carcinoma involves the TDLU, there is generally evidence of cellular proliferation as characterized by cellular stratification, loss of polarity and distension of the involved ducts and acini. In addition, the nuclei in carcinoma cells tend to show irregularly dispersed chromatin and variably prominent nucleoli. Finally, necrosis of varying degrees is often seen with carcinoma, and mitoses may be apparent (Fig. 16.2). Conversely, the epithelial cells in areas of radiation change show maintenance of cellular polarity and cohesion, lack of

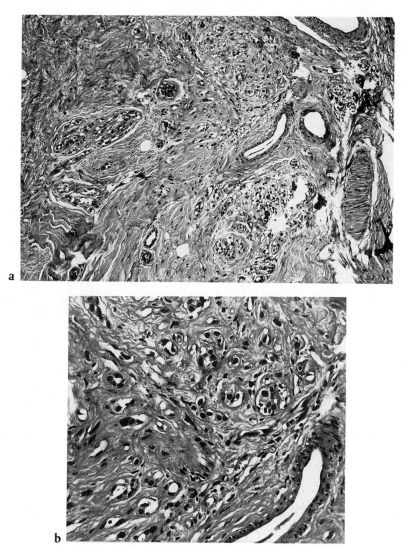

Fig. 16.3a, b Radiation-induced changes in terminal duct-lobular units. (a) Low power photomicrograph demonstrates several lobules with varying degrees of fibrosis and nuclear atypicality. (b) High power view demonstrates distorted acini, lined by atypical cells and entrapped in fibrous tissue, producing a pseudoinfiltrative appearance (a × 100; b × 270).

stratification, a diffuse homogeneous increase in chromatin, generally small or inconspicuous nucleoli, and no evidence of necrosis or mitotic activity. In some instances of radiation change, there may be extensive lobular fibrosis and atrophy with distortion of the lobular architecture. Entrapment of acini containing atypical epithelial cells may result in a pseudoinfiltrative pattern, thereby simulating invasive carcinoma. However, the lobulocentric configuration of such areas is usually apparent on low power examination (Fig. 16.3).

Additional pathological changes which are sometimes observed in non-neoplastic irradiated breast tissue include epithelial atypicality in large (extralobular) ducts, atypical fibroblasts in the stroma, and vascular changes such as myointimal proliferation in small arteries and prominent capillary endothelial cells (Schnitt et al 1984). However, these changes tend to be most prominent in cases in which the alterations in the TDLU are most marked. It is important to note that stromal fibrosis, a well-recognized feature of radiation effect in other organs, is so variable in both radiated and non-radiated breasts that it cannot by itself be considered a constant and reliable histological indicator of prior irradiation in the breast.

Tumour recurrence within the treated breast occurs in a small percentage of patients who undergo primary radiation therapy. These recurrences are most often seen in the vicinity of the original tumour and are not associated with the same grave prognosis as chest wall recurrences following mastectomy (Veronesi et al 1983; Osborne et al 1984; Sarrazin et al 1984). In fact, some studies suggest that an isolated recurrence in the treated breast does not adversely influence patient survival (Amalric et al 1982; Clark et al 1982). It is of interest to note that recurrences which are detected by mammography alone are typically composed predominantly or exclusively of intraductal carcinoma whereas recurrences which are detected by physical examination are most often infiltrating carcinomas (Schnitt et al 1985). Histologically, the recurrent tumours are usually similar in appearance to the initial lesion and rarely show morphological changes attributable to radiation effects (Schnitt et al 1985).

Patients who undergo primary radiation therapy for breast cancer require prolonged and careful follow-up to detect potentially curable local recurrences. The pathologist must be aware of the morphological alterations which occur in the therapeutically irradiated breast to provide accurate evaluations of these specimens.

REFERENCES

Amalric R, Santamaria F, Robert F et al 1982 Radiation therapy with or without primary limited surgery for operable breast cancer. A 20-year experience at the Marseilles cancer institute. Cancer 49: 30–34

Clark R M, Wilkinson R H, Mahoney L J, Reid J G, MacDonald W D 1982 Breast cancer: a 21-year experience with conservative surgery and radiation. Int J Radiat Oncol Biol Phys 8: 967–975

Clarke D, Curtis J L, Martinez A, Fajardo L, Goffinet D 1983 Fat necrosis of the breast simulating recurrent carcinoma after primary radiotherapy in the management of early stage breast carcinoma. Cancer 52: 442–445

Fajardo L F 1982 Pathology of radiation injury. Masson, New York

Haagensen C D 1986 Diseases of the breast, 3rd edn. Saunders, Philadelphia, p 954–971

Osborne M P, Ormiston N, Harmer C L, McKinna J A, Baker J, Greening W P 1984 Breast conservation in the treatment of early breast cancer. A 20-year follow-up. Cancer 53: 349–355

Sarrazin D, Le M, Rouesse J et al 1984 Conservative treatment versus mastectomy in breast cancer with macroscopic diameter of 20 millimeters or less. The experience of the Institut Gustave-Roussy. Cancer 53: 1209–1213

Schnitt S J, Connolly J L, Harris J R, Cohen R B 1984 Radiation-induced changes in the breast. Hum Pathol 15: 545–550

Schnitt S J, Connolly J L, Recht A, Silver B, Harris J R 1985 Breast relapse following primary radiation therapy for early breast cancer II. Detection, pathologic features and prognostic significance. Int J Radiat Oncol Biol Phys 11: 1277–1284

Stefanik D F, Brereton H D, Lee T C, Chun B K, Cigtay O, Dritschilo A 1982 Fat necrosis following breast irradiation for carcinoma: clinical presentation and diagnosis. Breast 8: 4–6

Veronesi U, DelVecchio M, Greco M et al 1983 Results of quadrantectomy, axillary dissection and radiotherapy (QUART) in T_1N_0 patients. In: Harris J R, Hellman S, Silen W (eds) Conservative management of breast cancer. Lippincott, Philadelphia, p 91–99

EXTENT OF INVASIVE DISEASE

The usual measure of the extent of invasive cancer is size of tumour. This is a valuable determinant of prognosis (Koscielny et al 1984) and a mandatory element in the defining features of an individual case. Size categories ordinarily considered have borders at measurements of 0.5, 1, 2 and 5 cm (Fisher et al 1984; Hartmann 1984). This is important information at the time of gross examination so that special care will be taken to record properly cancers approaching these limits. All too often smaller tumours cannot be adequately appreciated in the gross examination, and will need to be measured from histological slides. Because the shrinkage artefact of fixation and processing is not uniform, no generally applicable guidelines for correction are available, and estimates of size can be made directly from the histological sections.

A different problem is encountered when the invasive disease is only detected microscopically, often in the absence of a defined macroscopic lesion. Such changes are seen more frequently as a consequence of mammographic screening programmes (Patchefsky et al 1977) or biopsies for occult disease (Chetty et al 1983). The idea of 'minimal invasive cancer' was introduced by Gallager & Martin (1971) to incorporate invasive tumours with a volume no greater than that of a sphere 0.5 cm in diameter along with the non-invasive carcinomas (ductal and lobular) as a defined group of 'minimal breast cancers' with a high likelihood of survival. This upper size limit was established from a series of mammographically measurable carcinomas with extrapolation to a volume at which the probability of axillary metastases was less than 10%. Subsequent reports of minimal breast cancer (Wanebo et al 1974; Frazier et al 1977; Peters et al 1977; Nevin et al 1980) have verified this expectation in an experience with over 400 evaluable patients giving 95% disease-free survival for a median follow-up of five years (range one to 26 years). The American College of Surgeons' survey (Bedwani et al 1981) stressed the importance of nodal status. They reported 1423 patients with minimal invasive carcinoma measuring 1 cm or less in greatest diameter (8.4% of all cancers reported). Pathologically confirmed axillary lymph node metastases were present in 302 patients (21.2%), and the five year absolute survival with no evidence of disease was 70.3% for the lymph node negative group in contrast to 53.0% for the lymph node positive group. For the additional 323 patients (1.9%) with non-invasive disease the corresponding figure at five years was 74.3%. Acceptance of the concept and criteria for minimal breast cancer has been limited, and varied interpretations have been made of the tumour types to be included in the 'minimal' group (Wanebo et al 1974; Frazier et al 1977; Peters et al 1977). Hartmann (1984) has therefore made proposals for uniform definition of minimal breast cancer (MBC) to consist of in situ cancer (ductal or lobular type) and infiltrating carcinoma equal to or less than 1 cm in greatest diameter of any histological type, known as minimal invasive cancer (MIC). Wirman (1985) has recently reviewed this topic.

Still further difficulties exist in the definition of extent of invasion, and terms such as 'minimally invasive' or 'microinvasive' have been utilized to infer limitation in the extent of spread or aggression. Confusion has arisen because distinction has not always been made between *minimal invasive and microinvasive* although the latter is applied by some to mean limitation to a few fields detected by high power microscopy. Whilst the use of terms has been non-uniform, the recording of these cases with limited microscopic invasion is to be encouraged, whereby the practical survival value of identifying such foci and measurement of extent up to certain limits will eventually be determined with accrual of sufficient data. At present the relevance of such histological descriptions can only be stated as uncertain. This problem is not confined to the breast, as a recent account of experience in various organs shows (Burghardt & Holzer 1982). Studies with follow-up of such cases with minute invasive foci as defined either by size of invasive focus (foci), by percentage of tumour surface composed of invasive as opposed to in situ carcinoma (Silverberg & Chitale 1973; Patchefsky et al 1977), or by the number of microscopic fields with invasion will determine the utility of such assessments.

Our own experience leads us to believe in the importance of special considerations for cancers that are largely in situ but have microscopic foci of invasion, although few formal studies have been performed. Recording the measurement of the invasive focus separately seems the rational approach. Certainly, cases with a volume of invasive cancers considerably less than 0.5 cm diameter must be regarded as the least of the minimal invasive cancers, and never reported as simply 'cancers'. Also, note that overdiagnosis of focal invasion has frequently been the standard of practice in the past. We demand that invasion be present in more than a single collection of cells and that they must be outside a lobular unit or immediate periductal area, i.e. to be certain invasion is present it should be in interlobular tissue (Fig. 16.4a). Other distinguishing histological features are illustrated in Figure 16.4b–g

to demonstrate that microinvasion and its mimicry may take many guises. Their approximate size should be recorded, even if this entails a comment such as 'less than 0.1 mm'.

REFERENCES

Bedwani R, Vana J, Rosner D, Schmitz R L, Murphy G P 1981 Management and survival of female patients with 'minimal' breast cancer. As observed in the long term and short term surveys of the American College of Surgeons. Cancer 47: 2769–2778

Burghardt E, Holzer E (eds) 1982 Minimal invasive cancer (microcarcinoma). Clinics in Oncology, vol 1, no 2. Saunders, Philadelphia

Chetty U, Kirkpatrick A E, Anderson T J et al 1983 Localisation and excision of occult breast lesions. Br J Surg 70: 607–610

Fisher E R, Sass R, Fisher B et al 1984 Pathologic findings from the national surgical adjuvant project for breast cancers (protocol no 4). X. Discriminants for tenth year treatment failure. Cancer 53: 712–723

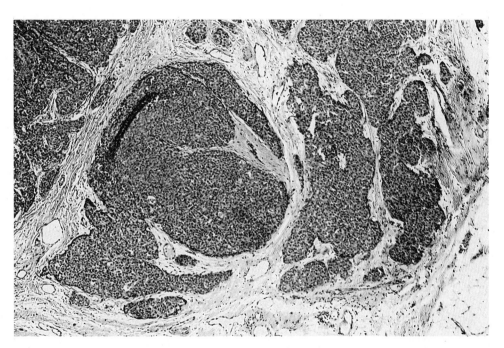

Fig. 16.4a Such a pattern of mammary parenchyma expanded and distorted by carcinoma in situ may make determination of 'microinvasion' difficult. In the absence of certainty that invasion is present, invasion should not be diagnosed. Here the distended units and smaller adjacent cell groups are identical, making invasion unlikely (× 60).

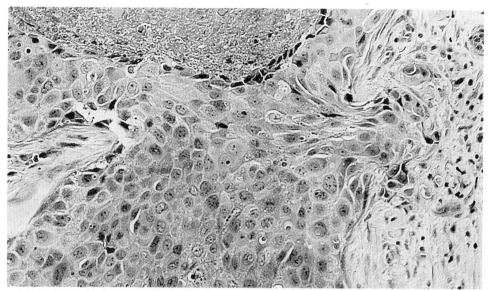

Fig. 16.4b This in situ carcinoma demonstrates a quite smoothly outlined irregularity at the right. Although basement membrane stains might demonstrate attenuation of that structure, such histological appearances cannot be interpreted as true invasion (× 250).

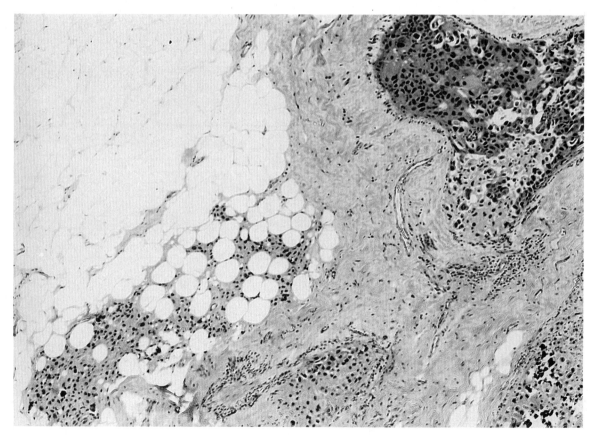

Fig. 16.4c The only focus of stromal invasion seen in this case of ductal carcinoma in situ is present in fat at the lower left. Interspersed cells between the fat cells in thick and thin cords can only be interpreted as stromal invasion ((× 80).

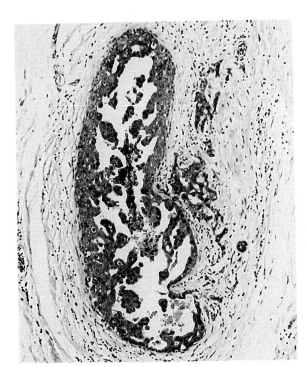

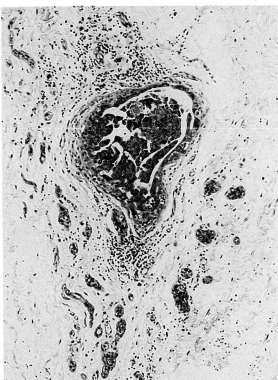

Fig. 16.4d These irregularly intersecting cords of breast carcinoma cells present to the right of the expanded duct cannot be explained as deformities of adjacent deformed or atrophic lobular units. Thus, when higher power examination demonstrates atypical nuclei, they must be accepted as a tiny focus of stromal invasion (× 80).

Fig. 16.4e Atrophic lobular or acinar elements are arrayed in an orderly and repeating serpentine fashion adjacent to the centrally placed ductal space which is largely filled with comedo carcinoma in situ. Even if atypical nuclei are present in these deformed lobular elements, they must be accepted as cancerization of lobules and not recognized as invasive breast carcinoma (× 80).

Frazier T G, Copeland E M, Gallager H S, Paulino D D, White E C 1977 Prognosis and treatment in minimal breast cancer. Am J Surg 139: 357–359

Gallager H S, Martin J E 1971 An orientation to the concept of minimal breast cancer. Cancer 28: 1505–1507

Hartmann W H 1984 Minimal breast cancer. Cancer 53: 681–684

Koscielny S, Tubiana M, Le M G et al 1984 Breast cancer: relationship between the size of the primary tumour and the probability of metastatic dissemination. Br J Cancer 49: 709–715

Patchefsky A S, Shaber G S, Schwartz G F, Feig S A, Nerlinger R E 1977 The pathology of breast cancer detected by mass population screening. Cancer 40: 1659–1670

Peters T G, Donegan W L, Burg E A 1977 Minimal breast cancer: a clinical appraisal. Ann Surg 186: 704–710

Silverberg S G, Chitale A R 1973 Assessment of significance of proportion of intraductal and infiltrating tumour growth in ductal carcinoma of the breast. Cancer 32: 830–837

Wanebo H J, Huvos A G, Urban J A 1974 Treatment of minimal breast cancer. Cancer 33: 349–357

Wirman J A 1985 The clinical significance of minimal breast cancer: a pathologist's viewpoint. C R C Crit Rev Oncol Hematol 3: 35–74

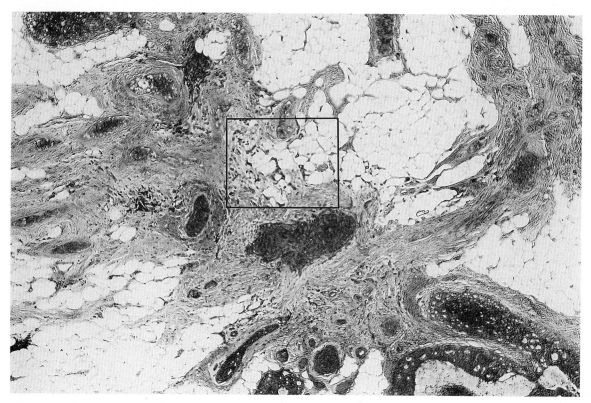

Fig. 16.4f This low power view of extensive ductal carcinoma in situ (large dark areas) with the periductal fibrosis has, in the central region, a tiny focus of stromal invasion seen at higher power in (**g**) (× 50).

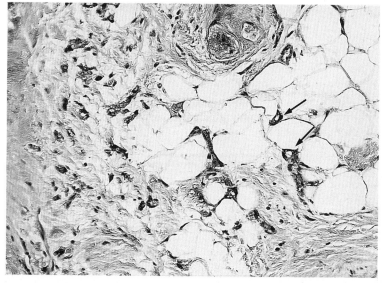

Fig. 16.4g Although atypical nuclei are not well seen, long, somewhat irregular collections of cells occasionally with intercellular lumen formation (arrow) are present. Several such areas were demonstrated in this case adjacent to areas of in situ carcinoma, without other disease within the breast or axilla (× 170).

VESSEL INVASION

Evaluation of vascular invasion of breast carcinoma has a chequered career. There has been much controversy concerning the histological certainty of this finding with great variability in incidence determinations. However, recent studies detailed below would indicate that such a finding may be validly determined and has prognostic significance.

For the most part, vascular invasion within the breast will be confined to lymphatics; however, blood vessels may be occasionally involved. As the certainty of differentiating lymphatic vessels from small veins is poor, vessel invasion is better left unspecified and understood to mean predominantly lymphatics and occasionally veins. The histological evaluation must avoid two evident pitfalls: the interpretation of intraductal tumour as being within a vessel and the interpretation of soft tissue spaces as vascular. The former is quite easily avoided if one does not accept tumour within spaces related to lobular units or within spaces histologically identical with adjacent ducts.

The fine and reduplicated pattern of elastica around many ducts will help avoid misinterpretations. Requiring that tumour cell emboli be within a space having an endothelial cell lining makes the histological determination of vascular invasion both sensitive and specific. Immunohistochemical techniques add to diagnostic certainty (Lee et al 1986). These spaces will most often be found adjacent to small blood-filled vessels and will be separated from mammary parenchymal elements by interlobular stroma in most cases (Fig. 16.5). The determination of vascular involvement should be made in a peritumoural location, and not from within the tumour mass. When artifactual tissue spaces without an endothelial lining (Fig. 16.6) are ignored, agreement in over 90% of cases of vascular invasion may be expected between pathologists (Fisher et al 1984).

Studies by Rosen et al (1981), Roses et al (1982) and Bettelheim et al (1984) have shown that the presence of carcinoma within peritumoural vessels is an important indicator of early recurrence in patients without lymph node metastases. There was at least a 20% difference in treatment failure between patients with and without peritumoural

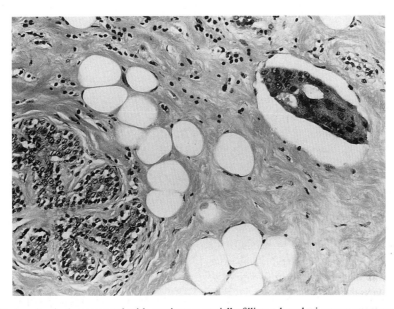

Fig. 16.5 Lymphatic invasion is demonstrated with carcinoma partially filling a lymphatic space at upper right. Note the space is within supporting connective tissue without differing ensheathing stroma, as a duct might have (× 200).

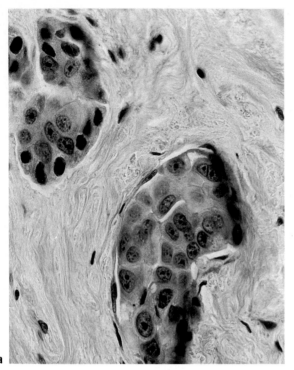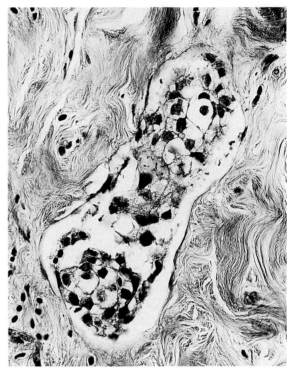

a   b

Fig. 16.6a, b Lymphatic invasion within the breast. Note that endothelial-lining cells protrude slightly into the space, and are not adjacent fibroblasts (**a** × 480; **b** × 400).

vascular invasion, favouring women without vascular invasion. Roses et al (1982) found peritumoural vascular invasion to be most predictive of recurrence as compared to many other histological features.

Davis et al (1985) have also demonstrated that peritumoural vessel invasion is an indicator of treatment failure in patients who have lymph node metastases. These investigators, using a very large multicentre study group, found vessel invasion by tumour cells in 59% of the patients. Different populations within the study (e.g. various treatment modalities or menopausal status) demonstrated a rate of death in patients with vessel invasion of 29–64%. The frequency of local or distant recurrence at four years after diagnosis was higher for women with, than for those without, vessel invasion (27% v. 18%). However, no difference in outcome was demonstrated between vessel invasion and no vessel invasion groups in postmenopausal women treated with endocrine therapy. In all other groups, the women with

vessel invasion fared less well. This study is an elegant demonstration of the utility of studying interaction of several variables, whether histological, therapeutic, etc.

REFERENCES

Bettelheim R, Penman H G, Thorton-Jones H, Neville A M 1984 Prognostic significance of peritumoral vascular invasion in breast cancer. Br J Cancer 50: 771–777

Davis B W, Gelber R, Goldhirsch A et al 1985 Prognostic significance of peritumoral vessel invasion in clinical trials of adjuvant therapy for breast cancer with axillary lymph node metastasis. Hum Pathol 16: 1212–1218

Fisher E R, Sass R, Fisher B et al 1984 Pathologic findings from the national surgical adjuvant breast project (protocol no 4). X. Discriminants for tenth year treatment failure. Cancer 53: 712–723

Lee A K C, DeLellis R A, Silverman M L, Wolfe H J 1986 Lymphatic and blood vessel invasion in breast carcinoma: a useful prognostic indicator? Hum Pathol 17: 984–987

Rosen P P, Saigo P E, Braun D W, Weathers E, DePalo A 1981 Predictors of recurrence in stage I (T1NoMo) breast carcinoma. Ann Surg 193: 15–25

Roses D F, Bell D A, Flotte T J, Taylor R, Ratich H, Dubin N 1982 Pathologic predictors of recurrence in stage I (T1NoMo) breast cancer. Am J Clin Pathol 78: 817–820

NECROSIS

Foci of necrotic tumour within invasive breast carcinomas may be large enough to be appreciated in gross appearance by evidencing dull areas sharply demarcated from the remainder of the tumour. Histologically, necrotic foci are recognized as they are elsewhere, by the loss of nuclear detail with karyorrhexis or extreme pyknosis progressing to complete loss of nuclear staining characteristics (Figs 16.7 and 16.8). Cytoplasmic detail is also lost. Small, occasional foci of necrotic carcinoma should not be considered as defining of the presence of this feature, particularly if it is being used as a prognostic indicator. Also, occasional loose (oedematous or myxoid), areas of fibrous tissue, suggestive of remote necrosis, do not qualify as necrosis for purposes of prognostication unless examples of ongoing necrosis are present in adjacent areas. Individual carcinomas

evidencing necrosis in the invasive component are regularly of high grade by both cytological and pattern criteria. Special types of mammary carcinoma usually do not have foci of necrosis, including variant types or special types mixed with no special type patterns. Only medullary carcinomas are excepted (Fisher et al 1978). Note that the characteristic necrosis of comedo carcinoma in situ should not be considered as evidence of necrosis in invasive portions of a tumour. When so defined, Carter et al (1978) found 40% of invasive carcinomas to have necrosis, while Fisher et al (1978) found 60% of carcinomas to have necrosis. However, the latter study included necrosis in non-invasive portions of the tumours. Hartmann (1986) has found an incidence of necrosis in invasive portions of carcinomas to be about 25% in tumours detected during screening.

Fisher et al (1978) noted that the presence of necrosis influenced treatment failure of breast cancer independent of tumour size, particularly when of marked degree. As necrosis was not

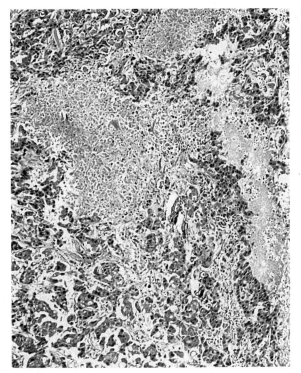

Fig. 16.7 Extensive necrosis of poorly differentiated breast cancer. Note viable cancer surrounds paler necrotic focus at upper left (× 60).

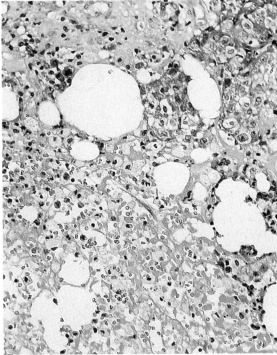

Fig. 16.8 Ghosted carcinoma cells predominate here as a reflection of necrosis. Note preservation of cells at upper right (× 200).

correlated with anatomically determined nodal status, necrosis gave independent prognostic usefulness. This study reported necrosis in 60% of invasive breast cancers, but included examples of necrosis in comedo in situ carcinoma as well as mild examples of necrosis.

The study of Carter et al (1978) defined tumour necrosis as infarct-like necrosis of groups of cells in the invasive portion of the carcinoma, and found it to be predictive of decreased survival at 10 years. This was particularly true in cases with lymph node metastases at initial treatment. Despite the close association of necrosis with other determinants of poor prognosis, specifically lack of special type characteristics and presence of high grade histological features, it is quite possible that necrosis is an independent determinant of poor prognosis. From the above cited studies it is probable that the presence of necrosis indicates a decreased five- and 10-year survival of 5–10%. Therefore, when well developed, this feature should be added to histopathological reports. However, when necrosis was evaluated in multi-stratified nodal positive groups in 10-year results (Fisher et al 1984) it did not represent a prognostic determinant in any nodal category (see Ch. 19). As necrosis is a feature closely correlated with nodal status, it may be particularly helpful in indicating pejorative clinical outcome when nodal status is unknown.

REFERENCES

Carter D, Elkins R C, Pipkin R D, Abbey H, Shepard R H 1978 Relationship of necrosis and tumour border to lymph node metastases and 10-year survival in carcinoma of the breast. Am J Surg Pathol 2: 39–46

Fisher E R, Palikar A S, Gregorio R M, Redmond C, Fisher B 1978 Pathologic findings from the national surgical adjuvant breast project (protocol no 4). IV. Significance of tumour necrosis. Hum Pathol 9: 523–530

Fisher E R, Sass R, Fisher B, et al 1984 Pathologic findings from the national surgical adjuvant project for breast cancers (protocol no 4). X. Discriminants for tenth year treatment failure. Cancer 53: 712–723

Hartmann W H 1986 Data from breast cancer detection and demonstration project. NCI/ACS. Personal communication

STEROID RECEPTORS

Histological correlates of oestrogen and progesterone receptor protein status in breast cancer have been sought, with only moderate success (DeSombre 1984). The practical importance of such a correlation would be in predicting responsiveness to hormonal manipulation when determination of oestrogen receptors by specific means might be unavailable, as well as the possibility that histological features might better predict responsiveness to hormonal manipulation in tumours with biochemically demonstrated receptors. There is a consistent, though imprecise, relationship between well-differentiated tumours and oestrogen receptor positivity (Millis 1980). Infiltrating lobular carcinomas were reported as almost regularly having oestrogen receptor (Rosen et al 1975), but later reports refuted that experience (Lesser et al 1981). Although marked lymphocytic infiltration is reported as being associated with decreased incidence of oestrogen receptor positivity (Lesser et al 1981; Chabon et al 1982), others disagree (McCarty et al 1980).

One particularly promising suggestion was that of Masters et al (1979), as well as Millis (1980), who reported that tumour elastosis was related to endocrine responsiveness, suggesting that tumours with oestrogen receptor without elastosis would respond clinically, similar to those without receptor. However, others have not found this relationship (Cooke 1982).

Through this somewhat conflicting body of information, the positive association of well-differentiated and low grade breast cancers with increased amount of oestrogen receptor and higher proportion of progesterone receptor positivity remains (McCarty et al 1980). It has also been found that survival predictability of estrogen receptor (ER) status alone is of little clinical utility; however, in conjunction with tumour stage, axillary metastases and histopathological grade ER is useful for identifying subpopulations at increased risk of tumour recurrence or mortality (Parl et al 1984).

REFERENCES

Chabon A B, Goldberg J D, Venet L 1982 Carcinoma of the breast: Interrelationships among histopathologic features, estrogen receptor activity, and age of the patient. Hum Pathol 14: 368–372

Cooke T 1982 The clinical application of oestrogen receptor analysis in early cancer of the breast. Ann Coll Surg Engl 64: 165–170

DeSombre E R 1984 Steroid receptors in breast cancer. In: McDivitt R W, Oberman H A, Ozzello L, Kaufman N (eds) The breast. Williams and Wilkins, Baltimore, p 149–174

Lesser M L, Rosen P P, Senie R T, Duthie K, Menendez-Botet C, Schwartz M K 1981 Estrogen and progesterone receptors in breast carcinoma: correlations with epidemiology and pathology. Cancer 48: 299–309

McCarty Jr K S, Barton T K, Fetter B F et al 1980 Correlation of estrogen and progesterone receptors with histologic differentiation in mammary carcinoma. Cancer 46: 2851–2858

Masters J R W, Millis R R, King R J B, Rubens R D 1979 Elastosis and response to endocrine therapy in human breast cancer. Br J Cancer 39: 536–539

Millis R R 1980 Correlation of hormone receptors with pathological features in human breast cancer. Cancer 46: 2869–2871

Parl F F, Schmidt B P, Dupont W D, Wagner R K 1984 Prognostic significance of estrogen receptor status in breast cancer in relation to tumor stage, axillary node metastasis, and histopathologic grading. Cancer 54: 2237–2242

Rosen P P, Menendez-Botet C J, Nisselbaum J S et al 1975 Pathological review of breast lesions analyzed for estrogen receptor protein. Cancer Res 35: 3187–3194

STROMA

Fibrosis

The density of fibrous tissue in the enveloping stroma of infiltrating carcinomas varies greatly from equivalence with uninvolved, adjacent tissue to great increases. Variability within an individual carcinoma, particularly as regards the oedematous or myxoid quality of stroma, is frequent (Fig. 16.9). Apart from being responsible for altered texture (imparting palpability) and being associated with the often present and characteristic stellate, gross shape, the degree of fibrosis in breast cancers has no clinical relevance beyond imparting palpability. Occasional carcinomas will have a great amount of central and frequently dense fibrous tissue which contains few or no carcinoma cells (Fig. 16.10). The outer aspects of such tumours are usually more cellular. Such tumours with only rare cancer cells in dense, abundant stroma present obvious problems in diagnosis by needle biopsy or aspiration.

Elastica

The presence within breast cancers of interstitial fibrillar material sharing staining qualities with elastin is quite frequent. Such foci are usually found in the central portion of the tumour mass. With haematoxylin and eosin staining they are hyaline and lightly haematoxylin staining (Figs 16.11 and 16.12). Various special stains for elastic tissue are positive including Verhoeff, aldehyde fuchsin and Congo red (Bogomoletz 1986).

Elastic fibres are found in two distinct patterns. One is found concentrically arranged as if remaining from an obliterated duct while the other presents as less conspicuous usually elongated fibrillar arrays (Parfrey & Doyle 1985).

The distribution may be sparse or aggregated (Figs 16.11 and 16.12). Several clinically useful associations for elastica have been suggested, primarily related to the more prominent and dense examples of the aggregated patterns. Presence of elastica, particularly in larger amounts, has been correlated with improved prognosis and oestrogen

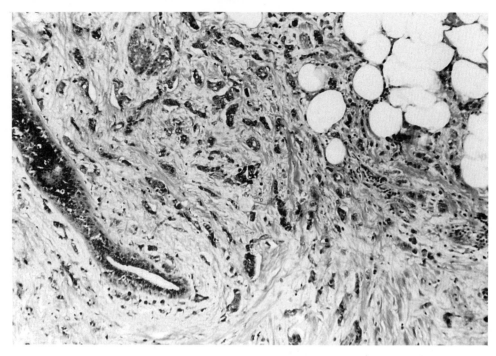

Fig. 16.9 Rounded groups of carcinoma cells are everywhere enveloped by a fibrous stroma, even in fat at upper right. Note oedematous stroma at left, particularly about the pre-existing duct which exits picture at upper left. The fibrous stroma is quite dense adjacent to and within fat (× 150).

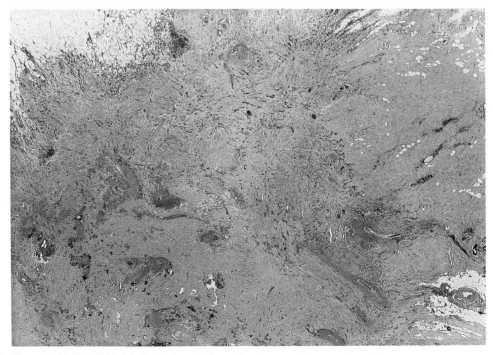

Fig. 16.10 The outer border of this lobular variant carcinoma is at upper left where clear fat is seen. Dark, thin strands, present in greatest number at border, are carcinoma cells in linear array. Somewhat dark clumps are elastica set in abundant fibrous stroma (× 13).

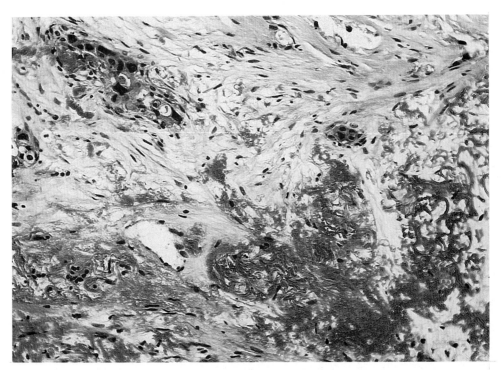

Fig. 16.11 The darker elastic material is seen primarily as sinuous or wavy fibrils within this breast cancer. Carcinoma cells are at upper left (× 225).

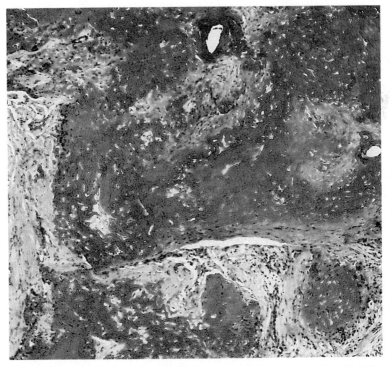

Fig. 16.12 Large clumps of hyaline elastic material are slightly refractile in this example of marked elastosis from the centre of a breast carcinoma (× 75).

receptor positivity (Masters et al 1979; Glaubitz et al 1984). Giri et al (1987) found greater clinical significance for the better developed elastotic changes at the centre of carcinomas. Whether these associations are independent or result from positive association with special cancer types, i.e. tubular and lobular, and low grade tumours, is not clear, but the latter association is currently favoured (Glaubitz et al 1984; Jacquemier et al 1984; Rasmussen et al 1985) (see also 'Steroid receptors').

Stromal giant cells

This rare feature of breast cancers has been recently highlighted in the literature and consists of a constellation of anatomical features which are almost regularly reported. However, specific clinical relevance of this pattern is not yet established. Fewer than 30 carcinomas with stromal giant cells have been documented in the literature, and few of these have had extended follow-up (Holland et al 1984). One case is described in a man (Bertrand et al 1986). The stromal giant cells may be sparse, leaving recognition of these cases to rest upon other features, specifically a rich vascularity adjacent to tumour islands (Agnantis & Rosen 1979) and a regular presence of tumour histological pattern, similar to that noted in Chapter 13 as *invasive cribriform* (Saout et al 1985).

Mammary carcinoma with stromal giant cells usually presents as a regularly rounded mass, mimicking medullary carcinoma, fibroadenoma or cyst by mammography. A distinctive gross feature is a brown colour due to the presence of haemosiderin in the vessel-rich stroma. Multinucleated giant cells are found adjacent to the islands of tumour cells, either directly applied or seeming to be separated by a narrow space (Fig. 16.13). The giant cells may also appear in spaces within the tumour cell groups (Fig. 16.14). Although osteoclasts are mimicked, the giant cells are best considered histiocytic (Sugano et al 1983; Holland et al 1984; Neilsen & Kiaer 1985), as first proposed by Factor et al (1977). Usually this exceptional stromal appearance is accompanied by crisply defined groupings of cohesive, invasive cancer cells with smoothly rounded intercellular spaces (Fig. 16.15). The terms 'adenocystic' and 'invasive cribriform' have been applied to this conformation (see Ch. 13). Careful studies by ultrastructure and by cytochemical analysis of mucin have not supported a designation of 'adenoid cystic' (Holland et al 1984). Many cases are associated with carcinoma in situ in the breast, most often lobular. The stromal giant cells may be found in lymph nodal and visceral metastases.

Mammary carcinoma with stromal giant cells has no known special prognostic significance; however, lymph node metastases are present frequently (50% of the cases reported by Holland et al 1984) and visceral metastases are reported (Agnantis & Rosen 1979). It is not clear, however, that cases with distant metastases had the wellfound epithelial islands described in later papers. Therefore, neither a favourable nor especially unfavourable prognosis may be accorded these cancers.

The average age at diagnosis may be younger than that for all breast cancers by at least five years. Although the incidence of carcinoma with stromal giant cells is unknown, largely because examples remain unrecognized unless giant cells are numerous, the incidence is probably not generally as high as the 1% figure found by Holland et al (1984).

Note that stromal giant cells may be found in benign conditions as well (Rosen 1979).

REFERENCES

Agnantis N T, Rosen P P 1979 Mammary carcinoma with osteoclast-like giant cells: a study of eight cases with follow-up data. Am J Clin Pathol 72: 383–389

Bertrand G, George P, Bertrand A F 1986 Carcinome mammaire a stroma-réaction giganto-cellulaire premier cas masculin. Ann Pathol 6: 144–147

Bogomoletz W V 1986 Elastosis in breast cancer. Pathol Annu 21 pt 2: 347–366

Factor S M, Biempica L, Ratner I, Ahuja K K, Biempica S 1977 Carcinoma of the breast with multinucleated reactive stromal giant cells. Virchows Arch (A) 374: 1–12

Giri D D, Lonsdale R N, Dangerfield V J M, et al 1987 Clinicopathological significance of intratumoural variations in elastosis grades and the oestrogen receptor status of human breast carcinomas. J Pathol 151: 297–303

Glaubitz L C, Bowen J H, Cox E B, McCarty Jr K S 1984 Elastosis in human breast cancer. Arch Pathol Lab Med 108: 27–30

Holland R, Urbain J G M, van Haelst M 1984 Mammary carcinoma with osteoclast-like giant cells. Cancer 53: 1963–1973

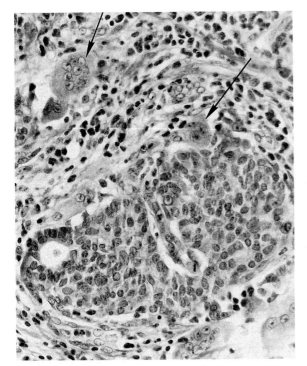

Fig. 16.13 Breast carcinoma with stromal giant cells. Note loose stroma rich in chronic inflammatory cells. Histiocytic giant cells are present at several locations (arrows) (× 250).

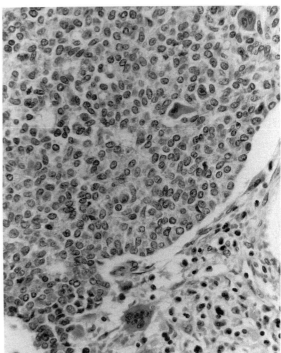

Fig. 16.14 Histiocytic giant cells (two) are within an epithelial island in this example of carcinoma with stromal giant cells (× 200).

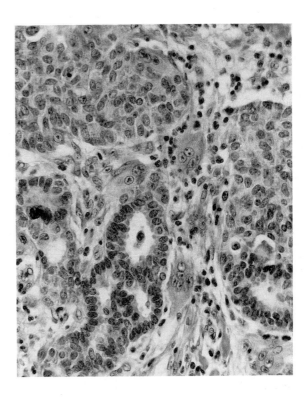

Fig. 16.15 Islands of carcinoma with stromal giant cells demonstrate the 'cribriform' feature of many of these neoplasms. Quite sharply demarcated spaces are present in the epithelial islands (× 250).

Jacquemier J, Lieutaud R, Martin P M 1984 Relationship of stromal elastosis to steroid receptors in human breast carcinoma. Recent Results Cancer Res 91: 169–175

Masters J R, Millis R R, King R J B, Rubens R D 1979 Elastosis and response to endocrine therapy in human breast cancer. Br J Cancer 39: 536–539

Neilsen B B, Kiaer H W 1985 Carcinoma of the breast with stromal multinucleated giant cells. Histopathology 9: 183–193

Parfrey N A, Doyle C T 1985 Original contributions: elastosis in benign and malignant breast disease. Hum Pathol 16: 674–676

Rasmussen B B, Pedersen B V, Thorpe S M, Rose C 1985 Elastosis in relation to prognosis in primary breast carcinoma. Cancer Res 45: 1428–1430

Rosen P P 1979 Multinucleated mammary stromal giant cell. A benign lesion that simulates invasive carcinoma. Cancer 44: 1305–1308

Saout L, Leduc M, Suy-Beng P T, Meignie P 1985 Presentation d'un nouveau cas de carcinome mammaire cribriforme associe a une reaction histocytaire giganto-cellulaire. Arch Anat Cytol Pathol 33: 58–61

Sugano I, Nagao K, Kondo Y, Nabeshima S, Murakami S 1983 Cytologic and ultrastructural studies of a rare breast carcinoma with osteoclast-like giant cells. Cancer 52: 74–78

CALCIFICATION

The frequent presence of microcalcifications in benign and malignant breast tissue has become of practical, diagnostic importance with the advent of diagnostic mammography. Indeed, many breast biopsies are occasioned by the presence of calcifications as detected by mammography, and approximately 50% of breast carcinomas will have mammographically detectable calcifications (Millis 1979). With the removal of these tissues, ideally the pathologist should be able to document that the tissue contains calcifications. However, this may be practically possible only with specimen radiography (Rosen et al 1974). In the majority of cases with cancer, a dominant mass will also be present, making identification of the lesion to be analysed relatively easy.

Histologically, the calcifications will vary from 10 μm to 500 μm in the great majority of cases (Millis et al 1976). A greater percentage of comedo carcinomas in situ will demonstrate calcification than any other carcinoma type, with invasive carcinomas of no special type making up the majority of carcinomas with calcifications (Millis et al 1976). Lobular carcinomas are rarely calcified (Bouropoulou et al 1984). The calcifications demonstrate many forms in benign and malignant tissues (Figs 16.16–16.19) with no known defining differential pattern as appreciated with the microscope. Calcifications are found in cysts, benign ducts, and often in sclerosed lobules.

REFERENCES

Bouropoulou V, Anastassiades O T, Kontogeorgos G, Rachmanides M, Gogas I 1984 Microcalcifications in breast carcinomas. A histological and histochemical study. Pathol Res Pract 179: 51–58

Millis R R 1979 Mammography. In: Azzopardi J G (ed) Problems in breast pathology. Saunders, Philadelphia, p 437–459

Millis R R, Davis R, Stacey A J 1976 The detection and significance of calcifications in the breast: a radiological and pathological study. Br J Radiol 49: 12–26

Rosen P P, Snyder R E, Robbins G 1974 Specimen radiology for nonpalpable breast lesions found by mammography: procedures and results. Cancer 34: 2028–2033

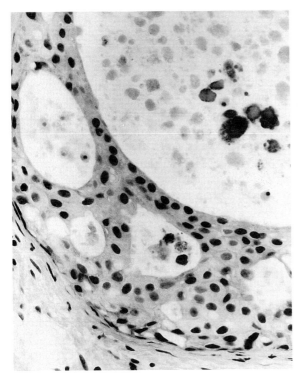

Fig. 16.16 Small, dark calcifications are seen in major lumen at right and in smaller, secondary lumen in this ductal carcinoma in situ (× 300).

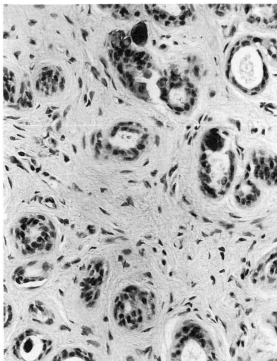

Fig. 16.17 This sclerosed, somewhat atrophic lobule has three rounded, dark calcific concretions. One is stromal at upper middle, one is in epithelium at middle right, and the last is in a lumen at lower left (× 240).

Fig. 16.18 The epithelium in this lobule with shattered, large calcifications demonstrates atypical features (× 225).

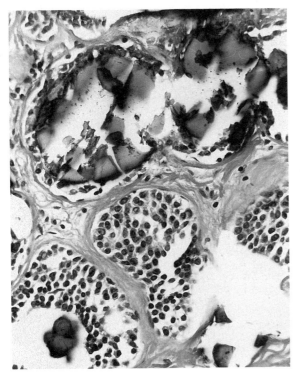

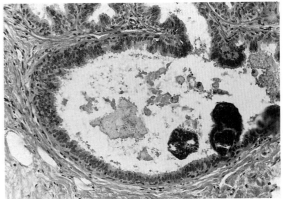

Fig. 16.19 Relatively large, laminated calcifications are present at lower right lumen of this small, benign cyst (× 125).

APOCRINE FEATURES

It has long been recognized that some breast cancers histologically resemble the apocrine-like changes which are so common in benign breast tissue. The confines of definition for accepting this change, and applying a designation of apocrine carcinoma, have varied from the use of strict criteria, recognizing 0.3–0.4% of breast cancers (Azzopardi 1979), to a much higher percentage if only eosinophilic tint to the cytoplasm is accepted as 'apocrine'. Frable & Kay (1968) demanded an identical appearance to apocrine glands and found an incidence of 1% of so-called apocrine tumours. Clinical follow-up of their cases revealed no difference from a controlled series of breast cancers. Fisher et al (1975) identified 2.2% of their 1000 cases as having oxyphilic granular cytoplasm, but they did not feel that this feature merited designation as a special type of cancer.

However, there are indications that histological resemblance to apocrine epithelium may have relevant physiological correlates. Miller et al (1985) found marked apocrine features in 12% of the series of breast cancers and reported a greater metabolism of testosterone precursors in these tumours. Mossler et al (1980) identified 0.4% of breast cancers as having uniformly fine, granular, pale, eosinophilic cytoplasm with apical cytoplasm projections, and demonstrated a high capacity, low affinity, non-saturable 4S progesterone-oestrogen binding protein as opposed to the usually demonstrable steroid receptor proteins of breast carcinomas.

Recently, localization of a unique 15 000 molecular weight glycoprotein present in normal apocrine cells (GCDFP15) has been studied in various breast cancer types (Mazoujian et al 1983; Eusebi et al 1984). This protein is found in many breast cancers and may even be found in lobular carcinomas (Eusebi et al 1984). Diffuse immunoreactivity of marked degree is confined to cancers with well-developed histological resemblance to apocrine cells (Eusebi et al 1986).

Apocrine features, then, may be found in varying degree by various techniques and histo-logical criteria in varying percentages of breast cancer with no known prognostic significance or clinical correlate save those suggested for steroid metabolism above.

If only finely granular eosinophilic cytoplasm is demanded, many breast cancers will have apocrine features (Fig. 16.20). A frequently presented problem in diagnosis is that moderately developed squamous features will closely resemble apocrine cytology (Fig. 16.21). Fortunately, no prognostic significance is ascribed to either feature. More stringent criteria would demand a copious cytoplasm which is eosinophilic and distinctly granular. Apical cytoplasmic protrusions or snouts might also be required by strict criteria (Fig. 16.22). A characteristic feature of apocrine change is the presence of PAS-diastase-resistant granules, and these are even less frequent in tumours than the regular eosinophilic granularity. We feel that the rare tumours demonstrating well-developed apocrine features throughout a predominant portion of the tumour should be reported as having marked apocrine features as a descriptive qualifier, and that apocrine carcinoma not be recognized as a special type of breast cancer.

REFERENCES

Azzopardi J 1979 Problems in breast pathology. Saunders, Philadelphia, p 341–344
Eusebi V, Betts C, Haagensen D E et al 1984 Apocrine differentiation in lobular carcinoma of the breast. Hum Pathol 15: 134–140
Eusebi V, Millis R R, Grazia M, Bussolati G, Azzopardi J G 1986 Apocrine carcinoma of the breast. A morphologic and immunocytochemical study. Am J Pathol 123: 532–541
Fisher E R, Gregorio R M, Fisher B et al 1975 The pathology of invasive breast cancer. A syllabus derived from findings of the national surgical adjuvant breast project (protocol no 4). Cancer 36: 1–85
Frable W J, Kay S 1968 Carcinoma of the breast. Histologic and clinical features of apocrine tumours. Cancer 21: 756–763
Mazoujian G, Pinkus G S, Davis S, Haagensen D E 1983 Immunohistochemistry of a gross cystic disease fluid protein (GCDFP–15) of the breast. Am J Pathol 110: 105–111
Miller W R, Telford J, Dixon J M, Shivas A A 1985 Androgen metabolism and apocrine differentiation in human breast cancer. Breast Cancer Res Treat 5: 67–73
Mossler J A, Barton T K, Brinkhous A D, McCarty K S, Moylan J A, McCarty Jr K S 1980 Apocrine differentiation in human mammary carcinoma. Cancer 46: 2463–2471

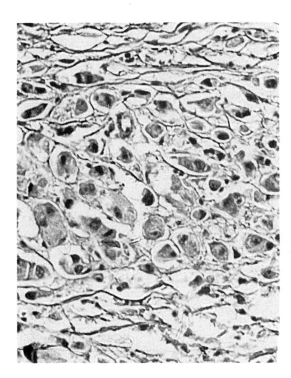

Fig. 16.20 Broad collections of breast cancer cells have relatively abundant cytoplasm which resembles apocrine change epithelium. This is a high grade, no special type carcinoma with cytoplasmic apocrine features (× 225).

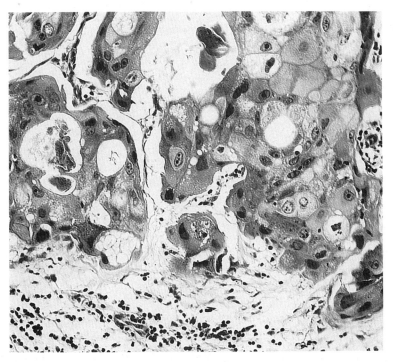

Fig. 16.21 Glassy cytoplasm, deeply eosinophilic and granular, suggests apocrine change. However, squamous features are also evident. Fortunately, no prognostic difference is indicated. Note that intercellular spaces are due to individual cell necrosis or keratinization in this carcinoma of no special type, high grade (× 400).

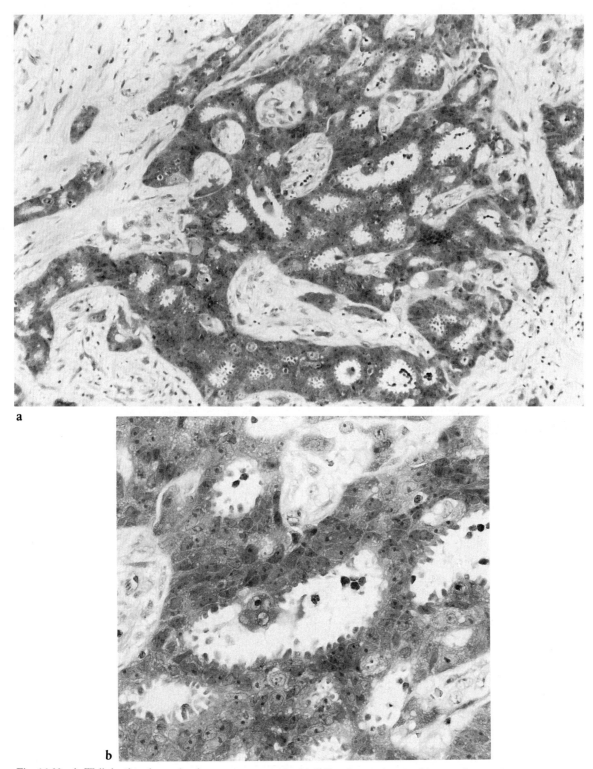

Fig. 16.22a, b Well-developed apocrine features are present in this infiltrating carcinoma of intermediate grade. Note well-developed apical 'snouts' projecting into well-developed glandular lumina (**a** × 200; **b** × 450).

ECCRINE FEATURES

It is of greater biological than nosological relevance that occasional breast neoplasms resemble those of eccrine sweat glands. After all, many tumours of eccrine glands have been named after their histological similarity to breast cancers (Wick & Coffin 1985). At this time, there is no impelling indication for the formal designation of any breast neoplasm after a similarly patterned tumour of eccrine derivation. This guideline is proposed with the exception of the useful diagnostic term 'syringomatous adenoma of the nipple' which is discussed in Chapter 18. It is of historical interest only that some more solid and clear cell patterns of papillary and usual hyperplasias in breast have been analogized to clear cell hidradenomas (Finck et al 1968). Fisher et al (1985) have commented that some breast neoplasms with orderly pattern and clear cytoplasm are analogous to eccrine acro-

spiromas (Johnson & Helwig 1969). Hertel et al (1976) have also presented a case of eccrine acrospiroma-like breast neoplasm as well as another adenoma of the breast resembling an eccrine spiradenoma. The practical importance of these rare cases lies in recognizing their benignancy.

One other pattern of breast neoplasm which can be mentioned is that which resembles the sclerosing sweat duct (syringomatous) carcinomas (Cooper 1986). These tumours of cutaneous adnexal origin may demonstrate dual pilar and eccrine differentiation (Nickoloff et al 1986). Also termed microcystic adnexal carcinoma, these cutaneous tumours are characterized by diffuse local infiltration and no demonstrated ability for distant metastasis. Histologically, there are tightly packed nests and cords of cells with occasional lumina which may contain keratin (Cooper 1986). Some nests have tapering formations resembling syringoma. Prognostic correlates of breast tumours with similar patterns (Figs 16.23 and 16.24) are unknown, but as they are similar in appearance

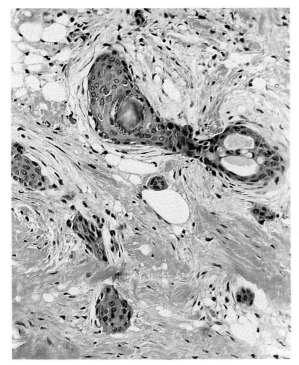

Fig. 16.23 Breast carcinoma resembles sclerosing carcinoma of sweat ducts with tightly packed aggregates of infiltrating cells. Note larger island with cyst formation at right and keratin formation at left (× 200).

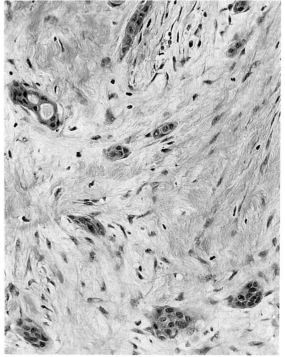

Fig. 16.24 Another area of same tumour as Figure 16.15 with decreased resemblance to sclerosing sweat duct (syringomatous) carcinomas. Syringomatous adenoma of the nipple is also mimicked (× 200).

to syringomatous adenomas of the nipple (Ch. 18) and as the cutaneous lesions are predominantly local problems, wide local excision would seem feasible.

REFERENCES

Cooper P H 1986 Sclerosing carcinomas of sweat ducts (microcystic adnexal carcinoma). Arch Dermatol 122: 261–264

Finck F M, Schwinn C P, Keasbey L E 1968 Clear cell hidradenoma of the breast. Cancer 22: 125–135

Fisher E R, Tavares J, Bulatao I S et al 1985 Glycogen-rich, clear cell breast cancer: with comments concerning other clear cell variants. Hum Pathol 16: 1085–1090

Hertel B F, Zaloudek C, Kempson R L 1976 Breast adenomas. Cancer 37: 2891–2905

Johnson B L, Helwig E B 1969 Eccrine acrospiroma. A clinicopathologic study. Hum Pathol 16: 1085–1090

Nickoloff B J, Fleischmann H E, Carmel J, Wood C C, Roth R J 1986 Microcystic adnexal carcinoma. Arch Dermatol 122: 290–294

Wick M R, Coffin C M 1985 Sweat gland and pilar carcinomas. In: Wick M R (ed) Pathology of unusual maliqnant cutaneous tumours. Dekker, New York ch 1, p 1–76

SQUAMOUS METAPLASIA

As is so often the case with adenocarcinomas having areas reminiscent of squamous epithelium, deciding when squamous alteration is present may be frustrating. Fortunately, this finding, no matter how stringently defined, has no prognostic significance in breast cancers. When stringently defined, squamous metaplasia is identified in about 4% of breast carcinomas (Fisher et al 1975). Such a demanding requirement for accepting the presence of squamous metaplasia includes sharply defined, eosinophilic cells with intercellular bridges and/or tight swirling formations (squamous pearls) with keratinization (Figs 16.25 and 16.26).

The preceding discussion of squamous carcinoma (Ch. 14) has noted the utility of reporting squamous features in carcinomas of no special type to aid in recognizing future metastases as consistent with the breast primary. How often the squamous features are presented in metastases has not been rigorously studied, but it is our impression that such features are less common in metastases.

REFERENCES

Fisher E R, Gregorio R M, Fisher B et al 1975 The pathology of invasive breast cancer. A syllabus derived from findings of the national surgical adjuvant breast project (protocol no. 4). Cancer 36: 1–85

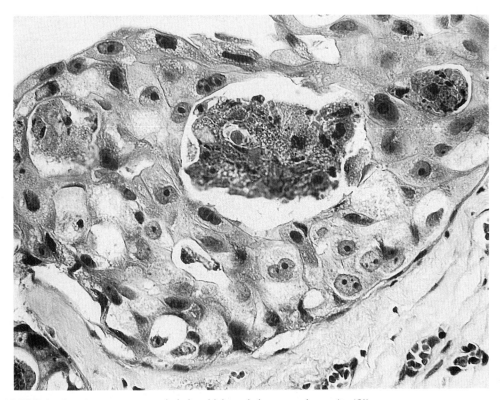

Fig. 16.25 Well-developed squamous metaplasia in a high grade breast carcinoma (× 450).

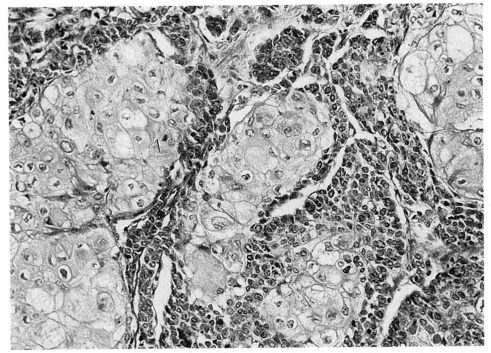

Fig. 16.26 Squamous metaplasia is evident in central portions of carcinoma islands in this tumour otherwise showing no differentiation. It is, therefore, a poorly differentiated carcinoma of no special type with squamous metaplasia (× 225).

Grading of invasive carcinoma of the breast

Background

From the earliest days of microscopical pathology it was recognized that malignant tumours differed in their degree of malignancy and that this was reflected in their morphological appearance (Hansemann 1890; Dennis 1891). The first formal analysis in carcinoma of the breast was carried out by Greenhough (1925), stimulated by the studies of Broders (1920, 1921) who found a good correlation between the loss of differentiation in squamous carcinomas of the lip and skin and clinical outcome. Greenhough (1925) examined tumours from patients undergoing radical mastectomy, and was able to divide them into three grades of malignancy based on an assessment of eight histological factors; the degree of glandular formation, epithelial secretion, the size of cells, the size of nuclei, variation in the size of both cells and nuclei, nuclear hyperchromatism and the mitotic activity. The number of cases was small but he showed a clear association between the histological grade of malignancy and 'cure', although the term 'cure' was not accurately defined (grade I, 19 cases — 68% cure; grade II, 33 cases — 33% cure; grade III, 21 cases — 0% cure). Similar findings were obtained by several workers (White 1927; Patey & Scarff 1928; Haagensen 1933) whilst others investigated more complex methods including assessment of stromal factors (Hueper & Schmitz 1929). Patey & Scarff (1928) followed the method of Greenhough, but attached most importance to tubule formation, variation in size of nuclei and mitotic and hyperchromatic figures. Scarff & Handley (1938), using the criteria derived by Patey & Scarff (1928), confirmed a clear correlation between histological grade and survival, 31% of patients with grade I tumours

being alive at 10 years compared with 13% of patients with grade III tumours.

Little interest was generated by these studies, possibly because at this time prognostic information was not used to determine the type of therapy received by a patient. It was not until 1950 that the concept of histological grading as an important prognostic factor was revived by Bloom (1950a, 1950b) in the United Kingdom. He made an extensive review of the literature and concluded that the best correlation with survival had been obtained in studies using methods derived from that originally devised by Greenhough (1925). In Bloom's method chief importance was placed on three factors: the degree of tubule formation, regularity in the size, shape and staining of nuclei, and hyperchromatism with mitotic activity. Each of the three factors was assessed subjectively as absent or present in slight, moderate or marked degree and the tumours were placed in three grades of malignancy, low, moderate and high. Grading was carried out in 470 cases; the five year survival ranged from 79% for grade I tumours to 25% for grade III tumours, whilst at 10 years the survival figures were 45% and 13% respectively. Bloom (1950a, 1950b) concluded that histological grading did provide a useful index of prognosis, but also stressed that prediction of survival was improved by combining grade with lymph node staging. Thus the five-year survival of 94% for patients with uninvolved axillary lymph nodes fell to 65% for those with involved lymph nodes in grade I tumours, and from 55% to 16% in grade III tumours. In a subsequent report, Bloom & Richardson (1957) extended Bloom's original study and also provided a refinement of the grading method. This took the form of a numerical scoring system. For each of the three histological factors examined the previous designation of slight, moderate and marked was replaced by a score of 1–3. This gave a total score of 3–9, and the grades were arbitrarily assigned as follows: grade I — 3, 4 or 5 points, grade II — 6 or 7 points, grade III — 8 or 9 points. The points system was not meant to ascribe a mathematical accuracy to the method, but to act as an aid to grading. Bloom & Richardson (1957) confirmed the association between grade and survival, and when follow-up on the same series of patients was later extended to 20 years the predictive ability was shown to persist (Bloom & Field 1971). The Bloom & Richardson method has now been used in a substantial number of studies (Wolff 1966; Hamlin 1968; Tough et al 1969; Champion et al 1972; Andersen et al 1981; Elston et al 1982; Parl & Dupont 1982; Elston, 1984) and in all it has been found to be both practical and useful in determining prognosis.

Alternative methods of histological grading in breast cancer have also been developed, such as that originally described by Black et al (1955) in the United States and designated as 'nuclear grading'. The method was in fact derived from the work of Bloom (1950a), but Black et al (1955) assessed tubular structures and nuclear appearances separately. They concluded that tubular differentiation did not contribute to the prediction of prognosis, but that the nuclear morphology did. Four grades were devised, based on the regularity of the nuclear outline, delicacy of chromatin strands, presence or absence of nucleoli and mitotic figures. Unfortunately, Black et al (1955) reversed the numerical order of the grades compared with Bloom's work, so that nuclear grades O and I apply to the poorly differentiated tumours and grade IV to the well-differentiated tumours. The nuclear grading method has been used extensively by Black and associates, and found to have a correlation with survival (Black & Speer 1957, 1959; Cutler et al 1963, 1969; Black et al 1975), although this was not supported by Kister et al (1969). The method devised by Hartveit (1971), based partly on examination of primary tumours and partly on necropsy material, uses cytological criteria such as definition of cell borders and nuclear/cytoplasmic ratio, but takes

no account of mitotic activity. Like the Black system the tumours with the best prognosis are grade III.

Comparisons of the various grading methods have been few. Eichner et al (1970) examined the Bloom & Richardson (1957) method and that of Black et al (1955). They found that the two methods gave similar correlations with survival at five-year follow-up, and concluded that both provided a useful means of estimating the neoplastic potential of breast tumours. Turner & Berry (1972) also evaluated the Bloom & Richardson method, but compared it with the system devised by Hartveit (1971). The Bloom & Richardson method was found to be more accurate in predicting prognosis in a series composed of both short-term and long-term survivors. Stenkvist et al (1979) undertook an analysis concentrating mainly on reproducibility, but also assessing interrelationships, using the WHO method (Bloom & Richardson 1957; Scarff & Torloni 1968), the Black method (Black & Speer 1957) and that of Hartveit (1971). They showed that the WHO and the Black method were closely related, and separated the tumours into three prognostic categories, whilst the Hartveit method gave no such stratification. The Bloom and Black methods appear to be superior to that of Hartveit in practical application and in correlation with prognosis. Fisher and associates have advocated a method which combines elements of both systems (Fisher et al 1975; Fisher 1977) by including the presence or absence of tubule formation with nuclear grade. They have shown a satisfactory correlation with survival (Fisher et al 1980), and more recently have introduced a further modification by considering the degree and type of tubule formation (Fisher et al 1984). However, it should be noted that approximately two-thirds of cases, even with the modified system, are placed in the poorly differentiated grade, so that stratification in this method is rather poor. This author has not carried out a large scale comparative survey but in a small pilot study found the Bloom method easier to use, and to give a better correlation with prognosis. The method, with the modifications used in the Nottingham/Tenovus breast study, is described in detail below.

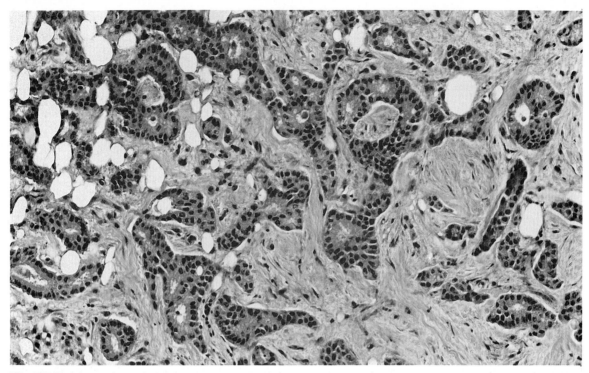

Fig. 17.1 Invasive carcinoma in which there is good tubular differentiation. Most of the tubules have clearly visible lumina. Tubule score — 1 point (× 196).

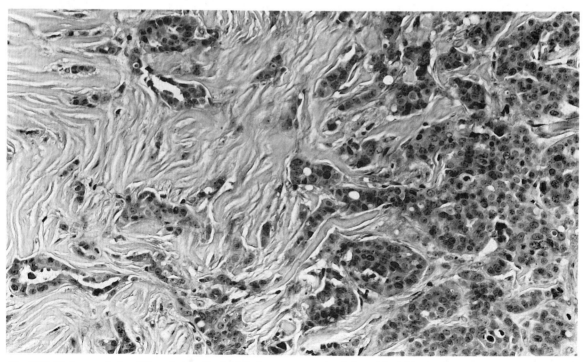

Fig. 17.2 Moderate tubular differentiation. To the left there are several tubules with visible lumina, but on the right more solid cords are formed. Tubule score — 2 points (× 196).

Methods

The first prerequisite for accurate histological grading is good, careful specimen preparation. Fixation in phosphate-buffered formalin gives perfectly adequate preservation but the best results are obtained if the tumour is sliced in the fresh state to allow good penetration of fixative. This may require special organization (for example, a research technician can be trained to sample tumours immediately after mastectomy following localization by the pathologist or surgeon with the advantage that specimens may also be deep frozen for hormone receptor assay or other studies), but the results will be greatly improved in comparison with the practice of immersing the whole breast unsliced in fixative. Blocks should be selected so as to give good representation of the whole tumour, and in particular the periphery. The number of blocks taken will depend on the size of the tumour; for a tumour of approximately 2 cm diameter two to four blocks would be appropriate. Careful processing is important, and sections should be cut at 4–6 μm; if sections are cut too thick, nuclear detail is obscured. Conventional staining with haematoxylin and eosin is sufficient and special stains are not required. Grading is only carried out in invasive carcinomas; tumours which are completely or predominantly in situ are not suitable for grading. The histological grade is obtained by analysis of the following three features, each of which is given a score of 1–3.

1. Tubule formation (Figs 17.1–17.3)

All parts of the tumour are scanned, and where the great majority is composed of formed tubules with clearly visible lumina a score of 1 point is given. In cases in which definite tubule formation is seen in moderate amounts but there are also clear areas of solid tumour growth, a score of 2 points is made. Where little or no tubule formation is seen, the cells growing in sheets or cords, the score is given as 3 points. With good fixation and processing clefts in tumour tissue due to shrinkage artefact should be reduced to a minimum. Their presence should not be mistaken for tubular structures.

2. Nuclear pleomorphism (Figs 17.4–17.6)

In this category an assessment is made of the variability of both size and shape of the tumour nuclei. Tumours in which nuclei are regular and show little variation in size and shape are given 1 point. Two points are given when a moderate variation is seen, without extremes of cell size or shape. Marked variation, particularly when very large and bizarre nuclei are present, scores 3 points. In the latter two categories nucleoli are often present, and multiple nucleoli in a nucleus favour a score of 3.

3. Mitotic rate (Fig. 17.7)

It is in this category that the present method differs most from that described by Bloom & Richardson (1957). They analysed the relative numbers of both hyperchromatic nuclei and mitotic figures. In practice it is often impossible to distinguish hyperchromatic nuclei from those which are simply pyknotic and also from lymphocytes within the tumour. Bloom & Richardson (1957) were rather imprecise in their allocation in this category, and a 'high power field' was not defined accurately. It is therefore recommended that hyperchromatic nuclei are ignored, and that points are allocated as follows, using a magnification of approximately 300 times. Less than 10 mitosis per 10 fields scores 1 point, 10–19 mitoses per 10 fields scores 2 points, and 20 or more mitoses per 10 fields scores 3 points. Mitotic activity is best assessed at the periphery of the tumour where active growth is most likely, and a minimum of 10 fields should be scanned. To obtain the overall tumour grade the scores for each category are added together, giving a possible total of 3–9 points. The grade is then allocated on the following basis:

1. 3–5 points: grade I — well differentiated
2. 6–7 points: grade II — moderately differentiated
3. 8–9 points: grade III — poorly differentiated.

It is recognized that the separation into three grades along these lines is arbitrary, and perhaps artificial, since it is likely that there is in fact a continuous scale of malignancy. However, as will be shown below, a good correlation with prognosis

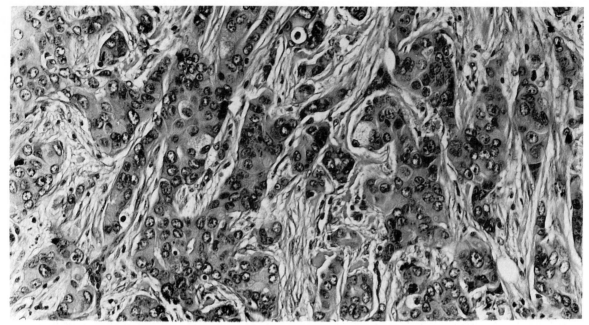

Fig. 17.3 This carcinoma is composed of solid cords and sheets of tumour cells, with no tubule formation. Tubule score — 3 points (× 196).

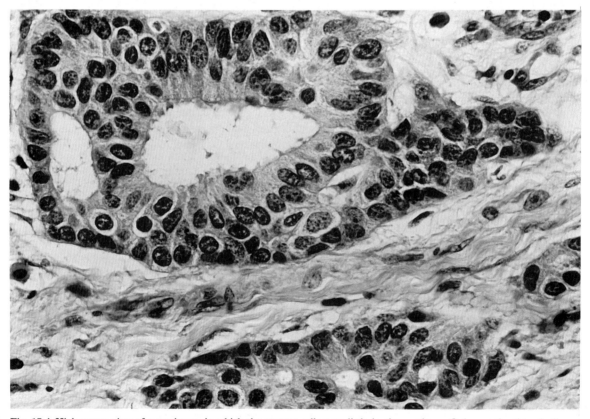

Fig. 17.4 High power view of a carcinoma in which the tumour cells vary little in size or shape. Only occasional nucleoli are visible. Variation score — 1 (× 490).

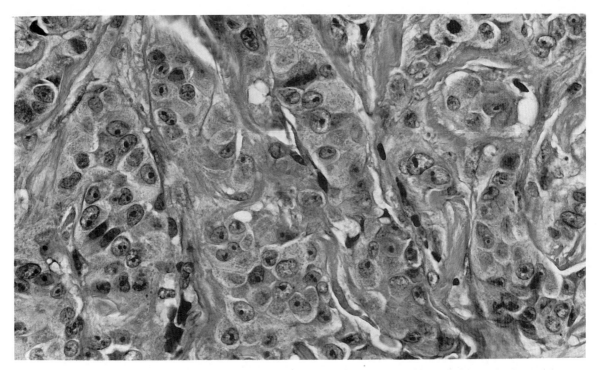

Fig. 17.5 In this tumour there is moderate variation in size and shape of nuclei. Many of the nuclei contain single nucleoli. Variation score — 2 (× 490)

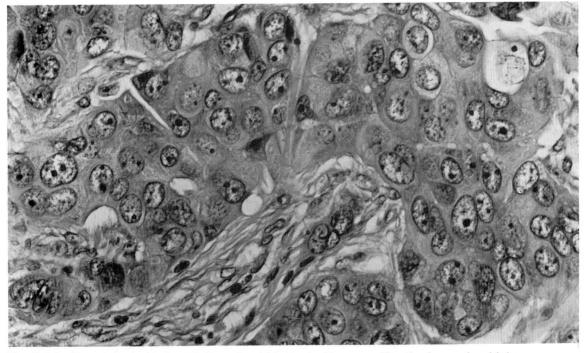

Fig. 17.6 A wide variation in the size and shape of nuclei is seen in this tumour. Note that in several nuclei there are two nucleoli. Variation score — 3 (× 490).

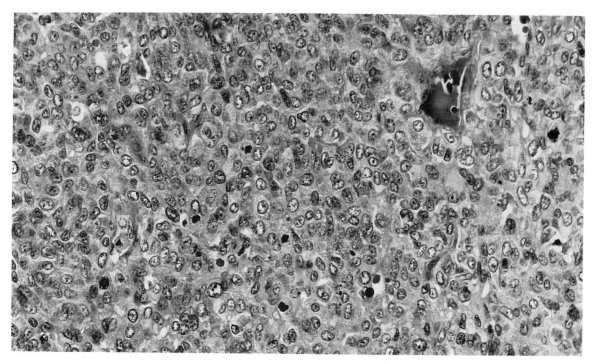

Fig. 17.7 A 'high power field' magnification of 300 times showing several mitotic figures. Mitosis count — 3 points (× 300).

is achieved. As Bloom & Richardson (1957) pointed out, the use of a numerical system is not meant to ascribe mathemetical accuracy to grading. Its main usefulness lies in the discipline it forces on the pathologist. Rather than giving an instinctive and subjective view of the degree of differentiation, the numerical system makes the pathologist assess each factor separately and think carefully about its relative value independently. Some degree of variation in appearance from one part of a tumour to another undoubtedly occurs, and this is the main reason for examining multiple blocks. Assessment of tubular differentiation is made on the overall appearances of the tumour, and so account is taken of any variation. Nuclear appearances are evaluated at the periphery of the tumour to obviate differences between the growing edge and the less active centre. In practice it has been found that variation is rarely significant enough to make a difference to the grade, and this is supported by other studies (Haagensen 1933; Bloom 1950a; Bloom & Richardson 1957; Tough et al 1969). If any difficulty is encountered then the nuclear appearances should be assessed in the least differentiated area.

Histological grading is based on a subjective assessment of microscopic appearances and difficulties in consistency and reproducibility are likely. This is reflected in the considerable variation in the relative proportions of each grade in reported series (Table 17.1). Some of the variation may be due to real differences in populations of patients studied, but other factors must also be considered. It is unfortunate that the majority of previous studies have been carried out by non-pathologists (e.g. Bloom & Richardson 1957; Wolff 1966; Tough et al 1969; Champion et al 1972) who, with respect, cannot have had the

Table 17.1 Comparison of the relative percentage of cases in each grade in different studies.

Study	Histological grade %		
	I	II	III
Bloom & Richardson (1957)	26	45	29
Wolff (1966)	33	33	34
Tough et al (1969)	11	51	38
Champion et al (1972)	23	52	25
Fisher et al (1980)	3	30	67
Fisher et al (1984)	11	23	66
Elston (1984)	17	37	46

depth of experience of a trained histopathologist. No information was given in these publications concerning the verification of results from double or cross-checking, essential in a subjective method. Inexperienced observers faced with a choice of three grades, have a tendency to 'play for safety' and allocate too high a proportion of cases to the middle grade. To achieve internal consistency in the Nottingham/Tenovus study tumours are graded independently by two experienced histopathologists, who now obtain 90% agreement on the first assessment. The remaining cases are re-examined independently and without knowledge of the previous results. If agreement is not achieved on this occasion the sections are further examined on a conference microscope by the two pathologists and agreement is reached by consensus. A similar degree of consistency was obtained by Fisher et al (1975), within one centre, and they also achieved only a 6% discrepancy by the same reviewer on different occasions (Fisher et al 1980). Reproducibility between different centres is more difficult to achieve. Cutler et al (1966), using nuclear grading, reported that 60% agreement was reached between an experienced observer and a pathologist who had not classified tumours previously. In the same study Black who devised the method, only obtained 70% agreement between his first and second readings. Stenkvist et al (1979) analysed the WHO, Black and Hartveit methods and concluded that all had a low inter- and intra-observer reproducibility. Interpretation of this latter study is difficult, because the authors give few details of their methods and no mention is made of their experience in breast cancer histology. A similar poor level of reproducibility was obtained by Delides et al (1982) using the WHO method. Rather more encouraging results have been obtained by the Yorkshire Breast Group. They have assessed the feasibility of histological grading on a regional basis, using the Bloom & Richardson method. The sections from each of 13 centres are examined independently by both the contributing pathologist and a co-ordinator. Preliminary results, based on 665 cases, show complete agreement between the two pathologists in 81% (Hopton 1980). This is a very high level of agreement considering the number of individuals who are participating. As Scarff & Torloni (1968) have pointed out, experience and dedication are essential requirements for accurate histological grading, and the method should only be undertaken by fully trained histopathologists. Results must always be double checked, preferably by a second pathologist but, if this is not possible, by the same pathologist on a separate occasion, without knowledge of the previous result. This is not a method which can be expected to yield good results from a casual approach.

Clinical significance and prognostic implications

The author has personal experience with histological grading in two large-scale studies, the Cancer Research Campaign Trial for early breast cancer, and the Nottingham/Tenovus Breast Cancer study. In the former, over 1500 tumours from 80 centres throughout the world were examined by a central panel of four pathologists. In the tenth year of follow-up a clear correlation between histological grade and prognosis was shown (Fig. 17.8), patients with well-differentiated tumours having a considerably better survival than those with poorly differentiated tumours (Elston et al 1982). The Nottingham/Tenovus study is based on a single surgical team and the pathological aspects are directed by a single pathologist (CWE). To date the results from 916 patients have been analysed. Once again there is a highly significant correlation with survival (Fig. 17.9). These results amply confirm previous reports and there can be no doubt that histological grade provides a good marker of prognosis. As suggested by Bloom (1950a) the predictive ability of histological grade is improved by its combination with lymph node stage. In the Nottingham/Tenovus study an attempt has been made to produce a composite prognostic index from an analysis of a number of factors. Initially, a group of patients with an extremely poor prognosis (death or major recurrence within 18 months of mastectomy) was identified, based on extensive local lymph node involvement (apex of axilla and/or internal mammary nodes), tumour size greater than 2 cm and histological grade II or III (Blamey et al

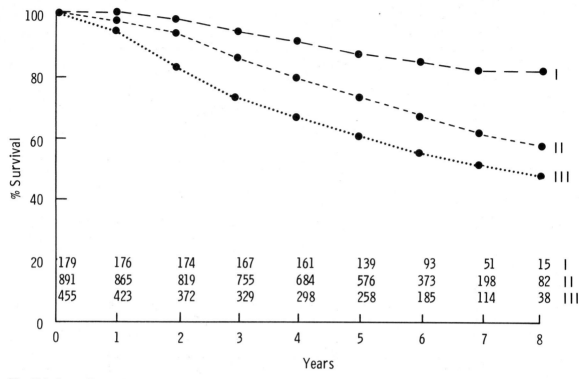

Fig. 17.8 Cancer Research Campaign trial for early breast cancer. Survival rates showing the correlation between histological grade and prognosis. X^2 for trend = 51.52, $P < 0.001$.

1979). When longer follow-up became available the data was analysed using the multiple regression technique of Cox (Cox 1972). In the Cox analysis individual factors are assessed independently whilst taking into account the weight of all the other factors. The only factors found to have a significant correlation with prognosis were tumour size, lymph node stage and histological grade (Haybittle et al 1982). Combination of these factors into a prognostic index, using the coefficients produced in the Cox analysis, permits stratification of patients into good, moderate and poor prognostic groups, having an annual mortality of 3%, 7% and 30% respectively (Todd et al 1987).

The correlation with prognosis supports the concept that histological grade provides a measure of tumour differentiation. Further evidence is obtained from kinetic studies of breast cancer using ^{3}H-thymidine uptake methods. It has been shown that tumours with a high labelling index (LI), indicating a rapid replication rate and thus, presumably, poorer differentiation, have a greater early relapse rate than those with a low LI (Meyer & Hixon 1979; Tubiana et al 1981). Tubiana et al (1981) further demonstrated a correlation between high LI and poor histological grade, the association with mitotic component of grade being particularly significant. Meyer et al (1977) have also correlated ^{3}H-thymidine uptake with a biochemical parameter, cytoplasmic oestradiol receptor (ER) content. They showed that tumours with a high LI tend to be ER negative, which complements the significant association between ER status and histological grade shown by Elston et al (1980), ER negative tumours usually being of poor grade (II or III). ER status correlates well with survival (Bishop et al 1979; Blamey et al 1980), but in the Nottingham/Tenovus index histological grade has a better predictive value

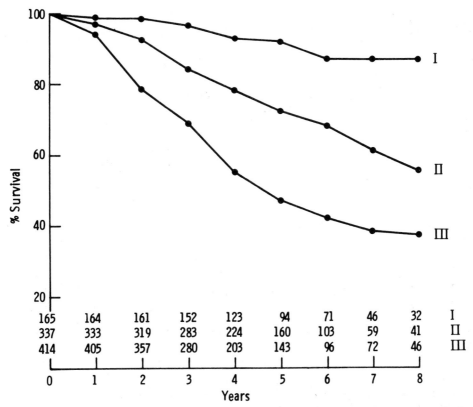

Fig. 17.9 Nottingham/Tenovus primary breast cancer study. Survival rates showing the correlation between histological grade and prognosis. $X^2 = 90.86$, $P < 0.0005$.

(Haybittle et al 1982). It is also relevant that assessment of DNA content, using both static cytometry (Auer et al 1984) and flow cytometry (Olszewski et al 1981; Tavares 1986; Dowle et al 1987) has demonstrated a significant correlation between DNA ploidy and histological grade. Tumours which are DNA diploid are more likely to be well differentiated, whilst DNA aneuploid tumours are usually poorly differentiated.

The methods of histological grading referred to in this chapter were devised before it was fully appreciated that carcinoma of the breast encompasses a variety of tumour types. In most published studies therefore, grading has been carried out on all the invasive carcinomas in a series, regardless of histological type. The correlation between tumour type and prognosis is discussed in some detail in Chapter 13. Briefly, special types, such as pure tubular, pure mucinous and invasive cribriform carcinoma carry an excel-

lent prognosis, whilst pure infiltrating lobular and medullary carcinomas appear to have an intermediate prognosis between the first group and the common infiltrating ductal carcinoma (no special type). It could be argued from such data that histological grading is only appropriate in the latter group of tumours, but a number of practical points require consideration. Tumour typing must be done with care, otherwise the wide range of recorded frequencies for special types, shown in Table 13.1, will result. Furthermore, up to a quarter of tumours in a series may be of mixed or combined type (Fisher et al 1975) and the prognostic significance of this group is unclear. Finally, if grading is restricted to the infiltrating ductal group, then at best 75% (Rosen 1979) and at worst only 53% (Fisher et al 1975) of cases will be included, and valuable prognostic data may be lost.

Since both histological grade and histological

type provide useful prognostic information it is clear that a reappraisal of these morphological methods of assessing tumour differentiation is required. In the Nottingham/Tenovus study we have shown that the mitotic count is the most powerful component of grade (Mann et al 1987). We are now engaged in a long term follow-up study to determine the relationship between the components of grade and type in the prediction of prognosis. It is hoped that in this way a combined index of differentiation will be produced which provides a more accurate guide to prognosis than is currently available when grade and type are assessed separately. The method for histological grading was first described over 50 years ago. Despite the fact that a clear correlation with survival has been demonstrated in numerous studies since then the method has largely been ignored by clinicians in their approach to therapeutic trials. Provided that grading is carried out by experienced pathologists following the guidelines described above, consistent and reproducible results will be obtained. There is good evidence that histological grade compares favourably with kinetic and biochemical parameters of differentiation and, until a more accurate histological predictor of prognosis becomes available, it should be used as part of a standard prognostic index in breast cancer, particularly where stratification of patients is required for therapeutic purposes.

Acknowledgements

I am grateful to the Working Party of the Cancer Research Campaign (Kings/Cambridge) Trial for early breast cancer for their permission to use the data shown in Figure 17.8, and to my colleagues in the Nottingham/Tenovus Primary Breast Cancer study for allowing me to use the data in Figure 17.9. My thanks are also due to Mr W. Brackenbury and Mr G. Gilbert for the photographs and to Mrs J. Rainbow for typing the manuscript.

REFERENCES

Andersen J A, Fischermann K, Hou-Jensen K et al 1981 Selection of high risk groups among prognostically favorable patients with breast cancer. Ann Surg 194: 1–3
Auer G, Eriksson E, Azavedo E, Caspersson T, Wallgren A 1984 Prognostic significance of nuclear DNA content in mammary adenocarcinoma in humans. Cancer Res 44: 394–396
Bishop H M, Blamey R W, Elston C W, Haybittle J L, Nicholson R I, Griffiths K 1979 Relationship of oestrogen-receptor status to survival in breast cancer. Lancet 2: 283–284
Black M M, Speer F D 1957 Nuclear structure in cancer tissues. Surg Gynecol Obstet 105: 97–102
Black M M, Speer F D 1959 Immunology of cancer. Int Abst Surg 109: 105–116
Black M M, Opler S R, Speer F D 1955 Survival in breast cancer cases in relation to structure of the primary tumor and regional lymph nodes. Surg Gynecol Obstet 100: 543–551
Black M M, Barclay T H C Hankey B F 1975 Prognosis in breast cancer utilizing histologic characteristics of the primary tumor. Cancer 36: 2048–2055
Blamey R W, Davies C J, Elston C W, Johnson J, Haybittle J L, Maynard P V 1979 Prognostic factors in breast cancer — the formation of a prognostic index. Clin Oncol 5: 1–10
Blamey R W, Bishop H M, Blake J R S et al 1980 Relationship between primary breast tumour receptor status and patient survival. Cancer 46: 2765–2769
Bloom H J G 1950a Prognosis in carcinoma of the breast. Br J Cancer 4: 259–288
Bloom H J G 1950b Further studies on prognosis of breast carcinoma. Br J Cancer 4: 347–367
Bloom H J G, Field J R 1971 Impact of tumor grade and host resistance on survival of women with breast cancer. Cancer 28: 1580–1589
Bloom H J G, Richardson W W 1957 Histologiccal grading and prognosis in breast cancer. Br J Cancer 11: 359–377
Broders A C 1920 Squamous-cell epithelioma of the lip. J A M A 74: 656–664
Broders A C 1921 Squamous cell epithelioma of the skin. Ann Surg 73: 141–160
Champion H R, Wallace I W J, Prescott R J, 1972 Histology in breast cancer prognosis. Br J Cancer 26: 129–138
Cox D R 1972 Regression models and life-tables. J R Stat Soc (B) 34: 187–220
Cutler S J, Black M M, Goldenberg I S 1963 Prognostic factors in cancer of the female breast. Cancer 16: 1589–1597
Cutler S J, Black M M, Friedell G H, Vidone R A, Goldenberg I S 1966 Prognostic factors in cancer of the female breast. II. Reproducibility of histopathologic classification. Cancer 19: 75–82
Cutler S J, Black M M, Mork T, Harvei S, Freeman C 1969 Further observations on prognostic factors in cancer of the female breast. Cancer 24: 653–667
Delides G S, Garas G, Georgouli G et al 1982 Intralaboratory variations in the grading of breast carcinoma. Arch Pathol Lab Med 106: 126–128
Dennis F S 1891 Recurrence of carcinoma of the breast. Trans Am Surg Assoc 9: 219–259
Dowle C S, Owainati A, Robins A et al 1987 The prognostic significance of the DNA content of human breast cancer. Br J Surg 74: 133–136

Eichner W J, Lemon H M, Friedell G H 1970 Tumor grade in the prognosis of breast cancer. Nebr Med J 55: 405–409

Elston C W 1984 The assessment of histological differentiation in breast cancer. Aust N Z J Surg 54: 11–15

Elston C W, Blamey R W, Johnson J, Bishop H M, Haybittle J L, Griffiths K 1980 The relationship of oestradiol receptor (ER) and histological tumour differentiation with prognosis in human primary breast carcinoma. In: Mouridsen H T, Palshof R (eds) Breast cancer — experimental and clinical aspects. Pergamon Press, Oxford, p 59–62

Elston C W, Gresham G A, Rao G S, Zebro T, Haybittle J L, Houghton J 1982 The cancer research campaign (Kings/Cambridge) trial for early breast cancer — pathological aspects. Br J Cancer 45: 655–669

Fisher E R 1977 Pathology of breast cancer. In: McGuire W L (ed) Breast cancer. Advances in research and treatment, vol 1. Current approaches to therapy. Churchill Livingstone, Edinburgh, ch 2, p 43–123

Fisher E R, Gregorio R M, Fisher B 1975 The pathology of invasive breast cancer. A syllabus derived from findings of the national surgical adjuvant breast project (protocol no 4). Cancer 36: 1–85

Fisher E R, Redmond C, Fisher B 1980 Histologic grading of breast cancer. Path Annu 15(1): 239–251

Fisher E R, Sass R, Fisher B et al 1984 Pathologic findings from the national surgical adjuvant project for breast cancer (protocol no 4). Discriminants for tenth year treatment failure. Cancer 53: 712–723

Greenhough R B 1925 Varying degrees of malignancy in cancer of the breast. J Cancer Res 9: 452–463

Haagensen C D 1933 The basis for the histologic grading of carcinoma of the breast. Am J Cancer 1: 285–327

Hamlin I M E 1968 Possible host resistance in carcinoma of the breast: a histological study. Br J Cancer 22: 383–401

Hansemann D von 1890 Ueber assymenstrische Zelltheilung in Epithel-krebsen und deren biologische Bedentung. Virchows Arch (A) 119: 299–326

Hartveit F 1971 Prognostic typing in breast cancer. Br Med J 4: 253–257

Haybittle J L, Blamey R W, Elston C W et al 1982 A prognostic index in primary breast cancer. Br J Cancer 45: 361–366

Hopton D 1980 Preliminary results of the pathological grading for Yorkshire breast cancer group patients. In: Yorkshire breast group symposium. The high risk patient with breast cancer. York, May 1980

Hueper W C, Schmitz H 1929 Relations of histological structure and clinical grouping to the prognosis of carcinomata of the breast and uterine cervix. Ann Surg 90: 993–999

Kister S J, Sommers S C, Haagensen C S, Friedell G H, Cooley E, Varma A 1969 Nuclear grading and sinus histiocytosis in cancer of the breast. Cancer 23: 570–575

Mann R, Ellis I O, Elston C W et al 1987 Evaluation of mitotic activity as a component of histological grade and its contribution to prognosis in primary breast carcinoma (submitted for publication)

Meyer J S, Hixon B 1979 Advanced stage and early relapse of breast carcinomas associated with high thymidine labelling indices. Cancer Res 39: 225–235

Meyer J S, Rao B R, Stevens S C, White W L 1977 Low incidence of oestrogen receptor in breast carcinomas with rapid rates of cellular replication Cancer 40: 2290–2298

Olszewski W, Darzynkiewicz Z, Rosen P P, Schwartz M, Melamed M 1981 Flow cytometry of breast carcinoma. 1. Relation of DNA ploidy level to histology and estrogen receptor. Cancer 48: 980–984

Parl F F Dupont W D 1982 A retrospective cohort study of histologic risk factors in breast cancer patients. Cancer 50: 2410–2416

Patey D H, Scarff R W 1928 The position of histology in the prognosis of carcinoma of the breast. Lancet 1: 801–804

Rosen P P 1979 The pathological classification of human mammary carcinoma: past, present and future. Ann Clin Lab Sci 9: 144–156

Scarff R W, Handley R S 1938 Prognosis in carcinoma of the breast. Lancet 2: 582–583

Scarff R W, Torloni H 1968 Histological typing of breast tumours (international histological classification of tumours, no 2). World Health Organization, Geneva

Stenkvist B, Westman-Naeser S, Vegelius J et al 1979 Analysis of reproducibility of subjective grading systems for breast carcinoma. J Clin Pathol 32: 979–985

Tavares A S 1986 Ploidy and histological types of mammary carcinoma. Eur J Cancer 3: 449–455

Todd J H, Dowle C, Williams M R et al 1987 A prognostic index in primary breast cancer. Br J Cancer (in Press)

Tough I C K, Carter D C, Fraser J, Bruce J 1969 Histological grading in breast cancer. Br J Cancer 23: 294–301

Tubiana M, Pejovic M J, Renaud et al 1981 Kinetic parameters and the course of the disease in breast cancer. Cancer 47: 937–943

Turner D, Berry C L 1972 A comparison of two methods of prognostic typing in breast cancer. J Clin Pathol 25: 1053–1055

White W C 1927 Late results of operation for carcinoma of the breast. Ann Surg 86: 695–701

Wolff B 1966 Histological grading in carcinoma of breast. Br J Cancer 20: 36–40

18

Non-intrinsic tumours

This chapter presents neoplasms other than those arising from breast parenchyma or specialized breast stroma which may present in biopsies of the breast. Those which have been chosen either occur with some frequency in the breast or produce the greatest histological similarity to intrinsic mammary neoplasms. Of course, peripheral nerve sheath tumours, etc. will occur in mammary tissue. Their proper diagnosis should provide no difficulty for the histopathologist. Some non-intrinsic neoplasms are discussed as part of differential diagnosis in other chapters, e.g. malignant melanoma with Paget's disease of the nipple. Sarcomas are included in Chapter 20, as are some benign lesions comprising a relevant differential diagnosis, e.g. haemangiomas with angiosarcoma.

Skin

Tumours of cutaneous origin presenting in the breast have relevance primarily to the region of the nipple where characteristic basal cell carcinomas (Davis & Patchefsky 1977) and related tumours (Bryant 1985) may occur, although they are rare. Clinical presentation mimics that of Paget's disease of the nipple (Sauven & Roberts 1983). There is little special importance to the knowledge that superficial cutaneous neoplasms may occur in skin overlying the breast, as they are easily separated from breast primaries by site of origin. However dermal tumours such as eccrine acrospiroma may present differential diagnostic problems (Ilie 1986). Sebaceous features may be seen in otherwise characteristic breast tumours (Tavassoli & Norris 1986).

A peculiar and unusual benign neoplasm of the nipple has recently been designated 'syringomatous adenoma of the nipple' (Rosen 1983). Previously included within the confines of definition of nipple adenoma (Doctor & Sirsat 1971), these interesting tumours are important to recognize as they may be easily confused with breast carcinomas, particularly tubular carcinomas.

Syringomatous adenoma of the nipple has no proven origin from the eccrine glands of the nipple, but the close resemblance to syringoma (a tumour of acknowledged skin appendage origin) and the restriction of such tumours to the nipple where eccrine glands are found make the assumption tenable and the term 'syringomatous' appropriate.

Syringomatous adenomas present clinically as localized nodules or plaques in the nipple. Rounded, oval and elongated solitary glandular elements infiltrate around the parenchymal elements of the nipple. They appear to have a normal relation to stroma, are less dilated and less angular than tubular carcinoma. The cells are small, regular, and cuboidal, usually present in several cell layers. Squamous metaplasia is frequent. Local recurrence after incomplete incision has been described (Rosen 1983). Eccrine-like mammary carcinomas are discussed in Chapter 16.

Granular cell tumours

Although rare, granular cell tumours (GCT) deserve a special place in histopathological differential diagnosis in the breast. This is not so much because of the difficulty of differentiating GCT from breast carcinomas, but because those unaware that GCT occur in breast may misinterpret these usually benign tumours as breast cancers.

In gross appearance, GCTs manifest the greatest mimicry of breast cancers. They are firm to hard, with rounded, slightly irregular borders which are fixed to surrounding tissues. Frequently noted is a gritty sensation on cutting — enhancing the mimicry of sclerosed carcinomas. Granular cell tumours are usually 1–3 cm in diameter when detected within the breast, and are smaller when found in the skin.

The average age at diagnosis is in the 30s, and is at least 10 years younger than for breast carcinoma (DeMay & Kay 1984). Granular cell tumours in breast will be found in an approximate ratio of one to every 1,000 breast cancers (Gordon et al 1985), and they are more common in blacks (Umansky & Bullock 1968). They occur more frequently in breast quadrants other than the upper outer. These peculiar tumours are found in many other body sites, with GCTs within the breast representing 6–8% of the total (DeMay & Kay 1984).

Regularly benign, GCTs are cured by local excision. However, there are rare malignant variants, recognized by large size, local invasion and pleomorphism. However, only one such tumour producing metastases has been described arising within the breast (DeMay & Kay 1984). Tissue of origin, long debated, is currently accepted as neural (Ingram et al 1984; Willen et al 1984). GCTs are comprised histologically of large cells in relatively distinct and usually rounded groups. Each cell has a small, dark, regular nucleus and an abundant, eosinophilic granularity to the cytoplasm (Fig. 18.1). Occasional cells will contain spherical inclusions, usually larger (2–10 microns) than the granules. These inclusions are also eosinophilic, but in addition are periodic acid-Schiff positive after diastase digestion.

Haematopoietic neoplasms

Virtually any neoplasm of haematopoietic elements may involve the breast. We will not attempt to be inclusive with regard to this broad and challenging area of oncology. However, certain topics are worthy of mention because of relatively frequent presentation of differential diagnostic challenge. The primary diagnostic dilemma is between lobular carcinoma, infiltrating type, and non-

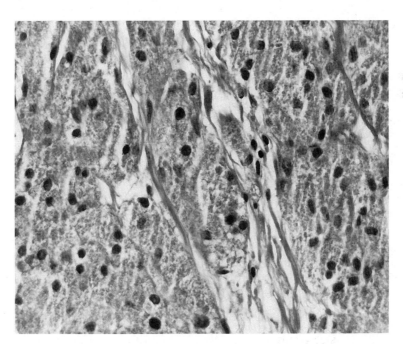

Fig. 18.1 Granular cell tumour with densely granular cytoplasm and irregular placement of nuclei. There is a rounded clustering of tumour cells (× 300).

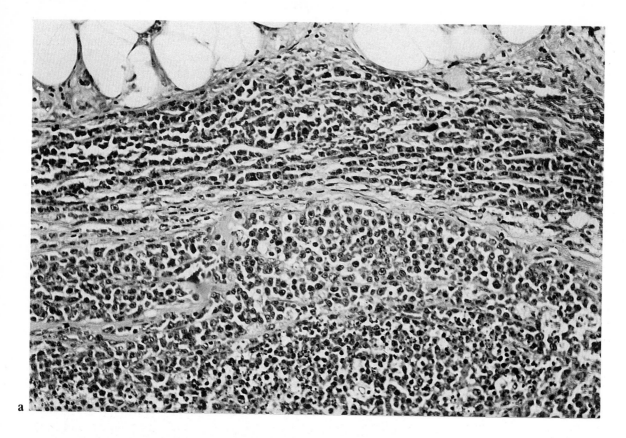

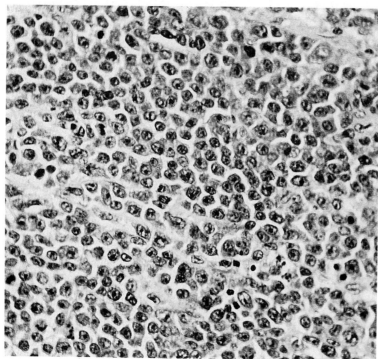

Fig. 18.2a,b Linear and more subtle circular orientation of cells suggests infiltrating lobular or poorly differentiated carcinoma in this well-defined breast mass. Higher power (**b**) shows central nuclear densities suggesting plasma cells. Electron microscopy and light chain immunocytochemistry supported plasmacytic features. Monoclonal cytoplasmic staining of immunoglobulin light chains was most defining. Diffuse bone marrow disease was simultaneously present in this elderly woman (**a** × 225; **b** × 450). (Courtesy of L. W. Rogers, A. D. Glick and J. Cousar.)

Hodgkin's lymphoma, leukaemic infiltration or myeloma.

Plasmacytoma and myeloma

Neoplasms of plasma cells, either isolated within the breast or as a localized manifestation of disseminated plasma cell myeloma, are unusual. However, these neoplasms represent an important bit of knowledge in the armamentarium of the diagnostic histopathologist. Without the fore-knowledge of their occurrence in breast, misdiagnosis of carcinoma will usually be rendered.

The familiar cytological features of plasma cells with eccentrically placed 'spoke wheel' nuclei are often subtle in neoplastic plasma cells. This indicates that breast neoplasms with diffuse patterns of infiltration (particularly solid and classical types of infiltrating lobular carcinoma) will often need ancillary studies for precise identification (Fig. 18.2) particularly if in situ epithelial disease is lacking. Routine mucin stains (p. 223) will often suffice to prove epithelial features. Methyl green pyronine stain, characteristically richly positive in largest portion of plasmacytic cytoplasm may, however, be somewhat positive in carcinoma cells. Electron microscopy and immunochemical studies of immunoglobulin and immunocyte markers may be necessary.

Most mammary plasmacytic neoplasms will be a manifestation of systemic disease, although a plasmacytic breast mass may present clinically prior to disease in bone. Apparently solitary plasmacytomas have also been discovered in the breast (Merino 1984; Kirschenbaum & Rhone 1985).

Non-Hodgkin's lymphoma

Most examples of mammary lymphoma have been recorded in the literature prior to the more current diagnostic approaches to lymphoid neoplasms. Of importance to the histopathologist challenged by an atypical lymphoid infiltrate in the breast are: (1) extranodal lymphomas do present in the breast, and (2) special studies of cell character-ization requiring other than routine sections may be required (Telesinghe & Anthony 1985).

Rare by any measure, mammary lymphomas constituted 0.12% of primary breast malignancies at the M. D. Anderson Hospital (Mambo et al 1977) and about 2% of extranodal lymphomas in an American survey (Freeman et al 1972). The same differential diagnostic considerations noted elsewhere in this chapter are relevant here. Often when fresh tissue is available, smears may be prepared both for later studies and immediate analysis. Such smears may make lymphoid character of the infiltrate more apparent. The diffuse and solid nature of the infiltrate is a histo-logically dominant feature (Fig. 18.3).

Prognosis of malignant lymphoma presenting in breast is generally, but not uniformly, poor (Mambo et al 1977; Obialero et al 1984; Tanaka et al 1984). When carefully confined to cases presenting with only localized breast disease, prognosis is good for most women (Dixon et al 1987). These cases may present with bilateral disease (Shpitz et al 1985).

Hodgkin's disease

Any presentation of Hodgkin's disease in the breast is rare, and it seems always associated with involvement of adjacent lymph node groups in the internal mammary chain or the neck. The pres-ence of Hodgkin's disease in the breast may be the primary presentation or may be an indicator of recurrence after therapy (Meis et al 1986).

Pseudolymphoma

Dense aggregates of lymphocytes effacing mammary architecture, and not demonstrating neoplastic features, are described (Fisher et al 1979; Lin et al 1980; Merino et al 1981). Pseudolymphoma or benign lymphocytic infiltration may be diagnosed when varied lymphoid cell types create a mass in the breast. As with similar events presenting else-where in the body, presence of germinal centres and regional variation in lymphocyte types will indicate a benign infiltrate. This simplistic state-ment should not be taken as one trivializing what may be a difficult differential diagnosis with lymphoma, but most cases are easily diagnosed. If broad areas of similar lymphoid cells are present, the special tools of lymphoma diagnosis will be necessary, and those sources referenced.

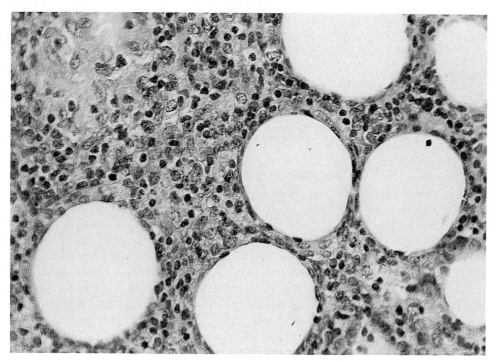

Fig. 18.3 A lymphocytic lymphoma of mixed small and large cells infiltrating mammary adipose tissue (× 400).

Leukaemia

Analogous with lymphoma, the complete histopathologist must always be aware that leukaemic infiltrates may be found within the breast. Usually, the foreknowledge that the patient has leukaemia will forewarn the diagnostician. One special situation deserves emphasis. Acute granulocytic leukaemia has long been known to produce soft tissue masses in clinical presentation or during the course of disease (Mason et al 1973). Indeed, these green tumours (chloroma, granulocytic sarcoma) which fade on exposure to air are part of the lore of anatomical and haematopathology.

The diffuse infiltration of neoplastic granulocytic precursors may recall many diagnostic possibilities under the microscope (Fig. 18.4). The nuclei are more irregular in shape than the infiltrating lobular carcinoma which is most closely simulated. Demonstration of the cytoplasmic esterase characteristic of myeloblasts is defining (Sears & Reid 1976). Differential diagnosis with haematoxylin and eosin is aided by recognition of scattered eosinophils in the leukaemic infiltrate.

Myeloid metaplasia may also present a tumour within the breast (Martinelli et al 1983).

Metastatic tumours

Virtually any malignant neoplasm, particularly those associated with widespread dissemination, may develop metastases within the breast. Most of these present late in the clinical course of disease (Nielsen et al 1981), and pulmonary and melanocytic malignancies are most frequent (McIntosh et al 1976). However, a series of metastatic cases based upon mammographical diagnosis contains 40% with no previous history of malignancy (McCrea et al 1983). These cases were approximately equally divided between haematological malignancies and solid tumours. The metastases often present as solitary masses, most frequently in the upper outer quadrant. Multiple lesions are surprisingly uncommon, although a diffuse spread sometimes having the

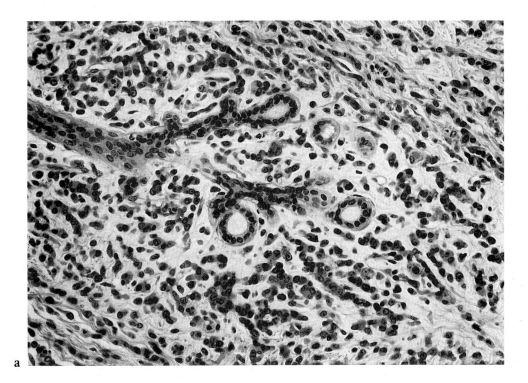

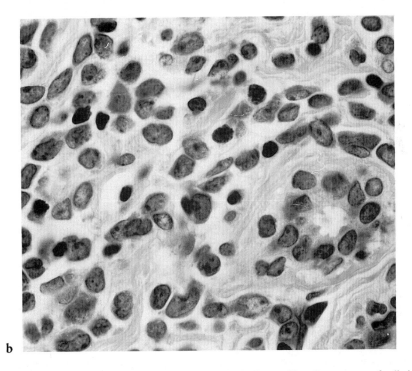

Fig. 18.4a,b Acute myelocytic leukaemia presented as a chloroma in the breast. Note linear arrays of cells in extralobular stroma at lower left of (a), and non-oriented infiltrates within the lobular unit. At higher power, cytological variability is evident. Only the prepared diagnostician and high quality slides will avoid a diagnosis of infiltrating lobular carcinoma (a × 200; b × 800). (Courtesy of R. L. Johnson.)

clinical appearance of an inflammatory carcinoma may be seen (McCrea et al 1983).

Considering the variety of histological appearances in primary breast neoplasms, differential diagnosis may entail special problems. Metastatic lesions may appear to have been imposed upon the breast with interspersed normal breast elements within the tumour, an appearance sometimes seen, of course, with tubular and lobular primary lesions of the breast but uncommon with other patterns of intrinsic mammary carcinomas. Associated in situ carcinoma is a strong supporting feature for a primary breast lesion; however, intraductal growth of metastatic lesions to the breast may be seen (Fig. 18.5). More extensive intralymphatic spread than invasive disease, particularly if lymphatic involvement is not primarily peritumoural, will be found more frequently in metastases than in primary breast cancers. This statement is most relevant when lymphatic spread is irregular, and excepts the diffuse lymphatic involvement of inflammatory breast carcinoma.

Several recurring clinical situations within the breast are relevant. It would seem from the number of case reports documenting metastases of carcinoid tumours of the gastrointestinal tract to the breast, that there is some propensity of these tumours to metastasize to the breast (Kashlan et al 1982). On the other hand, most of these case reports followed the first suggestion that carcinoid tumours may be primary within the breast. Thus, reporting of such cases may have been stimulated (Schürch et al 1980; Ordoñez et al 1985).

A breast mass may be the first symptom of rhabdomyosarcoma in children, particularly alveolar rhabdomyosarcoma (Gonzalez-Crussi & Black-Schaffer 1979; Howarth et al 1980). Girls with these lesions, presenting primarily in the early and mid-teenage years, soon demonstrated major disease elsewhere, usually in an extremity, buttock or retroperitoneal location. Carefully prepared histological material is mandatory for the correct differential diagnosis to be made by light microscopy. The alveolar rhabdomyosarcoma presents well-ordered groupings of somewhat spindled cells seemingly attached to a reticulin framework with loose cells often present in the centre of these aggregates. Cytoplasmic cross-striations are seldom evident by light microscopy and,

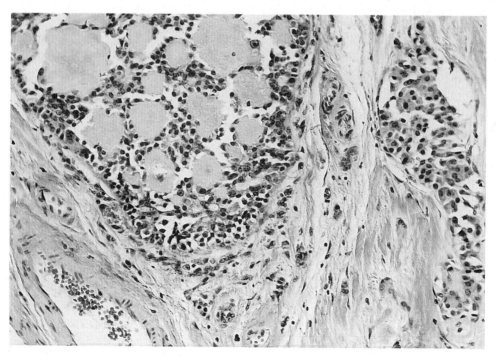

Fig. 18.5 This highly unusual example of metastasis to the breast has cancer cells in lymphatic at right and in a duct at upper left. Note small periductal vessels. The hyaline globes are amyloid within this medullary carcinoma of the thyroid (× 200).

particularly when the cells are not greatly enlarged, either carcinoma or lymphoma may be mimicked histologically.

Ovarian carcinoma has been convincingly described to involve the breast. Considering the propensity of breast cancer for involving the ovary, this can create a difficult diagnostic situation. Most of the metastases to the breast from the ovary have been high grade papillary carcinomas with multiple lesions presenting within the breast (Scotto et al 1985), a constellation of features inconsistent with a primary breast cancer.

Postmastectomy angiosarcoma

First described in 1948 (Stewart & Treves 1948), this rare but devastating complication of chronic lymphoedema forms an important part of the lore and clinical knowledge concerning breast cancer. Although many have long debated the precise cell type involved in these cases, recent studies with modern techniques (Miettinen et al 1983; McWilliam & Harris 1985) have proven the original contention of Stewart & Treves (1948) that these are endothelial sarcomas. It is apparent that carcinoma involving a lymphoedematous extremity as well as angiosarcoma in that setting may present a very similar gross and histological picture which may necessitate special studies for proper differential diagnosis (Schafler et al 1979; Hashimoto et al 1985). Note that angiosarcomas may occur in any chronic lymphoedematous extremity, and one of the first cases studied carefully by electron microscopy followed a lymph node dissection for melanoma (Gray et al 1966).

These angiosarcomas present in chronically lymphoedematous extremities usually at least 10 and frequently as many as 20 years or longer following initial mastectomy (Martin et al 1984). The initial presentation may be with small bluish, bruise-like areas evolving to aggressive tumour masses and distant metastases. Histological appearance is similar to that described for angiosarcoma in Chapter 20. It has never been clear whether these are truly lymphangiosarcomas or haemangiosarcomas, and it is thus preferable to term them angiosarcoma (Enzinger & Weiss 1983).

REFERENCES

Bryant J 1985 Fibroepithelioma of Pinkus overlying breast cancer. Arch Dermatol 121:310

Davis A B, Patchefsky A S 1977 Basal cell carcinoma of the nipple. Case report and review of the literature. Cancer 40: 1780–1781

DeMay R M, Kay S 1984 Granular cell tumor of the breast. Path Annu 19 (2): 121–148

Dixon J M, Lumsden A B, Krajewski A et al 1987 Primary lymphoma of the breast. Br J Surg 74: 214–217

Doctor V M, Sirsat M V 1971 Florid papillomatosis (adenoma) and other benign tumours of the nipple and areola. Br J Cancer 25: 1–9

Enzinger F M, Weiss S W 1983 Soft tissue tumors. Mosby, St Louis, p 422–449

Fisher E R, Palekar A S, Paulson J D, Golinger R 1979 Pseudolymphoma of breast. Cancer 44: 258–263

Freeman C, Berg J W, Cutler S J 1972 Occurrence and prognosis of extranodal lymphomas. Cancer 29: 252–260

Gonzalez-Crussi F, Black-Schaffer S 1979 Rhabdomyosarcoma of infancy and childhood. Am J Surg Pathol 3: 157–171

Gordon A B, Fisher C, Palmer B, Greening W P 1985 Granular cell tumours of the breast. Br J Surg Oncol 11: 269–273

Gray Jr G F, Gonzalez-Licea A, Hartmann W H, Woods Jr A C 1966 Angiosarcoma in lymphedema: an unusual case of Stewart-Treves syndrome. Bull Johns Hopkins Hosp 119: 117–128

Hashimoto K, Matsumoto M, Eto H, Lipinski J, LaFond A A 1985 Differentiation of metastatic breast carcinoma from Stewart-Treves angiosarcoma. Use of antikeratin and antidesmosome monoclonal antibodies and factor VIII-related antibodies. Arch Dermatol 121: 742–746

Howarth C B, Caces J N, Pratt C B 1980 Breast metastases in children with rhabdomyosarcoma. Cancer 40: 2520–2524

Ilie B 1986 Neoplasms in skin and subcutis over the breast, simulating breast neoplasms: case reports and literature review. J Surg Onc 31: 191–198

Ingram D L, Mossler J A, Snowhite J, Leight G S, McCarty Jr K S 1984 Granular cell tumors of the breast. Arch Pathol Lab Med 108: 897–901

Kashlan R B, Powell R W, Nolting S F 1982 Carcinoid and other tumors metastatic to the breast. J Surg Oncol 20: 25–30

Kirshenbaum G, Rhone D P 1985 Solitary extramedullary plasmacytoma of the breast with serum monoclonal protein: a case report and review of the literature. Am J Clin Pathol 83: 230–232

Lin J J, Farha G J, Taylor R J 1980 Pseudolymphomas of the breast. I. In a study of 8654 consecutive tylectomies and mastectomies. Cancer 45: 973–978

McCrea E S, Johnston C, Haney P J 1983 Metastases to the breast. Am J Roentgen 141: 685–690

McIntosh I H, Hooper A A, Millis R R, Greening W P 1976 Metastatic carcinoma within the breast. Clin Oncol 2: 393–401

McWilliam L J, Harris M 1985 Histogenesis of post-mastectomy angiosarcoma — an ultrastructural study. Histopathology 9: 331–343

Mambo N C, Burke J S, Butler J J 1977 Primary malignant lymphomas of the breast. Cancer 39: 2033–2040

Martin M B, Kon N D, Kawamoto E H, Myers R T, Sterchi J M 1984 Post mastectomy angiosarcoma. Am Surg 10: 541–545

Martinelli G, Santini D, Bazzocchi F, Pileri S, Casanova S 1983 Myeloid metaplasia of the breast. A lesion which clinically mimics carcinoma. Virchows Arch (A) 401: 203–207

Mason T E, Demaree R S, Margolis C I 1973 Granulocytic sarcoma (chloroma), two years preceding myelogenous leukemia. Cancer 31: 423–432

Meis J M, Butler J J, Osborne B M 1986 Hodgkin's disease involving the breast and chest wall. Cancer 57: 1859–1865

Merino M J 1984 Plasmacytoma of the breast. Arch Pathol Lab Med 108: 676–678

Merino M J, Joyner R E, Graham A 1981 Pseudolymphoma of the breast. Diagn Gynecol Obstet 3: 315–319

Miettinen M, Lehto V P, Virtanen I 1983 Postmastectomy angiosarcoma (Stewart-Treves syndrome). Light microscopic, immunohistological and ultrastructural characteristics of two cases. Am J Surg Pathol 7: 329–339

Nielsen M, Andersen J A, Henriksen F W et al 1981 Metastases to the breast from extramammary carcinomas. Acta Pathol Microbiol Scand (A) 89: 251–256

Obialero M, Zanetti P P, Dandria A, Francone C, Gagna G 1984 Il linfoma primitive della mammella. Min Med 75: 2815–2820

Ordoñez N G, Manning J T, Raymond A K 1985 Argentaffin endocrine carcinoma (carcinoid) of the pancreas with concomitant breast metastasis: an immunohistochemical and electron microscopic study. Hum Pathol 15: 746–751

Rosen P P 1983 Syringomatous adenoma of the nipple. Am J Surg Pathol 7: 739–745

Sauven P, Roberts A 1983 Basal cell carcinoma of the nipple. J R Soc Med 76: 699–701

Schafler K, McKenzie C G, Salm R 1979 Post-mastecomy lymphangiosarcoma — a reappraisal of the concept — a critical review and report of an illustrative case. Histopathology 3: 131–152.

Schürch W, Lamoureux E, Lefebvre R, Fauteux J-P 1980 Solitary breast metastasis: first manifestation of an occult carcinoid of the ileum. Virchows Arch (A) 386: 117–124

Scotto V, Masci P, Sbiroli C 1985 Breast metastasis of ovarian cancer during CIS-platinum therapy. Eur J Gynaecol Oncol 6: 62–65

Sears H F, Reid J 1976 Granulocytic sarcoma. Cancer 37: 1808–1813

Shpitz B, Witz M, Kaufman Z, Griffel B, Manor Y, Dinbar A 1985 Bilateral primary malignant lymphoma of the breast. Postgrad Med J 61: 729–731

Stewart F W, Treves N 1948 Lymphangiosarcoma in postmastectomy lymphoedema. A report of six cases in elephantiasis chirurgica. Cancer 1: 64–81

Tanaka T, Hsueh C L, Hayashi K et al 1984 Primary malignant lymphoma of the breast. With a review of 73 cases among Japanese subjects. Acta Pathol Jpn 34: 361–373

Tavassoli F A, Norris H J 1986 Mammary adenoid cystic carcinoma with sebaceous differentiation. Arch Pathol Lab Med 110: 1045–1053

Telesinghe P U, Anthony P P 1985 Primary lymphoma of the breast. Histopathology 9: 297–307

Umansky C, Bullock W K 1968 Granular cell myoblastoma of the breast. Ann Surg 168: 810–817

Willen R, Willen H, Galldin G, Albrechtsson U 1984 Granular cell tumour of the mammary gland simulating malignancy. Virchows Arch (A) 403: 391–400

19

Metastasis of breast cancer

REGIONAL LYMPH NODE METASTASES

Histological documentation of metastasis to regional lymph nodes remains the most valuable currently accepted determinant of prognosis in breast cancer (Fisher 1984; Fisher et al 1984). The many other prognostically useful features are most valuable as additive predictive factors in node negative or node positive groups, or as predictors of nodal metastases if the latter information is not available. For practical purposes nodal status is confined to evaluation of axillary nodes, although retrosternal (internal mammary) nodal evaluation adds marginally to prognostic implication (Veronesi et al 1983). Clinical evaluation of nodal status by palpation of axillary nodes is neither sensitive nor specific because of a 30% error rate in both positive and negative clinical impressions when tested by anatomical pathology.

Histologically, determination of metastatic carcinoma in lymph nodes usually presents no special challenge. With rare exceptions, the pattern dominating the primary carcinoma will be found in the nodal metastases (Sharkey & Greiner 1985). Smaller tumour deposits will be seen in subcapsular sinus and adjacent nodal tissue, and are sharply circumscribed from the nodal tissue (Fig. 19.1). A special circumstance does demand awareness during histological evaluation: many lobular and lobular variant carcinomas mimic histiocytes and thereby present difficulty in differential diagnosis. This mimicry is both cytological and situational as both cell types may be similar and each often fill subcapsular and medullary

sinuses diffusely (Fig. 19.2). The diagnostic uncertainty is enhanced in poorly prepared histological material. Subtle cues may help to resolve the diagnostic dilemma. Lobular carcinoma deposits in nodes often expand and distort medullary sinuses, appearing differently in one or another portion of a node, and the poorly cohesive cells may replace much of a node in a sheet-like fashion. On the other hand, histiocytes in nodal sinuses maintain a similar pattern throughout an individual lymph node. Special stains for mucosubstances (particularly the combined Alcian blue-PAS) will frequently be helpful (see Ch. 13) because a majority of lobular carcinoma cells will have some cells with cytoplasmic positivity.

Stroma around metastatic tumour is usually not well developed, although plentiful fibrous stroma is occasionally present (Fig. 19.3). Elastosis is virtually never seen to be associated with intranodal carcinoma.

An infrequent source of possible confusion with metastatic carcinoma is the presence of benign melanocytic naeval cells in the capsule of lymph nodes (Ridolfi et al 1977). In routine practice this occurrence is rare, but Wilkinson et al (1982) found naevus cells in 3% of axillary dissections when the material was sectioned serially. The naevus cells are often lightly pigmented and histologically characteristic of naevus cells seen in common intradermal nevi. Their confinement to the nodal capsule or fibrous extensions of the same makes differentiation from metastatic carcinoma relatively easy (Fig. 19.4). Rarely the melanocytes are spindled and deeply pigmented, allowing the designation of 'blue naevus' (Epstein et al 1984).

Other elements found rarely in axillary lymph

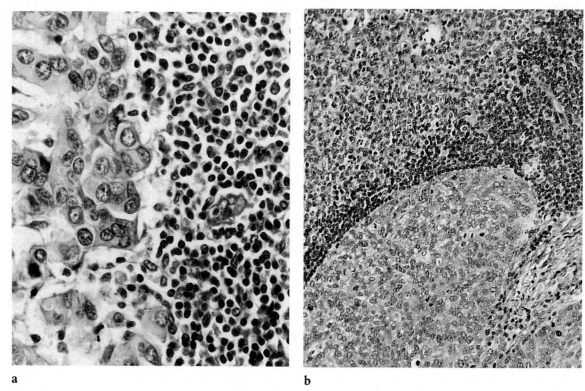

a   b

Fig. 19.1 (a) Somewhat cohesive tumour cells above are sharply demarcated from lymphocytes within the lymph node at right. (b) Highly cohesive breast carcinoma cells with low grade nuclei are at lower portion, sharply demarcated from lymphocytes and a germinal centre at upper left (**a** × 450; **b** × 200).

nodes are benign breast tissues (Turner & Millis 1980). These may present any of the patterns found elsewhere in the breast (Figs 19.5 and 19.6). Obviously, neoplasms may arise within this intranodal tissue, but it is rarely proven (Walker & Fechner 1982).

The presence or absence of metastases to axillary lymph nodes and the extent to which the lymph nodes are involved by metastatic disease are the most commonly used and the most reliable indicators for prognosis of patients with breast cancer. The extent of axillary lymph node involvement may be measured either by dividing the axilla into three levels according to the relationship to the pectoralis minor muscle or more simply by counting the number of lymph nodes involved by metastatic carcinoma. The former system is of greatest use and specificity when a standard radical mastectomy including both pectoralis muscles is available for examination.

One can, however, separately identify lymph nodes in the high and low axillary dissection from a modified radical mastectomy (without pectoralis muscles) and probably accomplish the same staging procedure. However, the number of lymph nodes involved is as useful a parameter in predicting survival.

With regard to the first techinique of documenting levels of involvement in the axilla, Berg & Robbins (1966) reported that the chance of 20-year postmastectomy survival with no axillary metastates was approximately 65%. If only axillary lymph nodes proximal to the pectoralis minor muscle were involved, the 20-year survival was reduced to 38%. With metastatic involvement of the lymph nodes in the middle of the axilla (below the pectoralis minor muscle) survival dropped to 30%, and if the high axilla (above the pectoralis minor muscle) was involved the 20-year survival rate fell to only 12%. The actuarial survival figures

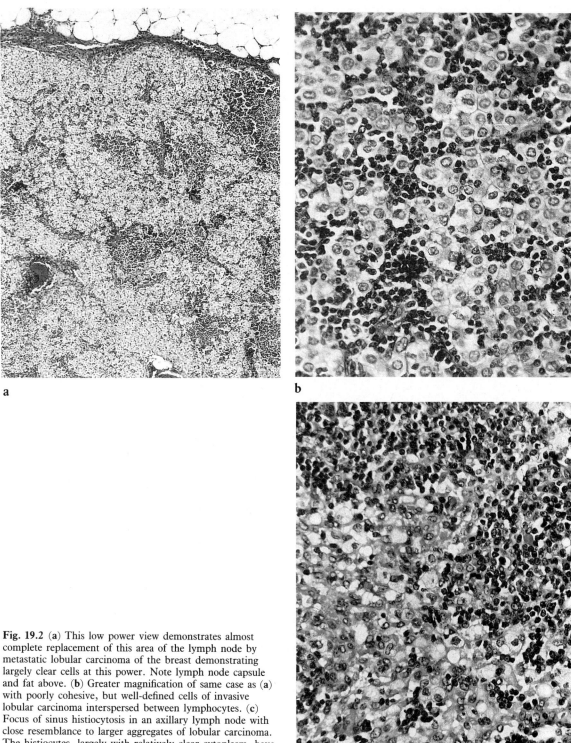

Fig. 19.2 (a) This low power view demonstrates almost complete replacement of this area of the lymph node by metastatic lobular carcinoma of the breast demonstrating largely clear cells at this power. Note lymph node capsule and fat above. (b) Greater magnification of same case as (a) with poorly cohesive, but well-defined cells of invasive lobular carcinoma interspersed between lymphocytes. (c) Focus of sinus histiocytosis in an axillary lymph node with close resemblance to larger aggregates of lobular carcinoma. The histiocytes, largely with relatively clear cytoplasm, have less well-defined cytoplasmic compartments than lobular carcinoma. Collections of lymphocytes are seen above and at upper right (a × 50; b,c × 320).

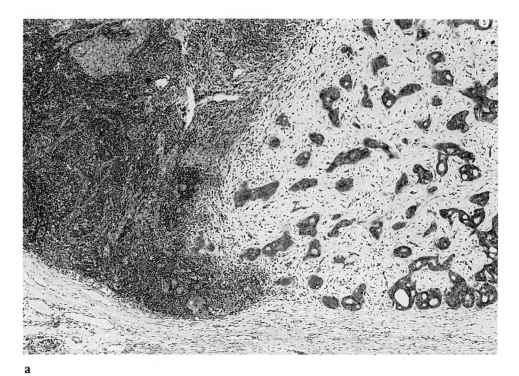

a

b

Fig. 19.3 (a) Also unusual, this metastatic deposit of breast carcinoma with well-defined glandular spaces has a well-defined and somewhat myxoid fibrous stroma around the glandular elements at right. Note at upper left a small collection of well-defined histiocytes in a medullary sinus of the lymph node. (b) Dense fibrous tissue surrounds glandular elements of a breast carcinoma (at right) metastatic to a lymph node (**a** × 60; **b** × 200).

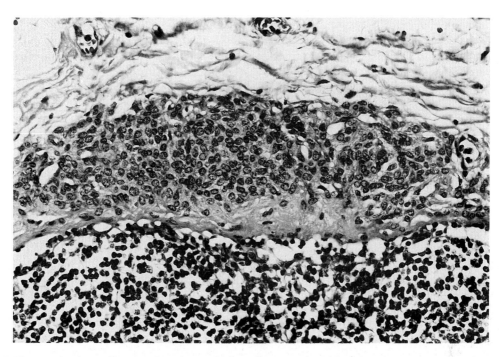

Fig. 19.4 The capsule of an axillary lymph node runs horizontally across the mid-portion of this photograph. At the upper portion of the capsule, abutting against the surrounding loose fibrous tissue at extreme upper portion of tissue, is a well-defined collection of benign melanocytic naeval cells ($\times$ 300).

at 30 years from this valuable series of patients (Adair et al 1974) were only slightly less in each group.

Survival figures based on the counting of number of lymph nodes involved are comparable (Smith et al 1977; Fisher et al 1984). Carefully analysed data from the National Surgical Adjuvant Breast Project (Fisher B et al 1983) have confirmed that the number of nodes involved by cancer provides valuable prognostic information, and that the mere documentation of node positivity or node negativity offers insufficient information with regard to disease-free survival and actuarial survival. At five years, women in this study treated by mastectomy had an 83% survival if no lymph nodes were involved and an 80% survival if one lymph node was involved at time of mastectomy. Women with two or three lymph nodes involved had a 65–70% five-year survival, and survival dropped to 54% if four to six lymph nodes were involved. Women with more than 12 lymph nodes involved had only a 28% survival at five years, although the number of women in this group is relatively small. Also of great interest

from this study is that the survival curves were becoming parallel at five years, indicating that the yearly incidence for treatment failure was becoming similar in all groups. Also, comparing the rate of failure per year, it was quite similar year after year for women with no or few lymph nodes involved and quite steep with most failures occurring in the first two or three years in women with greater numbers of nodes involved.

Skip areas, that is involvement of high axillary nodes without involvement of the lower axillary nodes, are very unusual (Rosen et al 1983), supporting the stance of Fisher et al (1981) that removal of the lower two levels of axillary node (low axillary dissection) achieves a satisfactory level of predictability with regard to nodal involvement. Veronesi et al (1987) found only 0.4% of node positive patients had metastases at the higher nodes when levels one and two were negative. Although somewhat controversial, an axillary nodal sampling (less extensive than dissection) approaches the predictive utility of a nodal dissection (Steele et al 1985).

A special consideration in lymph node involvement is the predictive importance of solitary micrometastases or occult metastases determined by serial sectioning of all lymph node material. It would seem that there is little practical or therapeutic significance to the finding of solitary micro-metastases whether by routine or extended histological sampling. In the study by Huvos et al (1971) patients with metastatic tumour deposits of less than 2 mm in diameter had an eight-year postmastectomy survival rate similar to that of

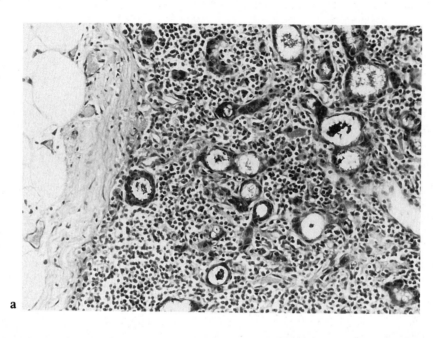

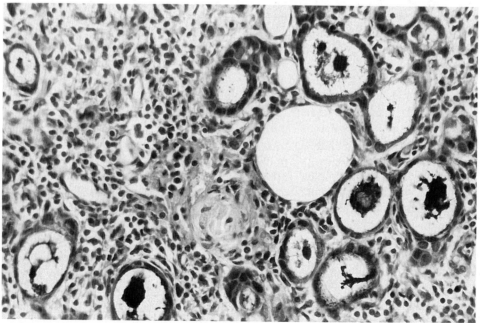

Fig. 19.5a–d Benign inclusions of epithelium in axillary lymph node. Note in (**a**) and (**b**) (same case) that the flattened cells of glands are dispersed irregularly in lymph node. Note benign cells in (**c**) and (**d**) (same case) (**a** × 150; **b** × 325; **c** × 125; **d** × 600). (**a,b** Courtesy of L. D. Richardson. **c,d** Courtesy of W. H. Hartmann.)

patients with no axillary metastases. Fisher et al (1978) indicated that micrometastases of under 1.3 mm in diameter were associated with a survival rate no different from that found in node-negative patients. Wilkinson et al (1982) found, by serial sectioning of lymph nodes, that an additional 17% of cases thought negative by

routine means would contain metastases. However, these women with occult lymph node metastases did not have a significantly poorer prognosis than those in whom such metastases were not found.

Another special consideration regarding nodal metastases is the patient who presents an unusual clinical pattern with metastases to lymph nodes in

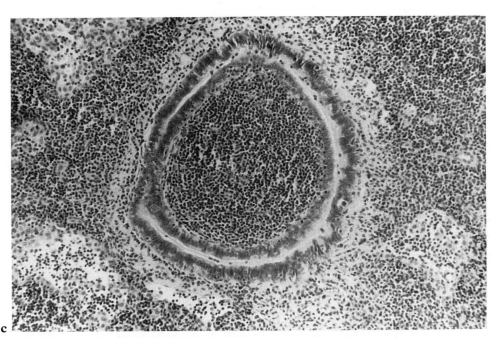

c

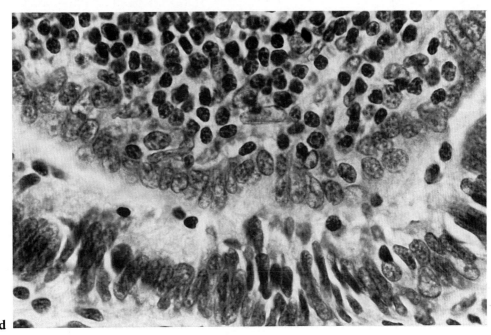

d

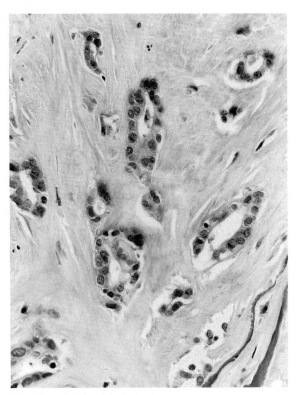

Fig. 19.6 Well-developed glandular formations are evident in this clinically solitary metastasis to bone from a breast carcinoma. A dense, fibrous stroma is present. Narrowed bony trabeculae are at lower right (× 200).

Histologically determined spread of metastatic mammary tumour from lymph nodal deposits into adjacent axillary tissue has long been considered to be an indicator of poor prognosis. However, Mambo & Gallager (1977) did not find an additive prognostic effect of this finding in women with four or more positive nodes. However, women with one to three positive nodes and extranodal extension of tumour did have a poorer prognosis than those with one to three positive nodes without this finding. Hartveit (1984) has recently reported that the presence of cancer cells in lymph node efferent vessels is a determinant of poor prognosis.

Patterns of reaction in lymph nodes have been evaluated for their likelihood of giving useful prognostic information, but are not generally accepted as having clinical utility. Of particular interest has been the prominence of histiocytes in nodal sinuses. However, a recent review of the National Surgical Adjuvant Breast Project data (Fisher E et al 1983) revealed no significant association between the presence or absence of any particular type of sinus histiocytosis of regional lymph nodes and five-year disease-free survival.

the axilla with an inapparent primary tumour within the breast. The first practical consideration in this situation is the documentation that the primary tumour is actually within the breast (Kemeny et al 1986). First of all women, particularly in age groups where breast cancer is relatively common, will very rarely have initial presentation of a carcinoma in the axilla which arises elsewhere than within the breast. If the histological pattern is consistent with breast primary, it may, with a certainty level of over 95%, be ascribed to a primary tumour in the breast in the absence of clinically detectable cancers elsewhere. This subject has been reviewed by Haupt et al (1985). They noted that many of these patients have a somewhat unusual tumour histology with sheets of large, pale and apocrine-like cells while others have more usual no special type or lobular patterns.

REFERENCES

Adair F, Berg J, Joubert L, Robbins G F 1974 Long term follow up of breast cancer patients: the 30-year report. Cancer 33: 1145–1150

Berg J W, Robbins G F 1966 Factors influencing short and long term survival of breast cancer patients. Surg Gynecol Obstet 122: 1311–1316

Epstein J I, Erlandson R A, Rosen P P 1984 Nodal blue nevi. Am J Surg Pathol 8: 907–915

Fisher E R 1984 The impact of pathology on the biologic, diagnostic, prognostic and therapeutic considerations in breast cancer. Surg Clin N Am 64: 1073–1093

Fisher E R, Palekar A S, Rockette H, Redmond C, Fisher B 1978 Pathologic findings from the national surgical adjuvant breast project (protocol no 4). V. Significance of axillary nodal micro and macrometastases. Cancer 42: 2032–2038

Fisher B, Wolmark N, Bauer M, Redmond C, Gebhardt M 1981 The accuracy of clinical nodal staging and of limited axillary dissection as a determinant of histologic nodal status in carcinoma of the breast. Surg Gynecol Obstet 152: 765–772

Fisher B, Bauer M, Wickerham D L, Redmond C K, Fisher E R 1983 Relation of number of positive axillary nodes to the prognosis of patients with primary breast cancer. Cancer 52: 1551–1557

Fisher E R, Kotwal N, Hermann C et al 1983 Types of tumor lymphoid response and sinus histiocytosis. Arch Pathol Lab Med 107: 222–227

Fisher E R, Sass R, Fisher B et al 1984 Pathologic findings from the national surgical adjuvant project for breast cancers (protocol no 4). X. Discriminants for tenth year treatment failure. Cancer 53: 712–723

Hartveit F 1984 Paranodal tumour in breast cancer: extranodal extension versus vascular spread. J Pathol 144: 253–256

Haupt H M, Rosen P P, Kinne D W 1985 Breast carcinoma presenting with axillary lymph node metastases. Am J Surg Pathol 9: 165–175

Huvos A G, Hutter R V P, Berg J W 1971 Significance of axillary macrometastases and micrometastases in mammary cancer. Ann Surg 173: 44–46

Kemeny M M, Rivera D E, Terz J J, Benfield J R 1986 Occult primary adenocarcinoma with axillary metastases. Am J Surg 152: 43–48

Mambo N C, Gallager H S 1977 Carcinoma of the breast: the prognostic significance of extranodal extension of axillary disease. Cancer 39: 2280–2285

Ridolfi R L, Rosen P P, Thaler H 1977 Nevus cell aggregates associated with lymph nodes: estimated frequency and clinical significance. Cancer 39: 164–171

Rosen P P, Lesser M L, Kinne D W, Beattie E J 1983 Discontinuous or 'skip' metastases in breast carcinoma. Ann Surg 197: 276–283

Sharkey F E, Greiner A S 1985 Morphologic identity of primary tumor and axillary metastases in breast carcinoma. Arch Pathol Lab Med 109: 256–259

Smith J A III, Gamez-Araujo J J, Gallager H S, White E C, McBride C M 1977 Carcinoma of the breast. Analysis of total lymph node involvement versus level of metastasis. Cancer 39: 527–532

Steele R J C, Forrest A P M, Gibson T, Stewart H, Chetty U 1985 The efficacy of lower axillary sampling in obtaining lymph node status in breast cancer: a controlled randomized trial. Br J Surg 72: 368–369

Turner D R, Millis R R 1980 Breast tissue inclusions in axillary lymph nodes. Histopathology 4: 631–636

Veronesi U, Cascinelli N, Bufalino R et al 1983 Risk of internal mammary lymph node metastases and its relevance on prognosis of breast cancer patients. Ann Surg 198: 681–684

Veronesi U, Rilke F, Luini A, Sacchini V, Galimberti V et al 1987 Distribution of axillary node metastases by level of invasion. Cancer 59: 682–687

Walker A N, Fechner R E 1982 Papillary carcinoma arising from ectopic breast tissue in an axillary lymph node. Diagn Gynecol Obstet 4: 141–145

Wilkinson E J, Hause L L, Hoffman R G et al 1982 Occult axillary lymph node metastases in invasive breast carcinoma: characteristics of the primary tumor and significance of the metastases. Path Annu 17: 67–91

INTRAMAMMARY METASTASES

Metastases of a breast carcinoma within the breast, or breasts, is a situation long discussed, and seldom formally studied. In the homolateral breast, this phenomenon is included with tumour multicentricity (see Ch. 16). The appearance of metastases in the opposite breast and its differentiation from a primary tumour is also discussed with bilaterality in Chapter 16. In summary, this latter event is uncommon, and is usually easily differentiated from a second primary carcinoma. The appearance of a second primary tumour is supported if it appears in the absence of distant metastases, is of lower grade or different type than the initial tumour, has an in situ component (other than lobular type), and is other than within the medial quadrants.

An unusual occurrence is the metastasis of carcinoma to intramammary lymph nodes (Lindfors et al 1986), an event which may have the same prognostic implication as metastasis to axillary nodes. Lymph nodes have been found within the breast in up to 28% of mastectomy specimens (Egan & McSweeney 1983).

REFERENCES

Egan R L, McSweeney M B 1983 Intramammary lymph nodes. Cancer 51: 1838–1842
Lindfors K K, Kopans D B, McCarthy K A, Koerner F C, Meyer J E 1986 Breast cancer metastasis to intramammary lymph nodes. Am J Roentgen 146: 133–136

SYSTEMIC METASTASES

Local skin, soft tissue and lymph node recurrences account for one-third of initial recurrence of breast cancer after therapy, with an additional approximately 10% presenting with ipsilateral pleural effusion. However, somewhat greater than 50% of women have distant metastases as the first sign of cancer recurrence. About 20% will have bone involvement only, somewhat greater than 10% pulmonary and 2–3% liver involvement only (Lee 1985). The remaining approximately 25% will have widespread metastases with only 1–2% of women presenting with initial evidence of recurrent disease in the central nervous system.

Histological patterns have little prognostic utility in this setting except in the recognition of histological consistency with metastases from a primary in the breast. One should not neglect the utility of reviewing the initial breast primary tumour, as the patterns of the primary and metastases are usually similar. Histological appearance of metastases from breast cancer is often quite characteristic with small, tightly cohesive groups of cells often appearing glandular (Figs 19.7–19.9). Another pattern of elongated clumps of tumour cells insinuated between bundles of collagen or smooth muscle is virtually diagnostic of metastatic mammary carcinoma, especially when intracytoplasmic lumina are evidenced (Fig. 19.9b). Well-developed patterns of tubular and cribriform carcinoma are virtually unheard of at distant sites. The mucinous pattern with extracellular mucin pools, metastatic from a breast primary, is also uncommon.

Of particular interest are the unusual metastatic sites and pattern of involvement seen with infiltrating lobular carcinoma. These carcinomas have an apparent predilection for metastases to the gastrointestinal tract and peritoneum where with the presence of their frequent clearly vacuolated and signet ring cytology they may closely mimic primary carcinomas of the gastrointestinal tract. As is also true for carcinoma of the stomach, this pattern of breast carcinoma may have sparsely scattered cells in tissue, rendering a diagnosis

Fig. 19.7 This metastasis to bone from a breast cancer forms glands and has, centrally, two intracytoplasmic vacuoles. The latter are clear spaces with central, lightly staining dots in this haematoxylin and eosin stain (× 800).

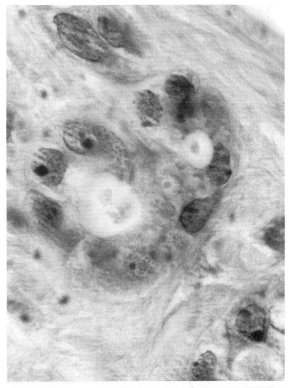

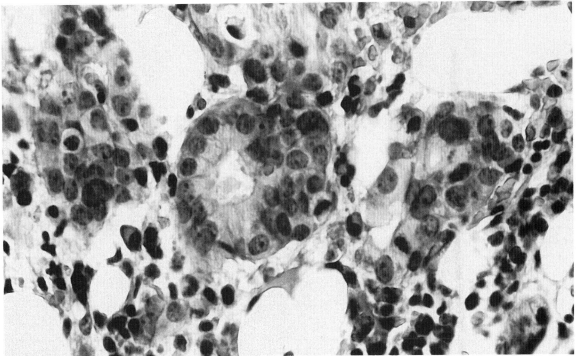

Fig. 19.8 In this needle biopsy specimen from bone marrow, glandular formations of metastatic breast cancer are present. One is obvious centrally, and more subtle, malignant cellular collections are present to left, right, and above the central malignant gland (× 650).

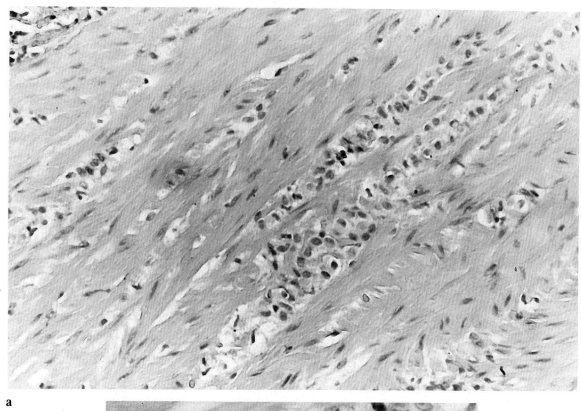

a

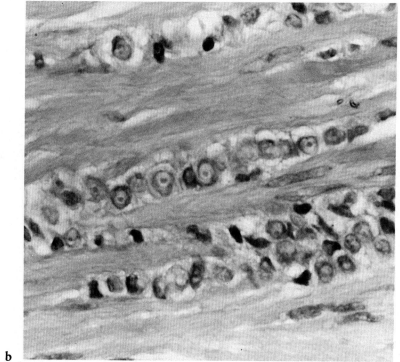

b

Fig. 19.9a,b Within a diffuse rectal wall metastasis this lobular carcinoma of breast is insinuated between muscle bundles. Many 'targetoid' intracytoplasmic lumina are evident in (**b**) (**a** × 225; **b** × 650).

difficult for those who are not prepared for this event with foreknowledge of the type of primary tumour (see Ch. 13, 'Infiltrating lobular carcinoma'). This unusual predilection seems to be shared by mixed or pleomorphic lobular variants, may produce metastases in the stomach mimicking a primary gastric cancer of linitis plastica type (Cormier et al 1980), and is perhaps particularly likely to occur in tumours with signet ring cells (Merino & LiVolsi 1981). This gastrointestinal and peritoneal involvement may produce a diffuse induration of the retroperitoneum and ureteral obstruction mimicking retroperitoneal fibrosis (Harris et al 1984). Such patterns of involvement may also favour the rare development of obstructive jaundice without extensive hepatic involvement (Engel et al 1980). It is also likely that most cases of diffuse infiltration of the meninges by metastatic breast cancer are associated with the infiltrating lobular type.

Approximately 20% of women with distant metastases will have them initially and dominantly in bone. These women have the longest life expectancy of women with distant metastases (Miller & Whitehill 1984; Sherry et al 1986). Histological material from bony metastases may be submitted to the histopathologist as part of a therapeutic procedure for fracture or impending fracture, or for diagnosis. The usual histological patterns of breast cancer may be expected. Because breast cancer metastases are usually lytic, bony trabeculae will not be broadened. Although detection of cancer cells may be made in smears of marrow aspirate, tissue sections of clot (Anner & Drewinko 1977) and biopsy are somewhat more often diagnostic.

Although clinical problems associated with metastases to bone usually involve focal lesions, rarely patients may experience marrow failure from extensive tumour invasion and myelofibrosis (Yablonski-Peretz et al 1985). Note should also be made of the possibility of multiple myeloma appearing in women after diagnosis of breast cancer (Savage & Garrett 1986), presenting obvious problems in differential diagnosis.

Metastatic carcinoma from the breast presenting as endometrial involvement, usually with bleeding, may be associated with either histological patterns of no special type or with lobular carcinoma (Kumar & Hart 1982; Rivel et al 1984; Piura et al 1985). Unusual presentations of metastatic disease other than those mentioned above, such as involvement of the bladder (Haid et al 1980) and endobronchial metastases, may be more common in breast cancer patients than in other malignancies (Albertini & Ekberg 1980; Kreisman et al 1983).

In keeping with the tendency of most metastases to demonstrate the pattern of original tumour, inflammatory carcinoma may metastasize to soft tissue presenting the same appearance at the metastatic site (Tschen & Apisarnthanarax 1981).

Endocrine organs are frequently involved by widespread breast carcinoma although rarely producing clinical difficulties except for occasional cases of pituitary disease. Patterns of metastases with regard to correlations of various sites of involvement are non-random and may reflect fundamental variance in metastatic capability (de la Monte et al 1984).

REFERENCES

Albertini R E, Ekberg N I 1980 Endobronchial metastasis in breast cancer. Thorax 35: 435–440

Anner R M, Drewinko B 1977 Frequency and significance of bone marrow involvement by metastatic solid tumors. Cancer 39: 1337–1344

Cormier W J, Gaffey T A, Welch J M, Welch J S, Edmonson J H 1980 Linitis plastica caused by metastatic lobular carcinoma of the breast. Mayo Clin Proc 55: 747–753

de la Monte S, Hutchins G M, Moore G W 1984 Endocrine organ metastases from breast carcinoma. Am J Pathol 114: 131–136

Engel J J, Trujillo Y, Spellberg M 1980 Metastatic carcinoma of the breast: a cause of obstructive jaundice. Gastroenterology 78: 132–135

Haid M, Ignatoff J, Khandeker J D, Graham J, Holland J 1980 Urinary bladder metastases from breast carcinoma. Cancer 46: 229–232

Harris M, Howell A, Chrissohou M, Swindell R I C, Hudson M, Sellwood R A 1984 A comparison of the metastatic pattern of infiltrating lobular carcinoma and infiltrating duct carcinoma of the breast. Br J Cancer 50: 23–30

Kreisman H, Wolkove N, Finkelstein H S, Cohen C, Margolese R, Frank H 1983 Breast cancer and thoracic metastases: review of 119 patients. Thorax 38: 175–179

Kumar N B, Hart W R 1982 Metastases to the uterine corpus from extragenital cancers: a clinicopathologic study of 63 cases. Cancer 50: 2163–2169

Lee Y-T N 1985 Patterns of metastasis and natural courses of breast carcinoma. Cancer Metastasis Rev 4: 153–172. Martinus Nijhoff, Boston

Merino M J, LiVolsi V A 1981 Signet ring carcinoma of the female breast: a clinicopathologic analysis of 24 cases. Cancer 48: 1830–1837

Miller F, Whitehill R 1984 Carcinoma of the breast metastatic to the skeleton. Clin Orthop 184: 121–127

Piura B, Bar-David J, Goldstein J 1985 Abnormal uterine bleeding as a presenting sign of metastatic signet ring cell carcinoma originating in the breast: case report. Br J Obstet Gynaecol 92: 645–648

Rivel J, Delmas J, Vital A et al 1984 Un cas de metastase uterine d'origine mammaire. Arch Anat Cytol Pathol 32: 45–47

Savage D, Garrett T J 1986 Multiple myeloma masquerading as metastatic breast cancer. Cancer 57: 923–924

Sherry M M, Greco F A, Johnson D H, Hainsworth J D 1986 Breast cancer with skeletal metastases at initial diagnosis: distinctive clinical characteristics and favorable prognosis. Cancer 58: 178–182

Tschen E H, Apisarnthanarax P 1981 Inflammatory metastatic carcinoma of the breast. Arch Dermatol 117: 120–121

Yablonski-Peretz T, Sulkes A, Polliack A, Weshler Z, Okon E, Catane R 1985 Secondary myelofibrosis with metastatic breast cancer simulating agnogenic myeloid metaplasia: report of a case and review of the literature. Med Pediatr Oncol 13: 92–96

Sarcomas of the breast

Primary sarcomas of the breast are rare. Yet the connective tissue investments and the parenchyma of the breast are capable of giving rise to many of the soft tissue sarcomas encountered at other sites. Usually the histological diagnosis is not difficult, as most mammary sarcomas can be categorized according to existing histological soft tissue classifications (Enzinger & Weiss 1983). Infrequently a given histological type of sarcoma creates a challenging differential diagnosis as it may resemble or be confused with a benign lesion, e.g. angiosarcoma. Cystosarcoma phyllodes, which occurs peculiarly within the breast, is a special problem, in part due to the terminology, but more importantly because of the histological difficulty in distinguishing some benign tumours from malignant ones. This chapter addresses these problems.

ANGIOSARCOMA

Terminology

Angiosarcoma is the preferred term for this highly malignant tumour of vasoformative tissue. Other common synonyms referred to in the literature include haemangiosarcoma, haemangioendotheliosarcoma, and capillary angiosarcoma.

Anatomical pathology

This tumour presents grossly as an ill-defined, unencapsulated, soft, spongy mass with dilated vascular channels. The average diameter was greater than 5 cm in most recent series (Stein-gaszner et al 1965; Donnell et al 1981; Merino et al 1983; Rainwater et al 1986). Haemorrhage and necrosis are common, especially in larger tumours. The neoplasm is usually located deep within the breast parenchyma. Occasionally, it may invade the pectoral fascia or extend to the skin surface producing a bluish discolouration. Rarely, the tumour may produce breast enlargement without a clinically discrete mass (Dunegan et al 1976).

Histologically, angiosarcomas are composed of anastomosing irregular vascular channels, lined by atypical endothelium supported by a delicate reticulin network or more dense framework. The endothelial cells are usually large, plump, and single layered (Figs 20.1–20.3). Cellular atypism may be mild. Mitoses are variable in number, but usually can be found after a careful search. Papillary projections lined by piled-up endothelial cells commonly project into the lumina. Cells within the stroma, similar to the vascular cells lining the vascular channels, are an important defining feature. The histological pattern of angiosarcoma is highly variable, occasionally within the same lesion.

The spectrum ranges from a well-differentiated angiosarcoma, superficially resembling a benign capillary haemangioma, to highly cellular tumours with less distinct vascular clefts as well as greatly dilated vascular channels. Higher grade lesions demonstrate spindle-shaped endothelial cells, extravasated red blood cells, haemosiderin-laden macrophages and chronic inflammation. These latter findings are related to haemorrhagic necrosis.

Donnell et al (1981) have stratified angiosarcomas into three categories grouped by histological appearance, apparently with prognostic

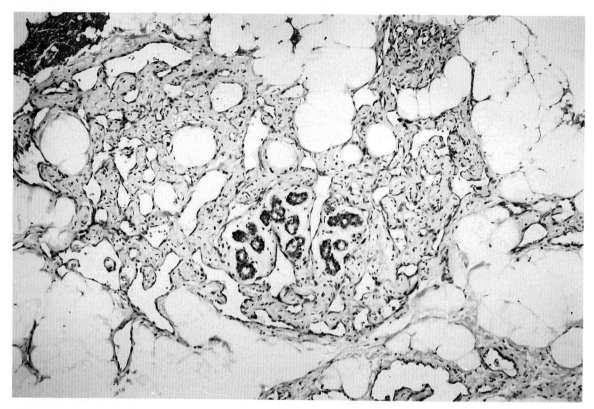

Fig. 20.1 Irregularly shaped vascular channels infiltrate diffusely and discontinously in this low grade angiosarcoma. Note lobular unit centrally with tapering angiosarcoma channels piercing it from above and below. Other sarcoma elements are present at each border of picture (× 120).

significance. The groups, I, II and III, correlate with tumours that are well differentiated, moderately differentiated, and poorly differentiated, respectively. All groups demonstrate hyperchromatic endothelial cells, interanastomosing vascular channels, and the presence of vessels within the breast parenchyma. Other histological features of group I cases include minimal endothelial tufting and rare or absent mitoses. Features common to group II cases were: the presence of endothelial tufting; focal papillary formations; minimal, if any, solid and spindle cell foci; and mitoses limited to papillary areas. The features of the group III cases were the following: the presence of prominent endothelial tufting; papillary formations; solid and spindle cell formation; numerous mitoses; and haemorrhagic necrosis.

Differential diagnosis

Angiosarcomas may resemble benign conditions, either organizing haematomas or benign haemangiomas. Haematomas are rarely encountered except in clearly documented cases of breast trauma or in mastectomy specimens preceded by a recent biopsy. The fact remains, however, that angiosarcoma may exhibit such a bland histological appearance that it resembles a haemangioma. Although Stewart (1950) stated that a benign angioma of the breast had never been documented to constitute a palpable or symptom-producing breast tumour, this is no longer true (Jozefczyk & Rosen 1985; Rosen 1985a). Therefore any palpable or symptomatic vascular lesion of the breast should be approached as if it were a sarcoma, until there is evidence to the contrary

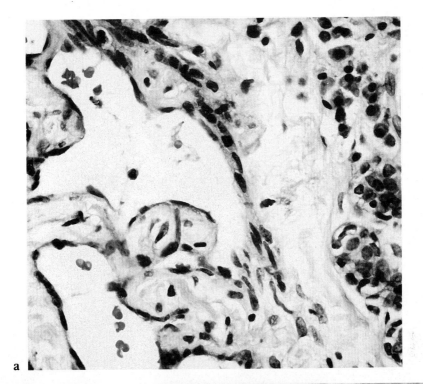

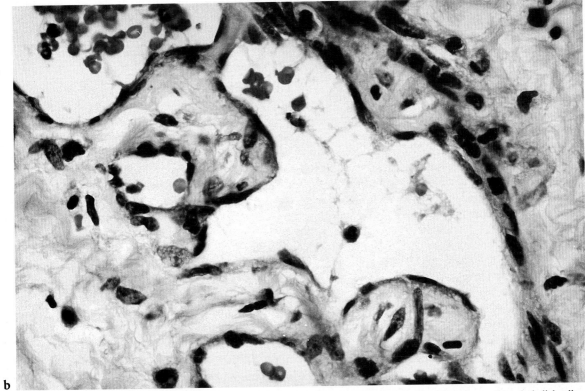

Fig. 20.2a, b Vascular spaces of low grade angiosarcoma are lined, almost continuously, by hyperchromatic endothelial cells. Note occasional similar cells in stroma (**a** × 450; **b** × 750).

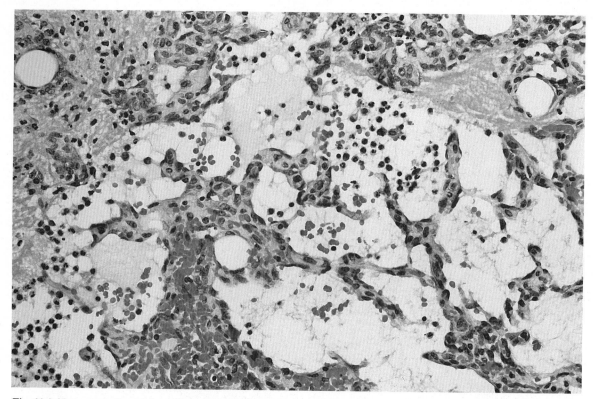

Fig. 20.3 Note poorly formed branching channels (largely clear with scattered erythrocytes) in this mammary angiosarcoma and obvious presence of neoplastic cells in stroma as well as endothelial location. Papillary tufts are suggested in blind-ending stromal elements (× 300).

(Dunegan et al 1976). Accordingly, benign vascular tumours of the breast have been categorized as haemangiomas, angiomatosis and venous haemangiomas.

Haemangiomas, in contradistinction to angiosarcomas, are usually incidental histological findings. These benign vascular tumours tend to be small lesions, usually with a diameter less than one lower power microscopic field. They are characteristically often perilobular in location and sharply circumscribed (Fig. 20.4). Some of the cases of Rosen & Ridolfi (1977) had a stromal or mixed stromal-lobular location. Despite the common usage of the term 'perilobular haemangioma', these lesions might better be termed simply haemangiomas as they may well occur both within as well as beyond lobular units (Nielson 1983). Lesueur et al (1983) found an 11% incidence of haemangiomas in a forensic autopsy study of the female breast. All except seven of the 32 lesions were less than 1.5 mm, while the two

largest haemangiomas were between 3–4 mm in size. Some women had multiple lesions; occasionally they occurred bilaterally. Histologically, these haemangiomas have uniform vascular spaces arranged close together with a scant connective tissue stroma. The endothelial cells show little or no atypia, although they may be plump and project slightly into the lumina. Such cells are not frequent, nor do they appear in adjacent stroma; both features of low grade angiosarcoma. Small haemangiomas are discrete, cohesive lesions, although they may have some irregular borders with extension of vessels into adjacent fatty or fibrous breast stroma. It should be noted that none of the lesions considered to be angiosarcoma by Donnell et al (1981) was of microscopic size. This fact, coupled with the histological criteria of angiosarcoma noted above, will enable the vast majority of angiosarcoma cases to be diagnosed correctly. The problem to be avoided is one of overdiagnosis of angiosarcoma in those slightly

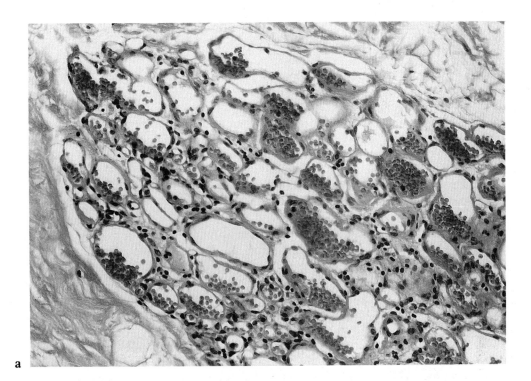

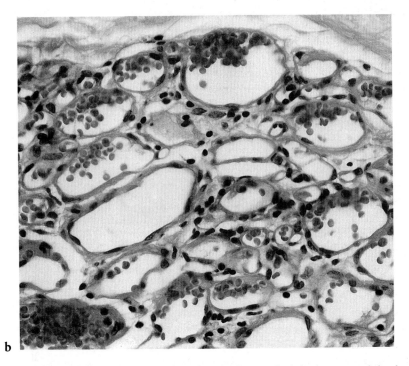

Fig. 20.4a, b This benign mammary stromal haemangioma is well circumscribed, having a smooth border with stroma at left, and above (**a**). Occasional plump endothelial cells are seen in (**b**) (**a** × 225; **b** × 370).

atypical vascular proliferations which exhibit some of the histological features common to angiosarcoma.

The distinction between a well-differentiated (group I) angiosarcoma and the rare lesion described as angiomatosis may require close scrutiny (Rosen 1985a). Angiomatosis demonstrates a diffuse growth of variably sized blood vessels that are distributed uniformly throughout the tumour. This contrasts with a well-differentiated angiosarcoma in which vessels have a heterogeneous distribution, being numerous and closely spaced in some zones, while being widely separated in others. Angiomatosis has been considered benign, yet conservative but complete excision is advisable in order to exclude the possibility of angiosarcoma. Although recognizing that this differential diagnosis is difficult, the problem is fortunately rare as only three cases have been reported by Rosen (1985a).

Various other benign vascular tumours have been described in the breast. A cystic hygroma, a benign tumour of lymphatic channels, has been described within the breast (Sieber & Sharkey 1986). Richly cellular and vascular angiolipomas of the subcutaneous tissue may be present in multiple (Brown et al 1982). Venous haemangiomas (Rosen et al 1985) and mammary subcutaneous vascular tumours (Rosen 1985b) are benign and show similar features to comparable soft tissue lesions occurring at other anatomical sites. Though extremely rare, a densely cellular haemangiopericytoma may resemble the solid areas of poorly differentiated angiosarcomas (Tavassoli & Weiss 1981).

Postmastectomy angiosarcoma is discussed in Chapter 18.

Clinical significance and prognostic implications

Angiosarcoma is the most aggressive and lethal of all the breast neoplasms, when reviewed collectively (Chen et al 1980). Younger women tend to be affected. The fact that some have been pregnant at the time of diagnosis raises the suspicion of hormone dependence. Two patients have been reported to develop cutaneous angiosarcomas occurring at the site of postmastectomy radiation exposure; this is a different disease, and should not be confused with mammary angiosarcoma (Otis et al 1986).

The initial recommended treatment is simple mastectomy, as axillary dissection has not been proven necessary, regardless of the histological appearance. The tumour does not metastasize to regional lymph nodes, but spreads haematogeneously to the contralateral breast, brain, lungs, bone and abdominal viscera. A few prolonged survivors are known, but local recurrences followed by death within three years is a usual course. The more recent use of adjuvant chemotherapy may be changing this dismal outcome, but the results are mixed. Although Donnell et al (1981) have implied prognostic significance to each of their three subgroups (see above), they have also suggested that prolonged survival may be partly related to the use of chemotherapy. Histological grading did not seem to correlate with patient survival in the Mayo Clinic series in which a slightly different grading system was applied (Rainwater et al 1986). Gross tumour size showed no correlation with survival in the series of Merino et al (1983) and Rainwater et al (1986). In summary, angiosarcoma remains a difficult histological diagnosis occasionally, and despite surgical and adjuvant therapy, long-term survivors are infrequent.

REFERENCES

Brown R W, Bhathal P S, Scott P R 1982 Multiple bilateral angiolipomas of the breast. Aust N Z J Surg 52: 614–616

Chen K T K, Kirkegaard D D, Bocian J J 1980 Angiosarcoma of the breast. Cancer 46: 368–371

Donnell R M, Rosen P P, Lieberman P H et al 1981 Angiosarcoma and other vascular tumours of the breast. Pathologic analysis as a guide to prognosis. Am J Surg Pathol 5: 629–642

Dunegan L J, Bobon H, Watson C G 1976 Angiosarcoma of the breast: a report of two cases and a review of the literature. Surgery 79: 57–59

Enzinger F M, Weiss S W 1983 Soft tissue tumours. Mosby, St Louis

Jozefczyk M A, Rosen P P 1985 Vascular tumors of the breast. II. Perilobular hemangiomas and hemangiomas. Am J Surg Pathol 9: 491–503

Lesueur G C, Brown R W, Bhathal P S 1983 Incidence of perilobular hemangioma in the female breast. Arch Pathol Lab Med 107: 308–310

Merino M J, Carter D, Berman M 1983 Angiosarcoma of the breast. Am J Surg Pathol 7: 53–60

Nielson B 1983 Haemangiomas of the breast. Pathol Res Pract 176: 253–257

Otis C N, Peschel R, McKhann C, Merino M J, Duray P H 1986 The rapid onset of cutaneous angiosarcoma after radiotherapy for breast carcinoma. Cancer 57: 2130–2134

Rainwater L M, Martin J K, Gaffey T A, van Heerden J A 1986 Angiosarcoma of the breast. Arch Surg 121: 669–672

Rosen P P 1985a Vascular tumors of the breast. III. Angiomatosis. Am J Surg Pathol 9: 652–658

Rosen P P 1985b Vascular tumors of the breast. V. Nonparenchymal haemangiomas of mammary subcutaneous tissues. Am J Surg Pathol 9: 723–729

Rosen P P, Ridolfi R L 1977 The perilobular hemangioma. A benign microscopic vascular lesion of the breast. Am J Clin Pathol 68: 21–23

Rosen P P, Jozefczyk M A, Boram L H 1985 Vascular tumours of the breast. IV. The venous hemangioma. Am J Surg Pathol 9: 659–665

Sieber P R, Sharkey F E 1986 Cystic hygroma of the breast. Arch Pathol Lab Med 110:353

Steingaszner L C, Enzinger F M, Taylor H B 1965 Hemangiosarcoma of the breast. Cancer 18: 352–361

Stewart F W 1950 Tumors of the breast. Altas of tumour pathology, section IX, fascicle 34. Armed Forces Institute of Pathology, Washington, D C, p 107

Tavassoli F A, Weiss S 1981 Hemangiopericytoma of the breast. Am J Surg Pathol 5: 745–752

PHYLLODES TUMOUR ('CYSTOSARCOMA PHYLLODES')

Terminology

The term cystosarcoma phyllodes has been in use since Müller introduced it in 1838 to describe a bulky breast tumour with a leaf-like gross appearance (Müller 1838). Although he believed the tumour was benign and should be separated from breast carcinoma, problems exist with the term since the lesion has an obvious malignant counterpart. To circumvent some of this confusion many institutions have signed out these tumours as 'cystosarcoma phyllodes, benign' or 'cystosarcoma phyllodes, malignant', depending on which was applicable. This facilitates a more logical therapeutic discussion of individual cases but at the same time condones the use of irrational verbiage of a 'benign sarcoma'. For decades pathologists have been loath to change this terminology, sanctioned by long usage. The recent revision of the World Health Organization classification of breast tumours has proposed the term 'phyllodes tumour' for the entity described by Müller 1838, thereby eliminating the word cystosarcoma (WHO 1981). 'Phyllodes tumour' is preferable since this term by itself has no inferred or explicit connotation of biological behaviour. Rather the pathologist should apply the appropriate qualification, 'benign', 'malignant', or 'borderline malignant', based upon the histological assessment of likely behaviour.

Anatomical pathology

The gross appearance of benign and malignant phyllodes tumours is similar. In early reports the tumours were of huge size but in modern series the average size is close to 5 cm in diameter (Pietruszka & Barnes 1978) with tumours 1–2 cm in diameter being common. They may form a round or oval mass that is commonly sharply circumscribed and encapsulated in half of the cases. Other tumours have a bosselated contour with pseudoencapsulation. The cut surface corre-

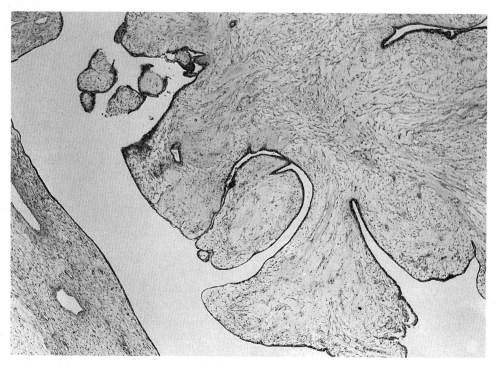

Fig. 20.5 Classic leaf-like projections of stroma are evident in this benign phyllodes tumour (× 40).

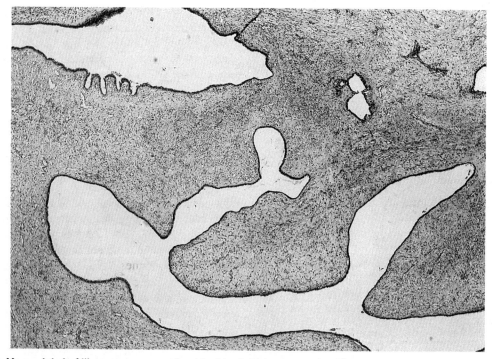

Fig. 20.6 More subtle leaf-like patterns are produced in this phyllodes tumour (× 40).

lates with the size of the tumour. Smaller phyllodes tumours are grey-white, glistening and fibrous. Larger tumours frequently contain clefts or cystic cavities. The cystic areas are usually serous or filled with serosanguinous fluid. Larger tumours are prone to haemorrhage, necrosis and other degenerative changes. Although size is an unreliable criterion of biological behavior, in two large series (Treves & Sunderland 1951; McDivitt et al 1967) benign phyllodes tumours were more commonly cystic than the malignant ones.

Histologically, the phyllodes tumour is composed of an extremely hypercellular stroma, accompanied by the proliferation of benign ductal structures. Phyllodes tumours at lower power resemble fibroadenomas except for enhanced intracanalicular growth pattern and the greater degree of stromal cellularity (Figs 20.5–20.8).

Norris & Taylor (1967) emphasized the unpredictable nature of phyllodes tumours if judged by a single criterion. This unpredictability is primarily in the direction of overdiagnosis of malignancy as evidenced by the 27 patients reported by Blumencranz & Gray (1978), with 13 of the phyllodes tumours diagnosed as malignant because of any combination of increased mitotic activity, invasive borders or marked pleomorphism. None of these women developed recurrences or metastases. Yet Hart et al (1978) have shown that phyllodes tumours can reliably be separated into benign and malignant categories by using several parameters. Malignant phyllodes tumours exhibit malignant stromal features, most commonly, cytological pleomorphism and an appreciable mitotic rate (Figs 20.9–20.12). In less obviously malignant cases, an infiltrating border is more indicative of a malignancy, or at least the possiblity of recurrence, than is a pushing border. An otherwise benign-appearing stroma may contain foci of bizarre giant cells that alone should not be interpreted as a criterion of malignancy. Recognition of malignancy depends upon thorough sampling of large lesions. Hypercellular areas generally display a pattern of fibrosarcoma, in which there is cytological anaplasia and substantial mitotic activity, enabling one to make a malignant diagnosis. The overgrowth of stroma in relation to epithelium is an important indicator of malignant behaviour (Ward & Evans 1986).

The malignant phyllodes tumour usually shows typical appearances associated with either fibrosarcoma or myxoliposarcoma. Occasionally less common patterns, such as rhabdomyosarcoma, chondrosarcoma and osteosarcoma, are encountered. Overgrowth of a purely sarcomatous element, losing its relation to epithelium, is probably the most determinant feature of malignant behaviour as revealed in recent series (Hart et al 1978; Pietruszka & Barnes 1978). One is particularly certain of malignant behaviour if the malignant portion is liposarcoma, rhabdomyosarcoma or other sarcomatous elements other than fibrosarcoma (Grigioni et al 1982).

The ductal elements are most often lined by a two-cell population similar to fibroadenomas. The typical canaliculi exhibit cuboidal epithelium resembling that in normal ducts. Variable ductal hyperplasia, adenosis and squamous metaplasia are associated with both benign and malignant tumours. Papillary epithelial hyperplasia can be disturbing, but coexisting carcinoma is rare. Haagensen's (1971) 84 phyllodes tumours contained three cases with concurrent lobular carcinoma in situ. However, other experience indicates ductal carcinoma in situ may be more common in phyllodes tumours (Grove & Kristensen 1986).

Differential diagnosis

Phyllodes tumours must be distinguished from fibroadenomas using the criteria set forth in Chapter 7. The term giant fibroadenoma is unacceptable as a synonym for a benign phyllodes tumour. That terminology tries to equate two different lesions that are quite distinct and separated by the differences in their stroma, not their size. The difference is that phyllodes tumours are characterized by a hypercellular stroma, especially that portion of the stroma adjacent to the epithelium, and by a well-developed leaf-like growth pattern.

Phyllodes tumours in the adolescent age group are rare and are likely to be confused with a giant fibroadenoma or juvenile fibroadenoma (Ashikari et al 1971; Nambiar & Kutty 1974; Pike & Oberman 1985). It cannot be overemphasized that size alone is not a diagnostic criterion for phyllodes tumour. The majority of both benign and malignant phyllodes tumours were under 5 cm in diameter in the series of McDivitt et al series (1967). A phyllodes tumour 1–2 cm in diameter does not insure benignancy. In the McDivitt et al (1967) study, 50% of malignant tumours were in the 1–4 cm range.

Irrespective of the patient's age, occasionally a fibroadenoma showing a hypercellular stroma and 'active' nuclei may be difficult to distinguish from a phyllodes tumour. When this occurs, the mitotic activity may help in differential diagnosis, as Fechner will allow fibroadenomas to have up to 3 mitoses/10 hpf (see Ch. 7).

This raises the question of how valuable are mitotic counts in evaluating phyllodes tumours? Clearly the histological evaluation of phyllodes tumours has been one of the most difficult areas in tumour pathology. No one advocates the diagnosis of benignancy versus malignancy to rest upon a single criterion, but multiple criteria such as utilized by Pietruszka & Barnes (1978) offers the best chance at correctly categorizing a tumour. Table 20.1 lists information derived from recent

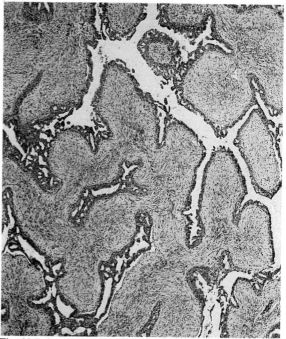

Fig. 20.7 An almost regularly branching pattern of cellular stroma is present in this phyllodes tumour (× 40).

Table 20.1 Comparison of various series of phyllodes tumours.

	Hart et al (1978)		Pietruszka & Barnes (1978)			Grigioni et al (1982)		
	Benign	Malignant	Benign	Borderline malignant	Malignant	Benign	Low grade sarcoma	High grade sarcoma
Number of patients	12	14	18	5	18	10	4	6
Infiltrating margins (% tumours)	17%	36%	17%	20%	68%	0	100%	100%
Stromal histology	Cellular fibrous	Fibro-sarcoma	Cellular fibrous	Fibro-sarcoma	Fibrosarcoma Liposarcoma Rhabdomyo-sarcoma Osteosarcoma Various types	Cellular fibrous	Fibrosarcoma	Fibrosarcoma Rhabdomyo-sarcoma Fibro/lipo-sarcoma Lipo/rhabdomyo-sarcoma
Mitoses per 10/hpf	<5 in 83%	>5 in 79%	0–4	5–9	10 or more	(0–4)★	(5–9)★	(10 or more)★
Local recurrences	2	4 (1 died from direct extension of tumour)	4	1 (died of direct lung invasion)	0	3	2	
Distant metastases	0	2	0	0	(2)†	0	0	(3)†

★Used categories of Pietruszka & Barnes (1978).
†All had heterologous elements, i.e. other than fibrosarcoma.

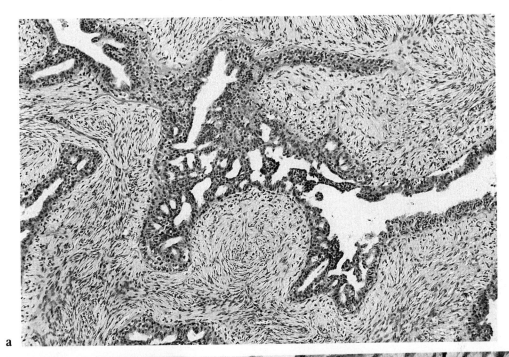

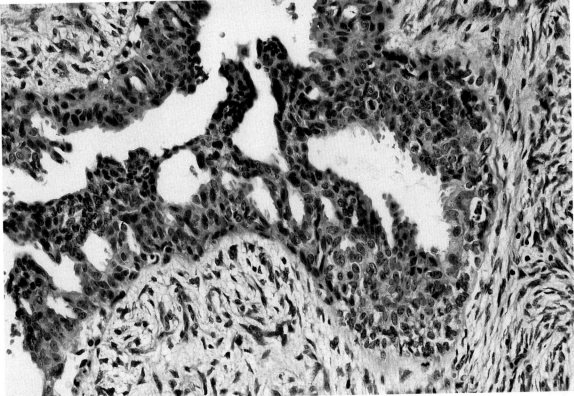

Fig. 20.8a, b Same case as Figure 20.7. Note at intermediate power (**a**) that the orientation of fibrous bundles maintains a relationship usually parallel to the epithelial–stromal junctions. At high power (**b**) the benign hyperplastic epithelium resembles that of gynaecomastia and the stroma has no definite features of malignancy (**a** × 100; **b** × 290).

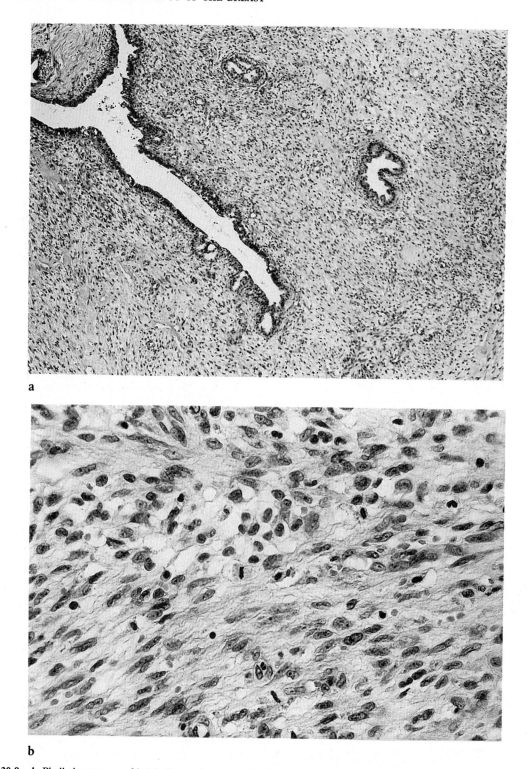

Fig. 20.9a, b Phyllodes tumour of borderline malignancy. Although stromal elements are not as closely related to epithelium as in benign phyllodes tumour, there was no broad overgrowth of fibrosarcomatous stroma in this tumour. Several mitoses without advanced nuclear atypia are appreciated at higher power (**a** × 75; **b** × 400).

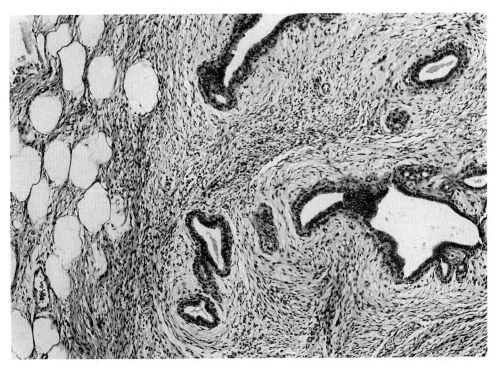

Fig. 20.10 Malignant phyllodes tumour demonstrates invasive character at left where stromal elements extends into fat (× 90).

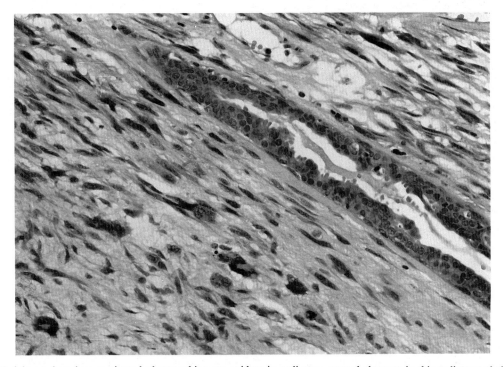

Fig. 20.11 Advanced nuclear atypia and pleomorphism are evident in malignant stromal elements in this malignant phyllodes tumour (× 370).

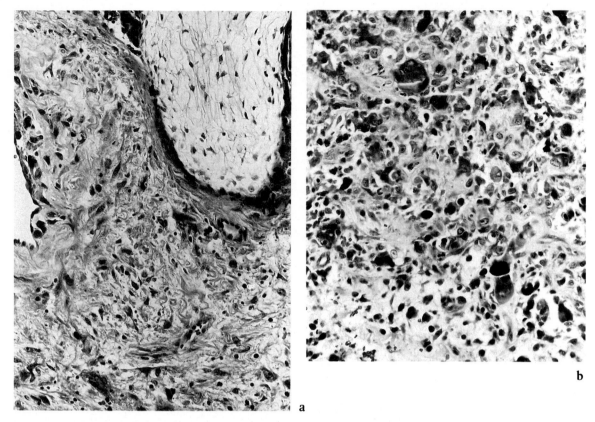

Fig. 20.12a, b Bizarre giant cells and spindle cells were focally present in this malignant phyllodes tumour. Note overgrowth of malignant stroma relative to benign stroma in (**a**), with benign stroma at upper right (**a** × 140; **b** × 200).

series of phyllodes tumours. A comparison shows that mitotic counts of malignant tumours consistently exceeded those classified as benign. Yet, mitotic figure counts are not infallible and are therefore not a defining feature of malignant behaviour if used alone. This point is illustrated in the case of a 13 cm malignant phyllodes tumour with a liposarcomatous stroma which metastasized to bone in the absence of detectable stromal mitoses (Spielmann et al 1985). In the same study of Spielmann et al (1985) seven non-metastasizing malignant phyllodes tumours had an average of 6 mitoses/10 hpf, while the average of the two metastasizing tumours in the series was 12 mitoses/10 hpf (23 for one case and zero for the liposarcoma that metastasized to bone). This series and those in Table 20.1 stress the need for a borderline category, in which metastases might occur, but are unlikely in most of these tumours

exhibiting a low grade fibrosarcoma appearance, and most will have 5–10 mitoses/10 hpf upon careful analysis. Rhabdomyosarcoma and liposarcoma are unfavourable histological types in the series of Grigioni et al (1982), giving rise to metastases and a mortality rate of 50% in their high grade cases. These tumours might be termed high grade sarcoma or definitely malignant. The high grade sarcomas include tumours with malignant components other than fibrosarcoma (Table 20.1).

Fibrosarcoma also is considered unfavourable histology when it is high grade and large areas of pure fibrosarcoma are present. Identifying tumours with unfavourable histology serves as a prognosticator, as these cases have a high likelihood of metastases, whereas most cases of phyllodes tumours customarily assigned to a malignant group have a low grade fibrosarcomatous stroma without overgrowth of a regular relationship to epithelium. These are best regarded as borderline malignant, as few of them will give rise to metastases.

Clinical significance and prognostic information

Phyllodes tumours are more common in women between 30 and 70 years, with the fifth decade having a higher percentage of tumours than any other decade. The mean age is about 10 years beyond that of fibroadenomas (Treves 1964). Although phyllodes tumours rarely occur in adolescents, they are usually benign, but a few notable exceptions of malignant phyllodes tumours with aggressive behaviour have been reported in this age group (Grigioni et al 1982; Kenda 1983a; Adami et al 1984). When lethal, malignant phyllodes tumours have metastasized haematogeneously, usually to the lungs, demonstrating only the stromal component in the metastases. Direct spread to the lungs through the thoracic wall (Hart et al 1978) and along nerve trunks to the brain stem (Grimes et al 1985) have been reported. There is poor correlation between malignant biological behaviour and those cases histologically classified as malignant. Hart et al (1978) classified 54% of their tumours as malignant, but only 23% of those died as a result of tumour. The authors acknowledged in their paper that some of the malignant cases would have been more appropriately classified as 'borderline malignant' and supported the concept of a 'low grade' malignant phyllodes tumour.

A retrospective review of published series of phyllodes tumours would appear to have a clear message: (1) some phyllodes tumours, although in the minority, are malignant at presentation and have the ability to metastasize and kill; (2) the majority of the tumours are benign and potentially curable by local excision when completely removed with a rim of uninvolved breast tissue; (3) a third subset exists: those phyllodes tumours considered to be of indeterminate biology, some of which recur, although most do not and few of which metastasize; and it is this third group which probably makes up at least the small majority of those tumours previously diagnosed as fully malignant, but which do not behave as such. For these reasons a borderline malignant or low grade sarcoma category of phyllodes tumours is justifiable. By placing some phyllodes tumours in this category, it would alert our surgical colleagues of the need to achieve clearance and reduce the risk of recurrence in a particular patient. It should be stressed that local recurrence per se is not an indicator of malignancy. Malignant transformation occurred in only two of the 28 recurrent benign phyllodes tumours (7%) reported by Hajdu et al (1976) and one patient died with metastatic disease. This is an apparently exceptional event as it is not recorded in most series.

The average interval between the diagnosis of primary benign and recurrent benign phyllodes tumours is two years (Hajdu et al 1976), but several years may lapse between recurrences. Phyllodes tumours by their very nature grow radially compressing the adjacent breast parenchyma creating a pseudocapsule through which invasive tongues of phyllodes stroma may permeate and grow into adjacent breast tissue.

Hence, if the tumour is enucleated or excised closely, these tongues may not be completely removed, placing the patient at risk for local recurrence. Appropriate therapy for all phyllodes tumours, as for any soft tissue tumour likely to recur, requires whatever operation is necessary to achieve complete removal including a surrounding rim of uninvolved breast tissue. In larger tumours, this may require simple mastectomy. Axillary dissection is not standard therapy, as lymph node metastases occur very rarely.

The primary reason for the borderline malignant category is to prevent overdiagnosis of malignancy. In light of current knowledge, it seems unjustifiable to give a fully malignant diagnostic term to lesions that only occasionally kill. The incidence of malignant phyllodes tumours is 0.18% of all malignant breast tumours as cited by Vorherr et al (1985). Two-year survival rates without recurrences are meaningful in malignant cases, as most recurrences occur by then. The review of Vorherr et al (1985) found a relative five-year survival rate of about 80% in those phyllodes tumours diagnosed histologically as malignant, but this figure includes borderline cases.

REFERENCES

Adami H O G, Hakelius L, Rimsten A, Willen R 1984 Malignant, locally recurring cystosarcoma phyllodes in an adolescent female. Acta Chir Scand 150: 93–100

Ashikari R, Farrow J H, O'Hara J 1971 Fibroadenomas in the breast of juveniles. Surg Gynecol Obstet 132: 259–262

Blumencranz P K, Gray G F 1978 Cystosarcoma phyllodes — clinical and pathological study. N Y State J Med 78: 623–627

Grigioni W F, Santini D, Grassigli A et al 1982 A clinico-pathologic study of cytosarcoma phyllodes. Twenty case reports. Arch Anat Cytol Pathol 30: 303–306

Grimes M M, Lattes R, Jaretzki A 1985 Cytosarcoma phyllodes — report of an unusual case, with death due to intraneural extension to the central nervous system. Cancer 56: 1691–1695

Grove A, Kristensen L D 1986 Intraductal carcinoma within a phyllodes tumor of the breast — a case report. Tumori 72: 187–190

Haagensen C D 1971 Diseases of the breast, 2nd edn. Saunders, Philadelphia, p 227–249

Hajdu S I, Espinosa M H, Robbins G F 1976 Recurrent cytosarcoma phyllodes — a clinicopathologic study of 32 cases. Cancer 38: 1402–1406

Hart W R, Bauer R C, Oberman H A 1978 Cystosarcoma phyllodes. A clinicopathologic study of twenty-six hypercellular periductal stromal tumours of the breast. Am J Clin Pathol 70: 211–216

Kenda J F N 1983 Fatal metastatic cystosarcoma phyllodes in a young woman. Arch Surg 118: 871–872

McDivitt R W, Urban J A, Farrow J H 1967 Cystosarcoma phyllodes. Johns Hopkins Med J 120: 33–45

Müller J 1838 Über den feinern Bau und die Formen der Krankhaften Geschwülste. Reimer, Berlin, p 54–60

Nambiar R, Kutty M K 1974 Giant fibroadenoma (cystosarcoma phyllodes) in adolescent females — a clinicopathological study. Br J Surg 61: 113–117

Norris H J, Taylor H B 1967 Relationship of histologic features to behavior of cystosarcoma phyllodes — analysis of ninety-four cases. Cancer 22: 22–28

Pietruszka M, Barnes L 1978 Cystosarcoma phyllodes — a clinicopathologic analysis of 42 cases. Cancer 41: 1974–1983

Pike A M, Oberman H A 1985 Juvenile (cellular) fibroadenoma. A clinico-pathologic study. Am J Surg Pathol 9: 730–736

Spielmann M, Toussaint C, Malcoste G et al 1985 Breast sarcomas — a retrospective study of 25 cases. Bull Cancer (Paris) 72: 202–209

Treves N 1964 A study of cystosarcoma phyllodes. Ann N Y Acad Sci 114: 922–936

Treves N, Sunderland D A 1951 Cytosarcoma of the breast; a malignant and a benign tumour. Cancer 4: 1286–1332

Vorherr H, Vorherr U F, Kutvirt D M, Key C R 1985 Cystosarcoma phyllodes — epidemiology, pathohistology, pathobiology, diagnosis, therapy, and survival. Arch Gynecol 236: 173–181

WHO 1981 International histological classification of tumours, 2nd edn. Histologic typing of breast tumours. World Health Organization, Geneva

Ward R M, Evans H L 1986 Cystosarcoma phyllodes. A clinicopathologic study of 26 cases. Cancer 58: 2282–2289

OTHER PRIMARY SARCOMAS

Other sarcomas of the breast arise so infrequently that the many reported series offer limited prognostic information because of the small number of patients, variable tumour classifications and non-uniform treatment modalities. Stromal sarcoma is a term that has been used inconsistently since its introduction by Berg et al (1962). It has been used on occasion in a generic sense to lump together all breast sarcomas exclusive of malignant phyllodes tumours. We do not support this usage, but agree with others that stromal sarcomas should be restricted to the exceptionally rare sarcomas arising from the specialized stroma of the breast (Callery et al 1985). We classify other mammary sarcomas histogenetically and attempt to assign a grade, as the prognosis of soft tissue tumours occurring at other sites correlates with histological grade and the presence or absence of necrosis (Costa et al 1984).

Pure liposarcomas of the breast are exceptionally rare, as many of the cases reviewed by Azzopardi (1979) proved to be malignant phyllodes tumours with liposarcomatous differentiation, which occurs rather commonly (Qizilbash 1976). Histologically, liposarcomas of the breast may show the same types of liposarcomas described at other sites (Kristensen & Kryger 1978). Tumours showing the pleomorphic liposarcoma pattern and infiltrating margins are more likely to recur (Austin & Dupree 1986).

Although pure fibrosarcoma is unusual in the breast, it is the most common type of sarcoma occurring outside the clinical setting of a phyllodes tumour (Barnes & Pietruszka 1977; Norris & Taylor 1968). An extremely difficult differential diagnosis is between a low grade fibrosarcoma and an infiltrating fibromatosis (Oberman 1965; Rosen et al 1978; Ali et al 1979). Fibromatosis is a locally infiltrating lesion incapable of metastases; however, as in other sites of the body, recurrences are common if the lesion is not carefully excised. Fibromatosis tends to be less cellular Wargotz et al and lacks the nuclear atypia characteristic of fibrosarcoma (Figs 20.13 and 20.14). Various

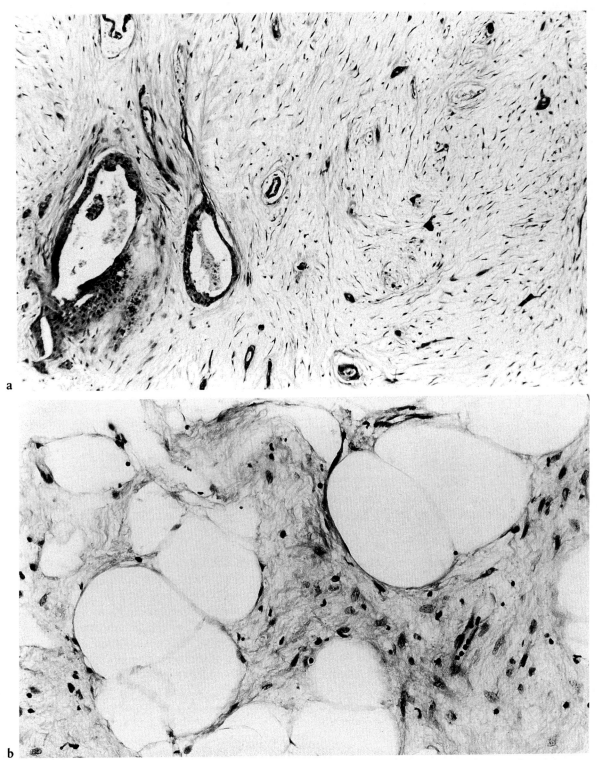

Fig. 20.13a, b These photographs of fibromatosis in the breast demonstrate in (**a**) the relatively hypocellular fibrous tissue enclosing and miniaturizing various parenchymal elements. In (**b**), infiltration of fat is apparent as are the nuclear features of enlarged, benign fibroblasts (**a** × 125; **b** × 325).

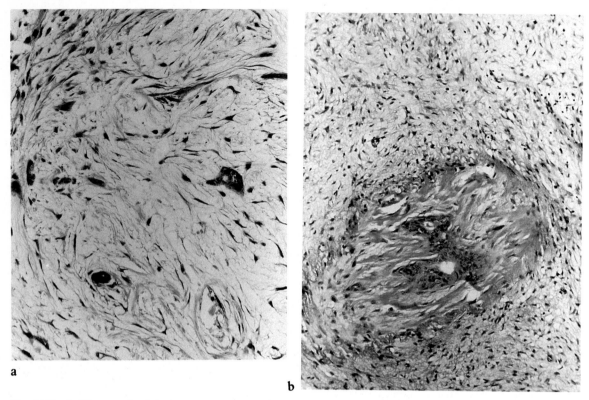

Fig. 20.14a, b Fibromatosis of the breast demonstrates miniaturized and enclosed epithelial elements in (a) (enlargement of an area in Figure 20.13a). Enclosed ductal elements may produce a benign and quite different periductal fibrous reaction as seen in (b) with infiltrating fibromatosis surrounding (a × 250; b × 125).

subtypes of malignant fibrous histiocytoma (Enzinger & Weiss 1983) occur in the breast, rarely following radiation therapy for carcinoma of the breast (Luzzatto et al 1986). The most important differential diagnosis when considering malignant fibrous histiocytoma is the separation from spindle cell carcinoma or carcinoma with sarcomatous metaplasia (see Ch. 14). Spindle cell proliferations in the breast, depending upon the merits of an individual case, may evoke a rather wide differential diagnosis ranging from various sarcomas to exceptionally rare, benign lesions such as fibromatosis, fasciitis and the so-called benign spindle cell breast tumour. This latter lesion, described by Toker et al (1981), is rare but has occurred slightly more often in males than in females; it has been compared to spindle cell lipomas and fibromas occurring at other sites, although the histogenesis of these spindle cell tumours remains unresolved (Böger 1984; Chan et al 1984).

An awareness of other uncommon benign mesenchymal breast tumours may prevent an inappropriate diagnosis of sarcoma in a given circumstance. Specifically, benign breast tumours may contain islands of cartilage (see 'Pleomorphic adenoma', Ch. 14) as well as malignant tumours of soft tissue and carcinomas with metaplasia (Ch. 14). Occasional benign lesions containing cartilage have been described as chondrolipomatous tumours (Dharkar & Kraft 1981) or as cartilaginous metaplasias in fibromas (Lawler 1969). Metcalf & Ellis (1985) have presented a similar benign tumour of mesenchymal tissues including fibrous, adipose, cartilaginous and smooth muscle elements as a choristoma. The important lesson is that histological benignancy may be accepted as such in these lesions. Smooth muscle tumours, both leiomyosarcomas (Chen et al 1981; Gobardhan 1984; Nielsen 1984) and leiomyomas (Nascimento et al 1979) have been described rarely. Although benign smooth muscle tumours may reach a large size or have irregular borders and cystic areas, they should not show necrosis, mitoses or significant cellular atypia (Chen et al 1981).

Despite the fact that tumours resembling pure osteosarcomas have been described (Savage et al 1984; Going et al 1986), separation of these from metaplastic carcinomas which have been totally replaced by the osteosarcomatous component may not be possible (see Ch. 14). 40% of the mammary osteosarcomas in the literature have a history of a pre-existing fibroadenoma or phyllodes tumour (Mertens et al 1982).

REFERENCES

Ali M, Fayemi A O, Braun E V, Remy R 1979 Fibromatosis of the breast. Am J Surg Pathol 3: 501–505

Austin R M, Dupree W B 1986 Liposarcoma of the breast: a clinicopathologic study of 20 cases. Hum Pathol 17: 906–913

Azzopardi J G 1979 Problems in breast pathology. In: Bennington J L (consulting ed) Major problems in pathology, vol II. Saunders, Philadelphia, p 367–368

Barnes L, Pietruszka M 1977 Sarcomas of the breast — a clinicopathologic analysis of ten cases. Cancer 40: 1577–1585

Berg J W, DeCrosse J J, Fracchia A A, Farrow J 1962 Stromal sarcomas of the breast. A unified approach to connective tissue sarcomas other than cystosarcoma phyllodes. Cancer 15: 418–424

Böger A 1984 Benign spindle cell tumor of the male breast. Pathol Res Pract 178: 395–398

Callery C D, Rosen P P, Kinne D W 1985 Sarcoma of the breast — a study of 32 patients with reappraisal of classification and therapy. Ann Surg 201: 527–532

Chan K, Ghadially F N, Alagaratnam T T 1984 Benign spindle cell tumour of breast — a variant of spindle cell lipoma or fibroma of breast? Pathology 16: 331–337

Chen K T K, Kuo T, Hoffman K D 1981 Leiomyosarcoma of the breast. Cancer 47: 1883–1886

Costa J, Wesley R A, Glatstein E, Rosenberg S A 1984 The grading of soft tissue tumors — results of a clinicohistopathologic correlation in a series of 163 cases. Cancer 53: 530–541

Dharkar D D, Kraft J R 1981 Benign chondrolipomatous tumour of the breast. Postgrad Med J 57: 129–131

Enzinger F M, Weiss S W 1983 Soft tissue tumours. Mosby, St Louis, p 154–198

Gobardhan A B 1984 Primary leiomyosarcoma of the breast. Neth J Surg 36: 116–118

Going J J, Lumsden A B, Anderson T J 1986 A classical osteogenic sarcoma of the breast: histology, immunohistochemistry and ultrastructure. Histopathology 10: 631–642

Kristensen P B, Kryger H 1978 Liposarcoma of the breast. Acta Chir Scand 144: 193–196

Lawler R G 1969 Cartilaginous metaplasia in a breast tumour. J Pathol 97: 385–387

Luzzatto R, Grossmann S, Scholl J G, Recktenvald M 1986 Postradiation pleomorphic malignant fibrous histiocytoma of the breast. Acta Cytol (Baltimore) 30: 48–50

Mertens H H, Langnickel D, Staedtler F 1982 Primary osteogenic sarcoma of the breast. Acta Cytol (Baltimore) 26: 512–516

Metcalf J S, Ellis B 1985 Choristoma of the breast. Hum Pathol 16: 739–740

Nascimento A G, Karas M, Rosen P P, Caron A G 1979 Leiomyoma of the nipple. Am J Surg Pathol 3: 151–154

Nielsen B B 1984 Leiomyosarcoma of the breast with late dissemination. Virchows Arch (A) 403: 241–245

Norris H J, Taylor H B 1968 Sarcomas and related mesenchymal tumours of the breast. Cancer 22: 22–28

Oberman H A 1965 Sarcomas of the breast. Cancer 18: 1233–1243

Qizilbash A H 1976 Cystosarcoma phyllodes with liposarcomatous stroma. Am J Clin Pathol 65: 321–327

Rosen Y, Papasozomenos S C, Gardner B 1978 Fibromatosis of the breast. Cancer 41: 1409–1413

Savage A P, Sagor G R, Dovey P 1984 Osteosarcoma of the breast: a case report with an unusual diagnostic feature. Clin Oncol 10: 295–298

Toker C, Tang C, Whitley J F, Berkheiser S W, Rachman R 1981 Benign spindle cell breast tumour. Cancer 48: 1615–1622

Wargotz E S, Norris H J, Austin R M, Enzinger F M 1987 Fibromatosis of the breast. A clinical and pathological study of 28 cases. Am J Surg Pathol 11: 38–45

Index